Surgery of Rheumatoid Arthritis

Contributors

Lewis D. Anderson
William H. Bickel
N. R. Boeve
Richard S. Bryan
Craig A. Campbell
D. Kay Clawson
F. Richard Convery
Richard L. Cruess
Roger Demers
Andre Derome
Martin A. Entin
Roger Gariepy
Alice L. Garrett
G. A. deGroot
Sig T. Hansen
R. W. Hehl
Malcolm Heppenstall
William N. Jones
Carroll A. Laurin
D. L. MacIntosh
Robert D. Midgley
Nelson S. Mitchell
Charles S. Neer II
Wylie T. Scott, Jr.
Nora Shepard
Edward H. Simmons
Alfred B. Swanson
Thomas K. F. Taylor
Borje Walldius
T. J. Waller
J. Watson-Farrar
Morris Ziff

Surgery of Rheumatoid Arthritis

edited by

Richard L. Cruess, M.D.

Orthopaedic Surgeon-in-Charge, Royal Victoria Hospital; Surgeon-in-Chief, Shriners' Hospital for Crippled Children, Montreal Unit; Associate Professor of Surgery, McGill University, Montreal, Quebec

and

Nelson S. Mitchell, M.D., C.M.

Assistant Orthopaedic Surgeon, Royal Victoria Hospital; Consultant, Shriners' Hospital for Crippled Children, Montreal Unit; Assistant Professor of Surgery, McGill University, Montreal, Quebec

J. B. Lippincott Company

Philadelphia • Toronto

Distributed in Great Britain by
Blackwell Scientific Publications
Oxford and Edinburgh

Standard Book Number 397-50283-4

Library of Congress Catalog Card Number 78—157907

Printed in the United States of America

1 3 4 2

Contributors

Lewis D. Anderson, M.D.
Associate Professor of Orthopaedic Surgery, University of Tennessee College of Medicine; Staff Member, Campbell Clinic; Memphis, Tennessee.

William H. Bickel, M.D., M.S. (Orth. Surg.), F.A.C.S.
Consultant, Department of Orthopaedics, Mayo Clinic; Professor of Orthopaedic Surgery, Mayo Graduate School of Medicine, University of Minnesota; Rochester, Minnesota.

N. R. Boeve, M.D.
Orthopaedic Research Department, Blodgett Memorial Hospital, Grand Rapids, Michigan.

Richard S. Bryan, M.D., M.S. (Orth. Surg.)
Consultant, Department of Orthopaedics, Mayo Clinic; Assistant Professor of Orthopaedic Surgery, Mayo Graduate School of Medicine, University of Minnesota; Rochester, Minnesota.

Craig A. Campbell, M.D.
Orthopaedic Resident, LAC-USC Medical Center, Los Angeles, California.

D. Kay Clawson, M.D.
Professor, Department of Orthopaedics, University of Washington School of Medicine, Seattle, Washington.

F. Richard Convery, M.D.
Associate Professor, Department of Orthopaedics, University of Washington School of Medicine, Seattle, Washington.

Richard L. Cruess, M.D.
Orthopaedic Surgeon-in-Charge, Royal Victoria Hospital; Surgeon-in-Chief, Shriners' Hospital for Crippled Children, Montreal Unit; Associate Professor of Surgery, McGill University; Montreal, Quebec.

Roger Demers, M.D., F.R.C.P.
Assistant Professor of Medicine, University of Montreal; Attending Physician, Department of Rheumatology, Hôtel-Dieu Hospital of Montreal.

André Derome, M.D., C.R.C.S. (C)
Assistant Professor of Surgery, Department of Orthopedic Surgery, University of Montreal; Attending Staff, Hôtel-Dieu Hospital of Montreal.

Martin A. Entin, M.D., C.M., M. Sc. (McGill), F.A.C.S.
Assistant Professor of Surgery, McGill University; Surgeon-in-Charge, Sub-Department of Plastic Surgery, Royal Victoria Hospital; Consultant in Plastic Surgery, Shriners' Hospital for Crippled Children; Montreal, Quebec.

Roger Gariepy, M.D., F.R.C.S. (C)
Head of Orthopaedics, Hotel Dieu Hospital, Montreal, Quebec.

Alice L. Garrett, M.D.
Associate Professor of Orthopaedic Surgery, College of Physicians and Surgeons, Columbia University, New York; Director of Surgical Services, New York State Rehabilitation Hospital, West Haverstraw, New York.

G. A. deGroot, M.D.
Orthopaedic Research Department, Blodgett Memorial Hospital, Grand Rapids, Michigan.

Sig T. Hansen, Jr., M.D.
Assistant Professor of Orthopaedics, University of Washington School of Medicine, Seattle, Washington.

R. W. Hehl, M.D.
Orthopaedic Research Department, Blodgett Memorial Hospital, Grand Rapids, Michigan.

Malcolm Edward Heppenstall, M.D.
College of Medicine, University of Tennessee; Campbell Clinic Foundation Residency Program; Memphis, Tennessee.

William N. Jones, M.D.
Associate Orthopaedic Surgeon, Massachusetts General Hospital; Clinical Instructor in Orthopaedic Surgery, Harvard Medical School; Boston, Massachusetts.

Carroll A. Laurin, M.D., F.A.C.S., F.R.C.S. (C)
Associate Professor of Experimental Surgery, McGill University; Associate Professor of Surgery, University of Montreal; Attending Surgeon, Hôtel-Dieu Hospital of Montreal.

D. L. MacIntosh, M.D., C.M., F.R.C.S. (C)
Staff Surgeon, Division of Orthopaedics, Toronto General Hospital; Assistant Professor of Surgery, Faculty of Medicine, University of Toronto; Toronto, Ontario.

Robert D. Midgley, M.D., C.M., F.R.C.S. (C)
Assistant Surgeon, Royal Victoria Hospital; Head, Division of Plastic Surgery, Queen Mary Veterans' Hospital; Consultant in Plastic Surgery, Queen Elizabeth Hospital; Assistant Professor of Surgery, McGill University; Montreal, Quebec.

Nelson S. Mitchell, M.D., C.M.
Assistant Orthopaedic Surgeon, Royal Victoria Hospital; Consultant, Shriners' Hospital for Crippled Children, Montreal Unit; Assistant Professor of Surgery, McGill University; Montreal, Quebec.

Charles S. Neer II, M.D.
Professor of Clinical Orthopaedic Surgery, College of Physicians and Surgeons, Columbia University; Attending Orthopaedic Surgeon, New York Orthopaedic Hospital, Columbia-Presbyterian Medical Center; New York, New York.

Wylie T. Scott, Jr., M.D.
Resident in Orthopaedic Surgery, Mayo Graduate School of Medicine, University of Minnesota, Rochester, Minnesota.

Nora Shepard
Orthopaedic Research Department, Royal Victoria Hospital, Montreal, Quebec.

Edward H. Simmons, M.D., B.Sc. (Med.), F.R.C.S. (C), M.S. (Tor.), F.A.C.S.
Clinical Teacher in Orthopaedic Surgery, Faculty of Medicine, University of Toronto; Attending Orthopaedic Surgeon, Toronto East General and Orthopaedic Hospital; Consulting Orthopaedic Surgeon, Ontario Society for Crippled Children's Centre; Consulting Orthopaedic Surgeon, Sunnybrook Hospital; Toronto, Ontario.

Alfred B. Swanson, M.D., F.A.C.S.
Chief, Orthopaedic Surgery Department; Chief, Orthopaedic Research Department; Blodgett Memorial Hospital, Grand Rapids, Michigan.

Thomas K. F. Taylor, F.R.C.S., F.R.C.S. (Ed), F.R.A.C.S., D. Phil. (Oxon)
Professor of Orthopaedic and Traumatic Surgery, University of Sydney; Director of Orthopaedic and Accident Services, Royal North Shore Hospital; Sydney, New South Wales, Australia.

Borje Walldius
Associate Professor; Assistant Head Surgeon; Orthopaedic Clinic, St. Goran Hospital, Stockholm, Sweden.

T. J. Waller, M.D.
Orthopaedic Research Department, Blodgett Memorial Hospital, Grand Rapids, Michigan.

J. Watson-Farrar, M.A., M.B. (Cantab), F.R.C.S. (Eng)
Consultant Orthopaedic Surgeon, Norfolk and Norwich Hospital; Orthopaedic Surgeon to the Artificial Limb Centre, Norwich, England; Consultant-in-Charge, Accident and Emergency Department; Member, British Orthopaedic Association; Member, S.I.C.O.T.

Morris Ziff, Ph.D., M.D.
Professor of Internal Medicine; Director of Rheumatic Diseases Unit; University of Texas Southwestern Medical School, Dallas, Texas.

Preface

During recent decades the medical profession has been altering its approach to rheumatoid arthritis. Originally it was felt that the disease was variable, but usually progressive, and that very little could be done to alter its course. At that time, surgeons were primarily involved in devising reconstructive procedures which would alleviate disabilities in the late stages of the disease. Recently there has been a vast improvement in the medical management of the rheumatoid patient; however, it has become apparent that, although symptoms can be influenced by sound medical management, the progress of the disease continues unabated. Consequently in many centers the team approach has been directed towards preventing deformities. Many surgical procedures have been developed and explored in an attempt to lessen eventual disabilities of the disease. Currently, many operations are available, and, at last, sufficient numbers of patients have been followed for an analysis to be made of the results of surgery which can offer the basis for a sound surgical approach to the disease.

This book attempts to outline recognized surgical procedures designed for the rheumatoid patient. Even more important, it tries to offer advice on the selection of the proper procedure for any given patient at any given stage of that patient's disease. It appears to the editors that this is the most difficult problem presently facing the surgeon treating rheumatoid arthritics. Although the book deals with established operative procedures only, it is obvious to all concerned that the field is changing rapidly. The development of better operations and newer implants of modern materials will undoubtedly necessitate a redefinition of the indications for, and approaches to, surgical intervention in rheumatoid arthritis.

Surgery of Rheumatoid Arthritis results from a course entitled "The Surgical Management of Rheumatoid Arthritis" which was given under the sponsorship of the Post-Graduate Board of the Royal Victoria Hospital and McGill University in Montreal in May 1970. The editors wish to express their appreciation to the Board and to its secretaries, Miss Susan Cushing and Mrs. Trudy Cusmariu.

Richard L. Cruess
Nelson S. Mitchell

Contents

Surgery of Rheumatoid Arthritis

CHAPTER 1

Pathogenesis of Rheumatoid Arthritis

MORRIS ZIFF, M.D.

Three major histological changes take place in the development of rheumatoid synovitis: proliferation of the synovial lining cells; infiltration of the deeper layer with mononuclear cells; and effusion in the synovial space, containing predominantly polymorphonuclear cells.

Under the electron microscope, the lining layer is seen to consist of three types of synovial cells: type A cells, which are phagocytic and take up particulate material and immune complexes from the synovial fluid; type B cells, which resemble fibroblasts and are believed to synthesize the protein and hyaluronic acid present in the synovial effusion; and type C or undifferentiated cells, which have the properties of both the type A and the type B cells.[2,8]

In the deeper regions of the synovial membrane, small lymphocytes make their way through the walls of capillaries and venules and surround them with dense infiltrates. Around some capillaries, lymphocytes predominate; however, around others, large numbers of plasma cells are seen. The dense nodules of lymphocytes and plasma cells appear to be actively engaged in an immune response. Large amounts of gamma globulin are synthesized.[10] Synthesis of the three common types—IgG, IgA and IgM—has been measured by incubating rheumatoid synovial membrane obtained at synovectomy with radioactively labeled amino acids. The amounts of immunoglobulin synthesized in the rheumatoid synovium are comparable to those made in human lymphoid tissue, indicating that the intensity of the immune response in rheumatoid synovium is comparable to that in lymphoid tissue.

Deposits of IgG, IgM and serum complement have been demonstrated in the rheumatoid synovium by the fluorescent antibody-staining method. The simultaneous presence of complement and immunoglobulin in tissue deposits indicates that these have been laid down in the form of antigen-antibody complexes.

In the synovial fluid, over 90 per cent of the cells are usually polymorphonuclear. The complement level in rheumatoid effusions is low, presumably as a result of having been bound by antigen-antibody complexes.[4,9]

Rheumatoid factors are also synthesized in rheumatoid synovial tissue.[3] They can be found in the synovial fluid as well as in the serum of patients with rheumatoid arthritis and are autoantibodies to human IgG. Not only do they react with human IgG, but they also cross-react with the IgG of a number of animal species, making it possible to test for rheumatoid factor with systems such as sheep cells coated with rabbit IgG.

The presence of rheumatoid factor seems to be correlated with the presence of subcutaneous nodules and bone erosion. It is almost always present in high titer in patients with rheumatoid vasculitis—a condition commonly associated with ischemic gangrene of the skin or peripheral neuropathy. There appears to be no direct correlation between the titer of rheumatoid factor and the day-to-day activity of the disease, though it is well established that patients with high titers of rheumatoid factor have a poorer prognosis than those with low or zero titers.

What does the presence of rheumatoid factor represent theoretically? The experiments of Abruzzo and Christian are of some interest in this connection.[1] When these authors injected heat-killed *Escherichia coli* into rabbits, antibodies to the *E. coli* developed in the usual manner. In response to repeated injections, however, an antibody to the rabbit IgG developed. This new antibody was a macroglobulin, or IgM, which had the properties of a rheumatoid factor. Presumably, the deformation of the rabbit IgG-*E. coli* antibody, as it was bound to the *E. coli* antigen, revealed antigenic sites inside the molecule to which the rabbit responded with autoantibody formation. By analogy, the implication from these experiments is that the patient with rheumatoid arthritis is undergoing continuous immunization by an unknown antigen which, like the *E. coli* in the rabbit, leads to the development of anti-IgG antibody.

It is now known that the rheumatoid factor occurs not only in the IgM form, but also in an IgG or lower molecular weight form. When host IgG combines with rheumatoid factor IgG, a complex is formed which effectively binds complement. Such IgG-Ig-C′ complexes are present in the synovial fluid and are thought to explain the low complement levels in rheumatoid synovial effusions.[13] It has been shown in our laboratory that these complexes are phagocytosed by both the type A and the type C synovial lining cells and the polymorphonuclear cells of the fluid.[6,7] The uptake of these complexes in the lysosomes of the phagocytic cells has been thought to bring about a release of lysosomal enzymes and other proteins. This may in turn stimulate further inflammation. The neutral and acid proteases released from the lysosomes may also participate in a proteolytic attack on the cartilage matrix.

The binding of complement by rheumatoid factor complexes activates the complement sequence and creates a C5, 6, 7 complex which is chemotactic for polymorphonuclear cells and attracts these cells from the synovial capillaries. This appears to be the principal basis for the predominance of polymorphonuclear cells in rheumatoid effusions.

There is another dimension to rheumatoid synovitis that has recently come into focus. This is the presence of macrophage migration inhibitory factors in the rheumatoid synovial fluid. Such factors have the capacity to immobilize macrophages and, presumably, to effect the accumulation of macrophages in chronic inflammatory reactions. The macrophage migration inhibitory factor (MIF) is ordinarily elaborated by lymphocytes undergoing blastic transformation as a result of contact with antigen. The elaboration of MIF is believed to be characteristic of the delayed hypersensitivity response. The presence of MIF in rheumatoid synovial fluid has been demonstrated in our laboratory and, presumably, is elaborated by lymphoblasts in the synovial membrane.[12] The identity of the antigen or immune complex which brings about the blastic transformation of these lymphocytes is not known. However, it seems clear that a substance which has the capacity to mediate a delayed hypersensitivity response and accumulate mononuclear cells is present in the synovial fluid.

The above discussion has dealt with the various aspects of rheumatoid synovitis which appear to be associated with an immunological response. These phenomena, which in essence represent major features of the pathogenesis of rheumatoid synovitis, are beginning to be reasonably well understood. What is not known is the identity of the initiating factor in the process. An autoimmune response based upon genetic susceptibility has often been postulated, but this has not been demonstrated. The possibility that the rheumatoid process is initiated by an exogenous agent, particularly an infectious agent, is deserving of serious consideration. The fact that patients with agammaglobulinemia are prone to a rheumatoid-like arthritis is very suggestive of this possibility. Another line of evidence is the occurrence of two spontaneous diseases of animals; namely, the disease of New Zealand black mice, and Aleutian mink disease. Both of these diseases resemble systemic lupus erythematosus, a related collagen vascular disease. There is good evidence that these diseases are caused by viral agents.

In the past, a number of unsuccessful attempts have been made to identify a viral agent in rheumatoid tissue. However, evidence has been obtained that rheumatoid synovial cells in tissue culture are resistant to rubella and Newcastle virus infection, and that non-rheumatoid cells are susceptible to both.[5,11] These findings have supported the possibility that latent viruses may persist in the rheumatoid synovial membrane.

REFERENCES

1. Abruzzo, J. L., and Christian, C. L.: The induction of a rheumatoid factor-like substance in rabbits. J. Exp. Med., *114*:791-806, 1961.
2. Barland, P., Novikoff, A., and Hamerman, D.: Fine structure and cytochemistry of the rheumatoid synovial membrane with special reference to lysosomes. Amer. J. Path., *44*:853-866, 1964.
3. Bartfeld, H., and Epstein, W. V.: Conference on rheumatoid factors and their biological significance. Ann. N.Y. Acad. Sci., *168*:1-207, 1969.
4. Fostiropoulos, G., Austen, K. F., and Bloch, K. J.: Total hemolytic complement (CH_{50}) and second component of complement ($C'2^{hu}$) activity in serum and synovial fluid. Arthritis Rheum., *8*:219-232, 1965.
5. Grayzel, A. I., and Beck, C.: Rubella infection of synovial cells and the resistance of cells derived from patients with rheumatoid arthritis. J. Exp. Med., *131*:367-373, 1970.
6. Hurd, E. R., LoSpalluto, J., and Ziff, M.: Formation of leukocyte inclusions in normal polymorphonuclear cells incubated with synovial fluid. Arthritis Rheum. *13*:724, 1970.
7. Kinsella, T., Baum, J., and Ziff, M.: Studies of isolated synovial lining cells of rheumatoid and non-rheumatoid synovial membranes. Arthritis Rheum. *13*:734, 1970.
8. Norton, W., and Ziff, M.: Electron microscopic observations on the rheumatoid synovial membrane. Arthritis Rheum., *9*:589, 1966.
9. Pekin, T., and Zvaifler, N.: Hemolytic complement in synovial fluid. J. Clin. Invest., *43*:1372-1382, 1964.
10. Smiley, J., Sachs, C., and Ziff, M.: *In vitro* synthesis of immunoglobulin by rheumatoid synovial membrane. J. Clin. Invest., *47*:624-632, 1968.
11. Smith, C., and Hamerman, D.: Significance of persistent differences between normal and rheumatoid synovial membrane cells in culture. Arthritis Rheum., *12*:639-645, 1969.
12. Stastny, P., and Ziff, M.: Macrophage migration inhibition and cytotoxicity in synovial fluids. Proc. Third Intl. Symp. Inflammation Club, Excerpta Medica (In press).
13. Winchester, R., Agnello, V., and Kunkel, H. G.: Gamma globulin complexes in synovial fluids of patients with rheumatoid arthritis. Partial characterization and relationship to lowered complement levels. Clin. Exptl. Immunol., *6*:689-706, 1970.

CHAPTER 2

The Effects of Synovectomy on Synovium and Cartilage in Rheumatoid Arthritis

NELSON MITCHELL, M.D., AND NORA SHEPARD

Many clinical reviews confirm that synovectomy is useful in relieving pain and in improving function in joints affected by rheumatoid arthritis.[4,8,12] There is some information available on the change in concentration of synovial fluid enzymes and immunological factors following this operation.[6] It was not known what effect synovectomy might have on the cartilage of rheumatoid joints; little was known about the recurrence of the disease in the regenerating synovium.

METHODS OF STUDY

The changes in grossly normal cartilage removed from patients at synovectomy for early rheumatoid arthritis have been studied by electron microscopy.[11] We subsequently performed direct surgical biopsies on ten patients at intervals of 3 weeks to 6 years after synovectomy. In each case samples of cartilage and synovium were removed for comparison with the original tissue. Three of these patients had had the operation 5 to 6 years before, and the original tissue was not available. However, since they were returning for synovectomy of the contralateral joints, the cartilage and synovium from these were considered comparable to the original tissue and were thus studied. Samples of cartilage and synovium were studied by both light and electron microscopy. In addition some samples of cartilage were incubated with 3H proline and radioautographs were made and studied.

The patients' ages ranged from 18 to 72 years. There were two men and eight women in the series. Seven had been on steroids prior to both operations and three had not. With the exception of one patient who had been followed for only 6 months at the time of biopsy, all the patients had been followed for a minimum of 1 year after biopsy. To date, eight of the ten patients have had a good clinical result without return of pain, effusion or other evidence of active disease in the joint. The other two patients, who underwent biopsies at 1 year and 1½ years after synovectomy, had been clinically free of the disease until the time of biopsy. At that time their synovia were found to have histological evidence of recurrence. Six months after biopsy one patient developed definite clinical evidence of recurrence and the other complained of some pain and swelling in the joint, indicating a probable return of the disease. It is to the eight clinically successful cases that we devote most of our attention.

CHANGES OBSERVED IN CARTILAGE AND SYNOVIUM

Two Months. The earliest changes noted in the synovium were seen 2 months after synovectomy. At this time, the diseased tissue had been replaced by a loose fibroblastic

This study was supported by a grant from the Canadian Arthritis and Rheumatism Society and the Medical Research Council.

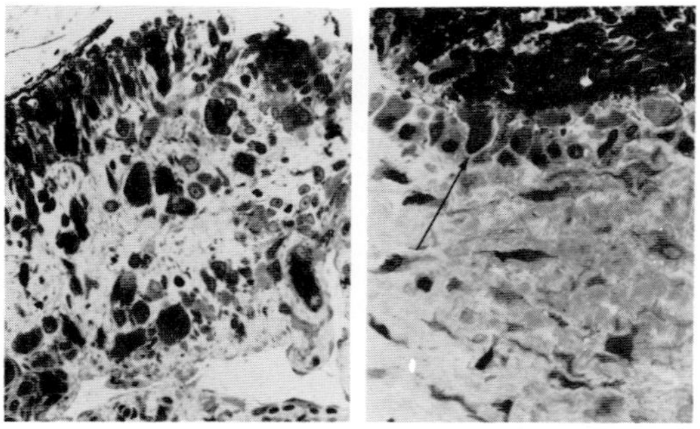

FIG. 2-1. (*Left*) Diseased synovium removed at the time of synovectomy. (*Right*) Nine weeks after synovectomy a layer of lining cells one cell thick lines the joint cavity (arrow). The deeper tissues contain collagen and fibroblasts. (×340)

stroma supporting a distinct layer of cells lining the joint cavity (Fig. 2-1). There was no evidence of inflammatory cell infiltration. At the time of synovectomy the lining cell population consisted almost entirely of A cells containing many lysosomes and phagolysosomes. At biopsy, electron microscopy showed that this had been replaced by a population of lining cells, some of which contained vacuoles and had cytoplasmic extensions resembling the A cell of normal synovium, while others had a cytoplasm occupied by rough endoplasmic reticulum resembling the B cells of normal synovium (Fig. 2-2). The large quantities of fibrin seen surrounding the cells at the time of synovectomy had disappeared.

The articular cartilage at the time of biopsy was little different from that at synovectomy. The changes described in rheumatoid arthritic cartilage were noted throughout both samples. Considerable amounts of pericellular material surrounded the cells, which had formed peripheral rims between this material and the normal matrix and had accumulated fat or lysosomes in their cytoplasm (Fig. 2-3). In many instances the cells appeared degenerate or even dead.

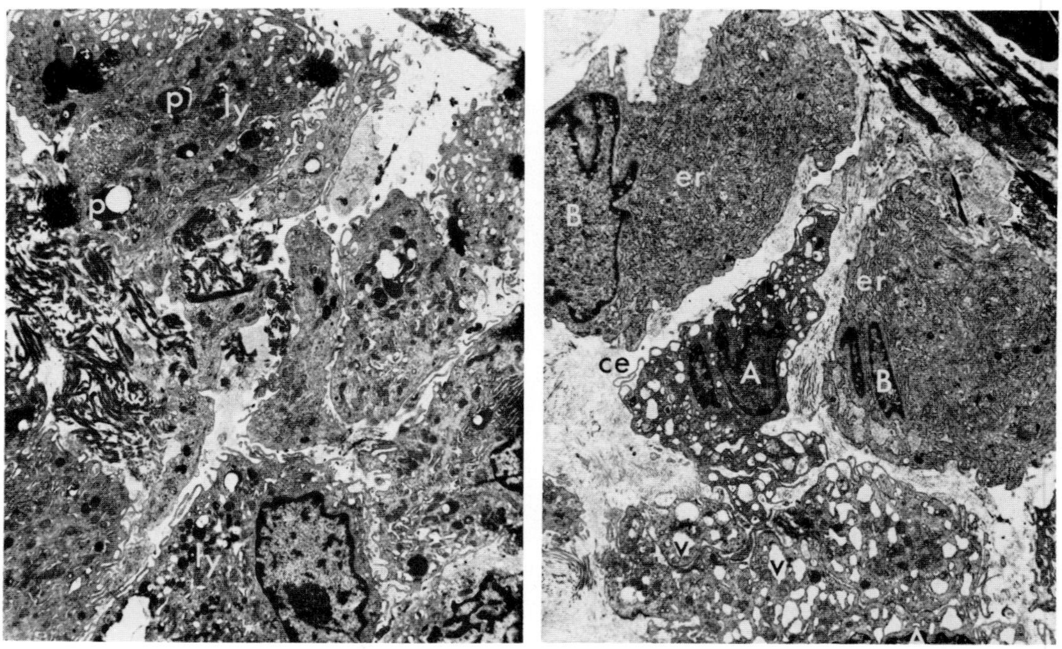

FIG. 2-2. (*Left*) Synovium removed at synovectomy. Cells containing phagolysosomes (p) and lysosomes (ly) are seen. (×3380) (*Right*) The regenerating membrane 9 weeks after synovectomy. Cells (A) containing vacuoles (v) and cytoplasmic extensions (ce) are noted in contrast to those (B) whose cytoplasm consists almost entirely of endoplasmic reticulum (er). (×3510)

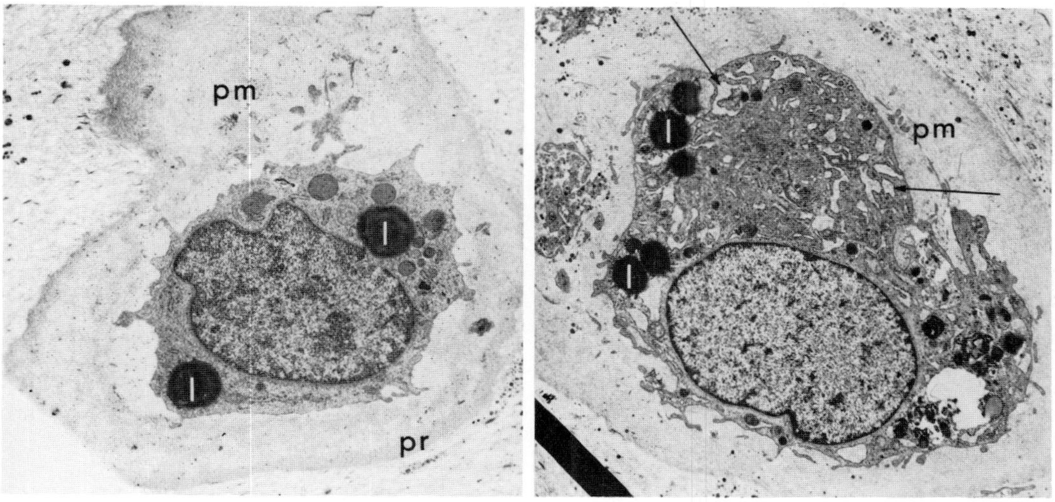

FIG. 2-3. (*Left*) A chondrocyte removed at synovectomy. Lipid (l) was found in the cytoplasm and the cell was surrounded by pericellular material (pm) bounded by a peripheral rime (pr). (×3870) (*Right*) Nine weeks after synovectomy intra-cellular lipid (l) and pericellular material (pm) were seen. Note the dilatation of the endoplasmic reticulum (arrows). (×4830)

Seven Months. Seven months after synovectomy the regenerating membrane was somewhat more cellular and the lining layer was two or three cells deep. The supporting stroma was made up of fibroblasts and showed no evidence of inflammatory cell infiltration (Fig. 2-4). Under the electron microsope the predominantly A cell population typical of rheumatoid synovium had been replaced by large uncrowded cells, among which both A and B cell types could be identified. The lysosomes and phagolysosomes, commonly seen in the rheumatoid synovium, had almost completely disappeared (Fig. 2-5).

The cells of the upper third of the articular cartilage, as seen under the electron microscope, contained smaller amounts of lipid and lysosomes after synovectomy. The Golgi zones were numerous and the endoplasmic reticulum was more abundant (Fig. 2-6). In the middle zone there was a tendency for the cells to show a dilatation of their endoplasmic reticulum, which was not observed in cartilage removed at synovectomy (Fig. 2-7). Radioautographs indicated that the diseased chondrocytes had absorbed little, if any, of the radioactive proline in contrast to the synovectomized tissue over whose cells many grains were seen (Fig. 2-8).

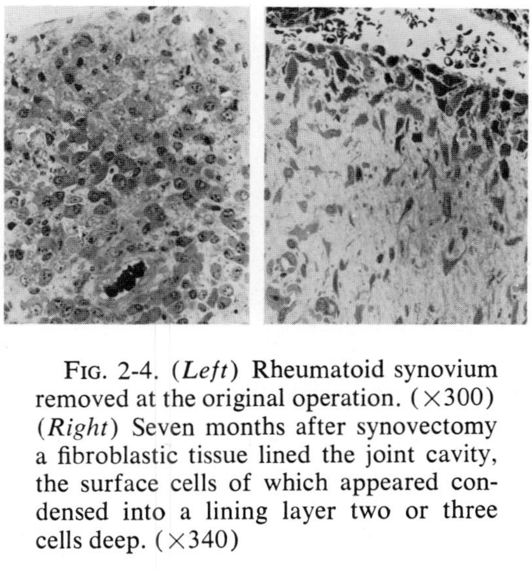

FIG. 2-4. (*Left*) Rheumatoid synovium removed at the original operation. (×300) (*Right*) Seven months after synovectomy a fibroblastic tissue lined the joint cavity, the surface cells of which appeared condensed into a lining layer two or three cells deep. (×340)

Twelve Months. The regenerated synovium 12 months after operation showed a scanty layer of lining cells supported by a stroma which had now become almost entirely collagenous (Fig. 2-9). Under the electron microscope the A cell synovium of

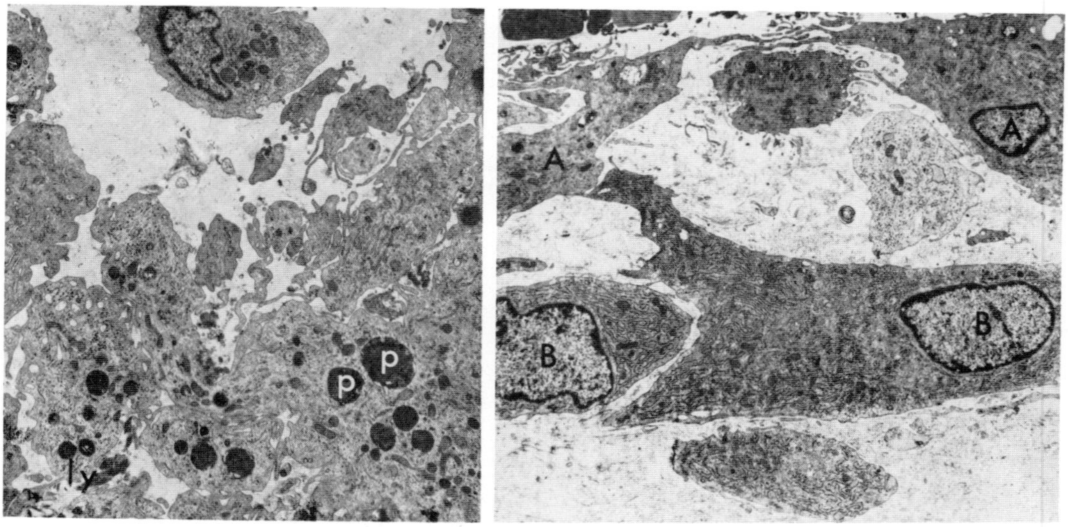

FIG. 2-5. (*Left*) Diseased synovium made up entirely of cells possessing vacuoles, cytoplasmic extensions, phagolysosomes (p) and smaller lysosomes (ly). (×5685) (*Right*) The joint cavity 7 months after synovectomy was lined by cells (A) which had vacuoles and cytoplasmic extensions, while other cells (B) had a cytoplasm occupied entirely by endoplasmic reticulum. (×4160)

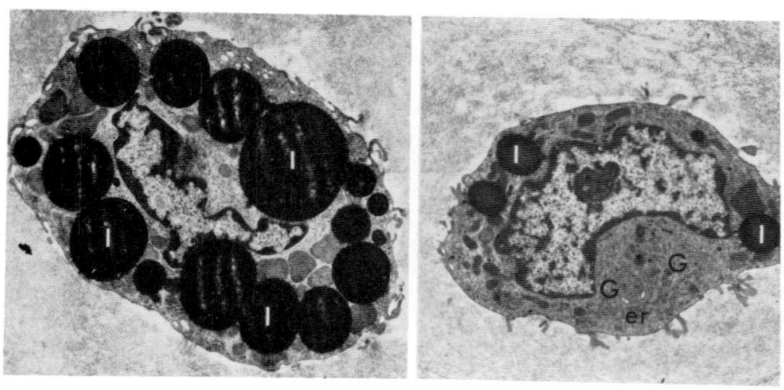

FIG. 2-6. (*Left*) A chondrocyte near the joint surface at the time of synovectomy. Note the large accumulation of lipid (l). (×8379) (*Right*), A chondrocyte from the same area 7 months later showing lipids (l), a Golgi (G), and endoplasmic reticulum (er) in the cytoplasm. (×8027)

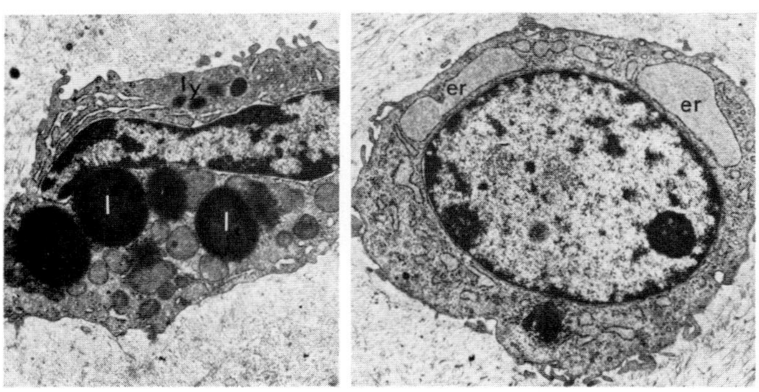

FIG. 2-7. (*Left*), Chondrocyte from the middle zones removed at operation. Lipids (l) and lysosomes (ly) are noted. (×8208) (*Right*) Chondrocyte from the same area 7 months later. The endoplasmic reticulum (er) is dilated. (×9570)

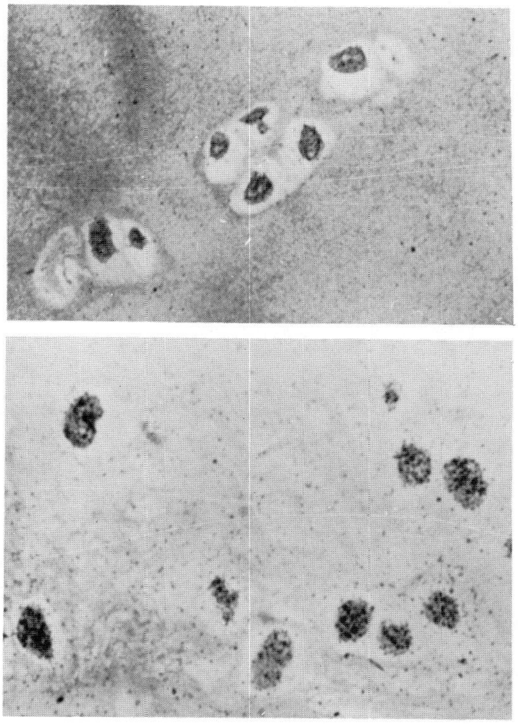

FIG. 2-8. (*Top*) Chondrocytes from rheumatoid cartilage removed at synovectomy showing pericellular spaces with little if any uptake of radioactive proline. (×400) (*Bottom*) The cartilage at the time of biopsy shows loss of pericellular space and abundant uptake of proline. (×400)

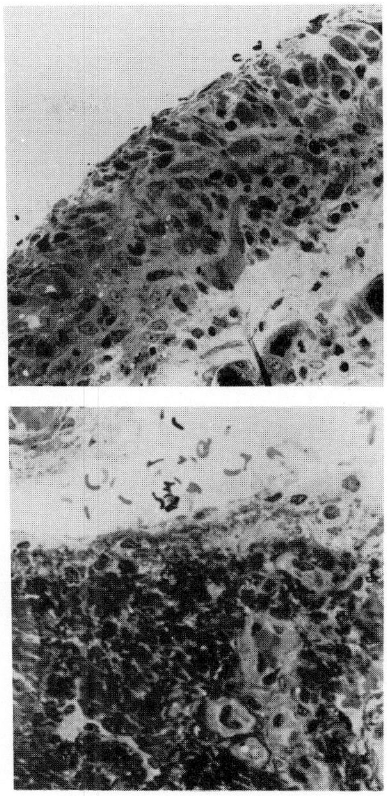

FIG. 2-9. (*Top*) Synovium removed at synovectomy. (×400) (*Bottom*) Regenerated membrane 1 year later shows infrequent cells at the joint surface with abundant collagenous tissue below. (×340)

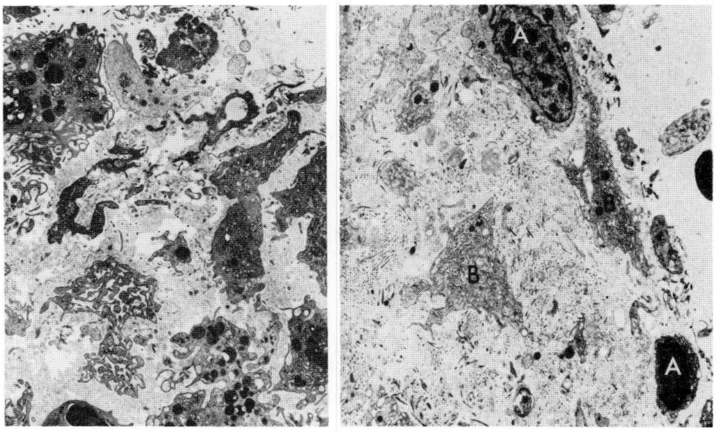

FIG. 2-10. (*Left*) Crowded cells containing many lysosomes and showing vacuoles and cytoplasmic extensions make up the synovium removed at synovectomy. (×4400) (*Right*) One year later the lining population consisted of cells (A) containing vacuoles and some lysosomes, while other cells (B) had cytoplasm made up of endoplasmic reticulum. (×3500)

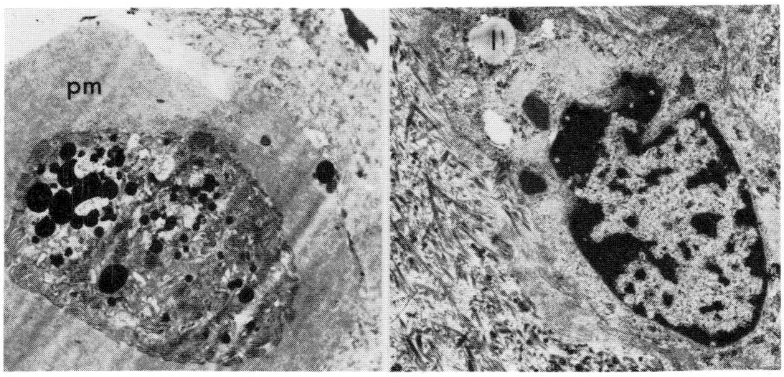

Fig. 2-11. (*Left*) A surface chondrocyte at synovectomy showing an accumulation of dense material, probably fat and lysosomes, surrounded by a considerable amount of pericellular material (pm). (×5600) (*Right*) One year later cells from the same area showed little lipid (l) and a disappearance of the pericellular material. (×10,560)

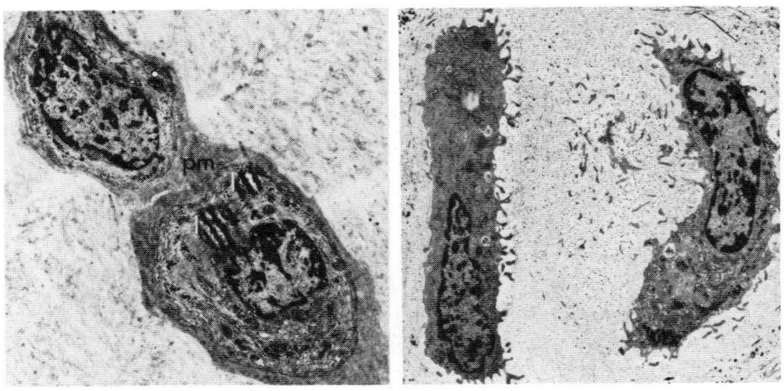

Fig. 2-12. (*Left*) A pair of chondrocytes from the deepest zone at synovectomy. Lipid (l) and pericellular material (pm) are noted. (×6400) (*Right*) A pair of chondrocytes at the time of biopsy. The lipid had disappeared and the area surrounding the chondrocytes is made up of matrix which appears normal for this level. (×6400)

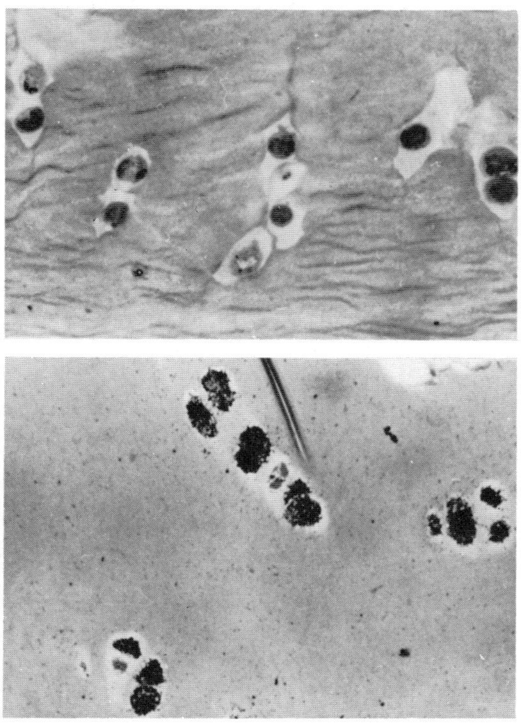

Fig. 2-13. (*Top*) Chondrocytes from rheumatoid cartilage showing scanty uptake of radioactive proline. (×400) (*Bottom*) One year after synovectomy large pericellular spaces have disappeared and many grains overlie the cells. (×400)

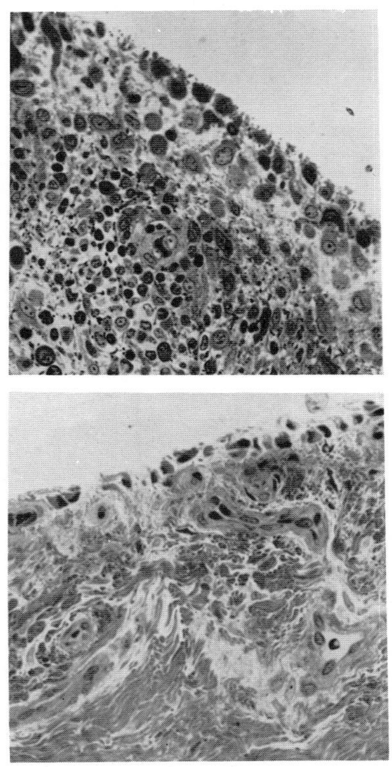

Fig. 2-14. (*Top*) Diseased synovium removed at synovectomy. (×340) (*Bottom*) Synovium biopsied 5 years later shows a single layer of lining cells supported by a dense collagenous tissue. (×300)

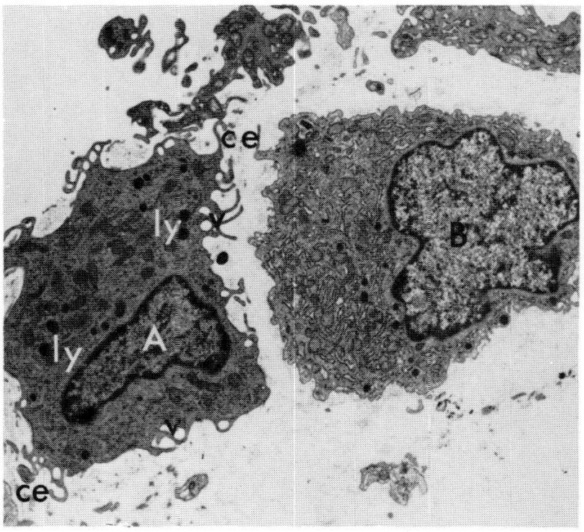

FIG. 2-15. The lining cells consisted of equal numbers of cells (A) containing vacuoles (V) and occasional lysosomes (ly) and possessing cytoplasmic extensions (ce) and cells (B) whose cytoplasm contained primarily endoplasmic reticulum. (×5685)

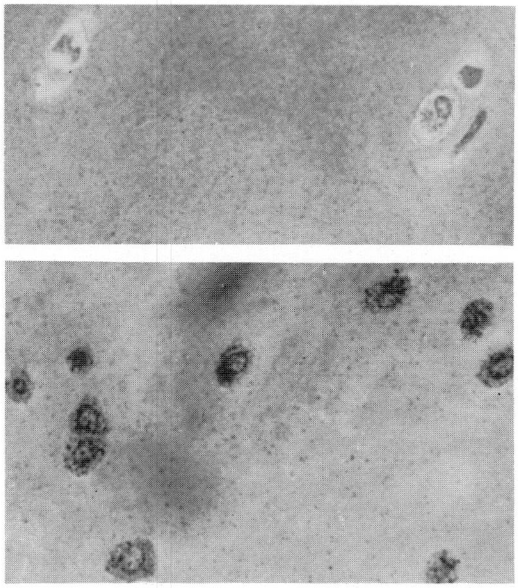

FIG. 2-17. (*Top*) Cartilage removed at the time of the original synovectomy shows little uptake of proline by the chondrocytes. (×400) (*Bottom*) Five years after synovectomy absorption has increased, and the pericellular spaces have diminished. (×400)

the diseased tissue had been replaced by cells showing characteristics of both cell types (Fig. 2-10). Chondrocytes near the surface of the cartilage at the time of synovectomy contained large amounts of fat and were surrounded by some pericellular material. One year later, cells from the same region showed little if any fat or lysosomes, and the pericellular space had become much smaller (Fig. 2-11). Similar observations were made in the middle and deeper zones, where the chondrocytes were indistinguishable from normal cells at the time of biopsy (Fig. 2-12). The autoradiographs demonstrated little, if any, absorption of proline by the rheumatoid chondrocytes. One year after synovectomy, however, the pericellular spaces had become smaller and the uptake was abundant (Fig. 2-13).

Five Years. Five years after synovectomy the synovial membrane was very similar to that seen at 1 year. There was still a scanty

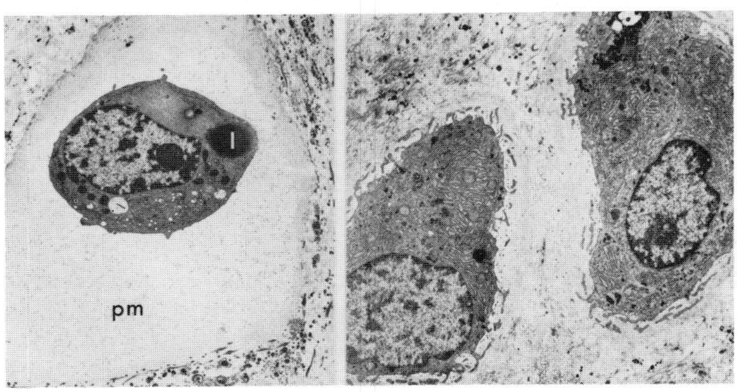

FIG. 2-16. (*Left*) A chondrocyte from the deepest zone of the diseased cartilage showing lipid (l) and a large pericellular space (pm). (×5060) (*Right*) Deep chondrocytes 5 years after synovectomy. (×4840)

layer of lining cells supported by dense collagenous subsynovial tissue (Fig. 2-14). Viewed through the electron microscope the lining cells were uncrowded and showed equal proportions of A and B cell types (Fig. 2-15). The cartilage cells of all zones, including the deepest, contained considerable amounts of endoplasmic reticulum. There were few lysosomes, and these cells were not surrounded by large pericellular spaces (Fig. 2-16). The synovectomized chondrocytes showed considerably greater affinity for proline as compared to the diseased cartilage (Fig. 2-17).

SIGNIFICANCE OF OBSERVED CHANGES

Ten patients had synovial and cartilage biopsies from 3 weeks to 6 years following synovectomy. In each instance the biopsy was compared with the diseased tissue. Eight of these patients have had no clinical signs of recurrence one year after biopsy. Two patients who had had no clinical evidence of recurrence at the time of biopsy, subsequently developed signs of the disease. Of the two clinical failures, both were female and both had positive rheumatoid serology. One had been on steroids and one had not. Of the eight successful cases, six women and two men, one of the men and one of the women did not have positive serology. One of the men and one of the women had never taken steroids and the remainder all had. Although this series is small, it does not appear that age, sex, rheumatoid serology or steroid intake had any appreciable effect on the changes found in the cartilage after synovectomy.

Histological studies showed that in the successful cases the diseased membrane was replaced after about 2 months by a membrane containing lining cells demonstrating characteristics of the A and B cell types.[2] Studies of synovial regeneration have indicated that complete regeneration takes about 6 weeks in rabbits.[9,10] In our patients the regenerating lining layer was initially supported by a loose stroma of fibroblasts. This stroma, beginning at 7 months, and continuing on to the end of the study (6 years) showed an increasing tendency to become densely collagenous. As more time elapsed the lining cells, which were initially numerous, became fewer in number. The predominantly A cell population lining the rheumatoid joint gave way to a population of equal numbers of A and B cells by the time of biopsy. The high intracellular content of phagolysosomes and lysosomes was not seen in the regenerated lining cells. In none of the clinically successful cases was the subsynovial inflammatory cell infiltration typical of rheumatoid disease seen in the regenerated membrane. Fibrin accumulation around the cells had likewise disappeared. Although the regenerated synovium, because of its scanty cellular content and predominantly collagenous base, is not typical of normal synovium in most areas of the joint, it would seem, nevertheless, that histologically this new membrane represents an improvement on that which was removed. It may be that the successful formation of a collagenous joint lining provides some barrier to the ingrowth of proliferative rheumatoid tissue.

With the exception of a tendency to dilatation of the endoplasmic reticulum, no significant changes could be found in the chondrocytes at 3 weeks and 2 months following synovectomy. At 1 year, however, the elongated surface cells, which had not been found in the diseased cartilage, had reappeared. A reduction of lysosomes was similarly noted. In the deeper cells lysosomes and large pericellular spaces had also disappeared. Five and 6 years after synovectomy, cartilage cells appeared quite different from the diseased cells and were morphologically identical to the normal chondrocytes.

None of the patients in this report had shown gross evidence of pannus at the time of the original operation. The cartilage, both at the time of synovectomy and at biopsy, looked normal to the naked eye. The ultramorphological changes in the chondrocytes in these patients were not then due to an overlying pannus but must have been mediated indirectly by such things as enzymes, reduction of hyaluronate protein or pH changes.[1,3,5] All of these originate primarily in the synovium. Removal of the synovium and its successful replacement by a tissue free of disease apparently results in improvement in chondrocyte morphology. It is interesting to note that not until an identifiable synovial membrane has reappeared do the chondrocytes show any real evidence of such improved morphology. This occurred seven months after synovectomy in this series.

The surface chondrocytes were not found in the diseased joints but appeared after synovectomy. This could occur either by metaplasia of deeper cells which were pushed closer to the surface following an erosion of some of the cartilage, or it could occur by duplication of these cells to produce an immature type which could then undergo metaplasia to form the surface cell. Mitotic figures are rarely seen in cartilage and a previous attempt to demonstrate tritiated thymidine uptake by incubated cartilage as a measure of mitosis failed in both diseased and synovectomized cartilage.*

Coincident with an improvement in morphology there appeared to be a change in chondrocyte function with regard to the uptake of proline. Repo and Mitchell† have shown that in normal animals proline will ultimately become incorporated into the collagen fraction of the matrix. It seems that this is a normal maintenance function of adult chondrocytes. The uptake of proline by the rheumatoid cartilage was markedly reduced but after synovectomy the radioactive proline was again found in abundance in these chondrocytes. Improvement in morphology would appear to be substantiated by an improved chondrocyte function.

Not all patients have a satisfactory clinical result from synovectomy. Of those that do, the ones who maintain this clinically improved picture for the longest time have the greatest chance of reversing some of the morphological and perhaps functional cartilage alterations caused by the disease. Similarly, those patients who maintain a good clinical result are likely to possess joint lining cells having many of the features of normal synovial cells and they will be supported by an envelope of dense collagenous tissue. It is suggested that this stroma may be a relatively infertile ground for the aggressive infiltration of rheumatoid inflammatory cells.

* Mitchell, N., and Shepard, N. Unpublished work.

† Repo, R. U., and Mitchell, N. Unpublished work.

REFERENCES

1. Arai, M.: Catalyze activity of synovial fluid in joint diseases. Tohoku J. Exp. Med., *91*: 35-40, 1967.
2. Barland, P., Novikoff, A. B., and Hamerman, D.: Electron microscopy of the human synovial membrane. J. Cell. Biol., *14*:207-220, 1962.
3. ———: Lysosomes in the synovial membrane in rheumatoid arthritis: a mechanism for cartilage erosion. Trans. Ass. Amer. Physicians, *77*:239-247, 1964.
4. Barnes, C. G., and Mason, R. M.: Synovectomy of the knee joint in rheumatoid arthritis. Ann. Phys. Med., *IX* (3), 1966.
5. Barnett, C. H.: Wear and tear in joints. J. Bone Joint Surg. [Brit.], *38*:567-575, 1958.
6. Cracchiolo, A., and Barnett, E. V.: Immunologic changes in a synovial fluid following synovectomy of the knee for rheumatoid arthritis. J. Bone Joint Surg., *51*: 475-486, 1969.
7. Evanson, J. N., Jeffrey, J. J., and Krane, S. M.: Human collagenase: identification and characterization of an enzyme from rheumatoid synovium in culture. Science, *158*:499-502, 1967.

8. Gariépy, R., Demers, R., and Laurin, C. A.: The prophylactic effects of synovectomy of the knee in rheumatoid arthritis. Canad. Med. Ass. J., *94*:1349-1352, 1966.
9. Mitchell, N., and Blackwell, P.: The electron microscopy of regenerating synovium after subtotal synovectomy in rabbits. J. Bone Joint Surg., *50*:675-686, 1968.
10. Mitchell, N., and Cruess, R. L.: Synovial regeneration after synovectomy. Canad. J. Surg., *10*:234-239, 1967.
11. Mitchell, N., and Shepard, N.: The ultramorphology of articular cartilage in early rheumatoid arthritis. J. Bone Joint Surg., *52*:1405-1423, 1970.
12. Swett, P. O.: Review of synovectomy. J. Bone Joint Surg., *20*:68-76, 1938.

CHAPTER 3

Synovectomy of the Knee in Rheumatoid Arthritis

Carroll A. Laurin, M.D., Roger Gariépy, M.D., Roger Demers, M.D., and André Derome, M.D.

The history of synovectomy began almost a hundred years ago when Volkmann, in 1877, performed the first synovectomy of the knee on a patient suffering from tuberculosis.[3] Almost 23 years elapsed before Mignon attempted the operation on a rheumatoid knee.[2] Synovectomies were then performed for a variety of conditions, and for many years surgeons were intermittently enthusiastic or disappointed with the operation. Swett was the first on this continent to publish a well-documented series to justify more than a passing interest in an operation which had yet to have clear indications and a sound understanding of the expected results.[4]

The purpose of this review is to clarify the role that a surgical synovectomy can play in the treatment of rheumatoid arthritis, an acknowledgedly unpredictable disease. It is based on 123 synovectomies of the knee performed for rheumatoid arthritis (Table 3-1). Of these patients, seven died, 13 were lost to follow-up, and 51 were excluded because the follow-up period was less than 2 years. Fifty-two synovectomies had an adequate follow-up period and were interviewed in person and examined by us.

Table 3-1. Follow-Up Status of 123 Knee Synovectomies for Rheumatoid Arthritis

Follow-Up Status	*Number of Patients*
Adequate follow-up and personal interview	52
Follow-up less than two years (excluded from study)	51
Lost to follow-up	13
Dead	7
Total	123

Seven of the 52 synovectomies were bilateral; the series contained nine men and 31 women. The operations were all performed in the same hospital* by three surgeons (R.G., A.D., C.A.L.), using essentially the same surgical technique and postoperative regimen along the lines originally conceived by the senior surgeon (R.G.). The average period of observation was 6½ years, with a range varying from 2 to 12 years. There were no children in this group of patients, whose ages ranged from 25 years to 71, with an average of 46 years.

INDICATIONS AND CONTRAINDICATIONS FOR A SYNOVECTOMY

The classical, and admittedly theoretical, indication for a surgical synovectomy is a chronically painful and swollen joint that does not respond to a sound medical regimen. It is indeed relatively easy to define the theoretical indications for the operation; the clinical application of these criteria can at times be more difficult. What is a "sound medical regimen"? How long should one persist before resorting to surgery? Ideally the final decision should be made

* Department of Orthopaedic Surgery and Rheumatology, Hotel-Dieu Hospital, Montreal.

jointly by a rheumatologist and a surgeon or by a person who is familiar with what each specialty can offer for the rheumatoid knee. The judicious use of anti-inflammatory drugs, a fair trial with gold salts or systemic or intra-articular cortisone must be tempered with sound medical judgment and excellent systemic care, considering the physical and emotional condition of the patient.

In view of the unpredictable and varying evolution of the disease, it is tempting to evade the question of how long one should continue with the medical treatment of a chronically painful and swollen joint before surgery is proposed. Two factors can assist the physician in his decision: the duration of the unsuccessful medical treatment and the physical examination of the involved joint.

Surgery should be contemplated after 6 months of sound but unsuccessful treatment. The clinical criteria of an unsatisfactory response to treatment are pain, persistent effusion, and a clinically palpable synovial membrane; the indications for surgery are almost imperative if, furthermore, a mild flexion deformity of the knee exists. Indeed, a mild (less than 15°) knee flexion deformity which develops in spite of adequate treatment should probably be considered to be an absolute indication for synovectomy. If this deformity appears or persists, in spite of an acceptable control of the subjective complaint of pain, one must assume that organic and potentially irreversible changes are developing in that joint. A painful flexion deformity will usually correct itself as the effusion regresses and as the acute congestion is medically controlled. If the deformity persists in the absence of pain, one is faced with a disease that is progressing in spite of adequate treatment, and the indications for surgery are that much stronger.

The gradual development of a mild flexion deformity must not, of course, be confused with the serious flexion deformities noted in more advanced cases of rheumatoid arthritis; the authors merely wish to point out the importance of a mild deformity as an indication for surgery.

Clinical Indications for Synovectomy

1. Six months of sound but unsuccessful medical treatment.
2. Persistent pain.
3. Intermittent or constant effusion.
4. Clinically palpable synovial membrane.
5. Appearance or persistence of a mild knee joint deformity.
6. Early radiological evidence of joint involvement.

A clear concept of the pathology of this systemic disease is essential to properly comprehend the indications and the purpose of this operation. Rheumatoid arthritis is a systemic disease of unknown etiology whose first clinical manifestations are due to synovial lesions. The ideal candidate for a synovectomy is a patient whose disease is essentially, and primarily, at the synovial phase. Since this synovial period is theoretically reversible, either by spontaneous remission or adequate medical treatment, the clinical decision can be difficult. However, what may begin as mere synovial congestion, with pain, effusion and restriction of motion, may gradually deteriorate as the synovial disease becomes more widespread. The abnormal synovial membrane can indeed become obstructive, invasive, and destructive, affecting cartilage and ligaments. Ideally, a synovectomy should have been performed before that phase.

The clinical and pathological considerations that favor a good result following a synovectomy have been described as the synovial phase. Knee joint motion and stability are preserved, x-ray signs are minimal, and the general condition of the patient is adequate. The patient's medical condition, however, must not take precedence over his motivation. Results are better if he is willing and able to cooperate fully

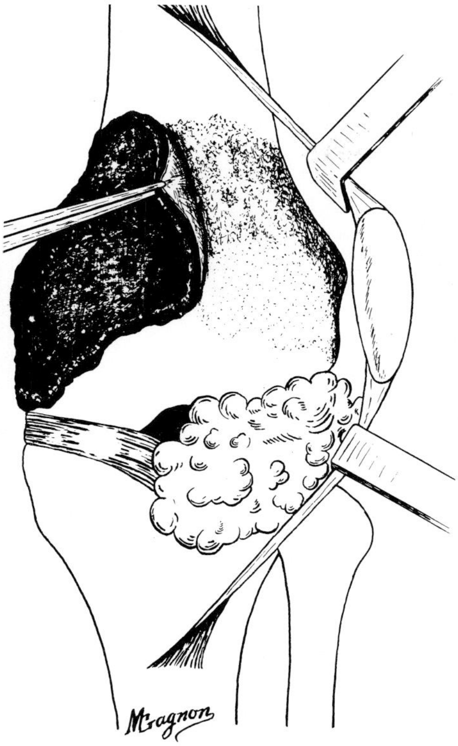

A

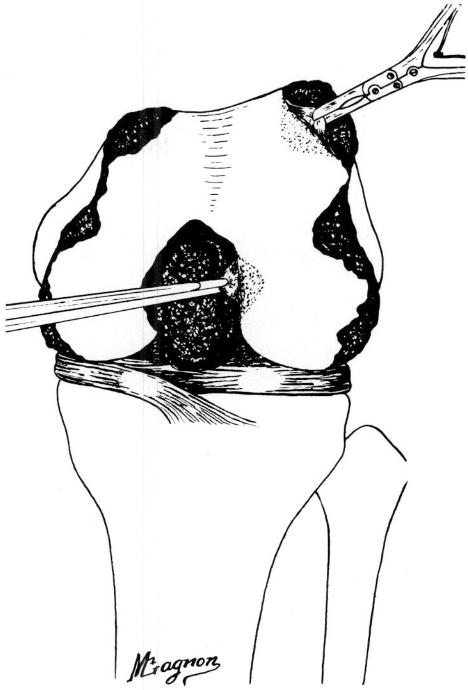

C

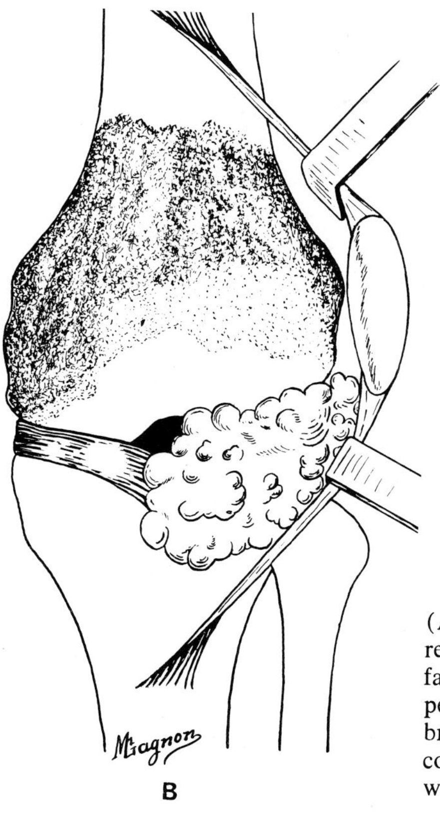

B

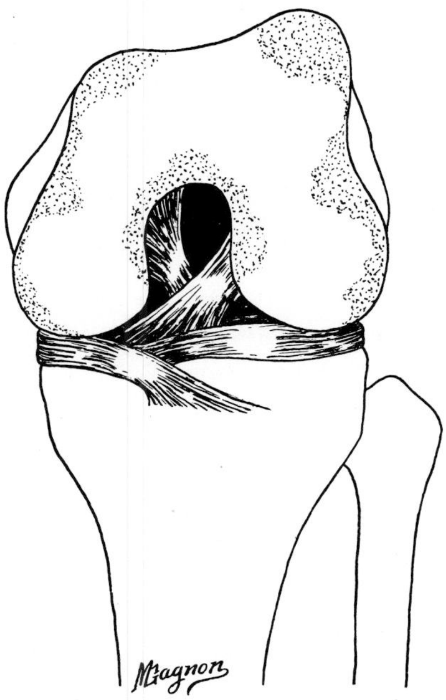

D

FIG. 3-1. The surgical steps of the synovial dissection: (A) Synovectomy of medial and lateral patello-femoral recesses (Steps 1 and 2); (B) partial ablation of the fat pad (Step 3, not yet performed); (C) removal of perichondral pannus using rongeurs (Step 4) and debridement of intercondylar notch (Step 5); (D) intercondylar dissection completed: note abnormal cartilage where perichondral pannus has been removed.

during the convalescence period, if he has the upper extremities to use crutches, the hips to permit early ambulation, and the desire to participate actively in the postoperative physiotherapy program. The patient must obviously be considered holistically and as a member of the therapeutic team.

The ideal candidate for a synovectomy described in the above paragraph is, in actual practice, so rare that one might even question his existence. Unfortunately, most patients are referred for surgery when it has become obvious that further medical treatment will be disappointing. By that time the knee joint has usually sustained irreversible damage. While such a delay undoubtedly prejudices the possible role of a synovectomy, the operation may still be proposed in spite of clinical evidence that the local disease has evolved beyond the synovial phase. Such clinical signs and findings need not be contraindicative to surgery. They represent what are admittedly not ideal conditions for a synovectomy, yet such candidates can be improved by the operation. Thus, mild joint deformities or early cartilage damage need not necessarily prejudice a surgeon against a synovectomy; under such circumstances, the operation is more correctly called a joint debridement. Similarly, a chronically elevated sedimentation rate is not a contraindication to surgery. However, in a clinically florid phase of the disease the operation should obviously be delayed until the systemic condition of the patient is better controlled. In this respect, it is germane to mention that the operation has not, in the authors' experience, precipitated any systemic exacerbation of the disease. The age of the patient is not, by itself, an adverse factor; it is rather the age of the *disease* that is important. If the associated systemic lesions and the adjacent articulations permit adequate cooperation, the operation can succeed in a well-motivated patient, even in his late sixties.

SURGICAL TECHNIQUE

Surgical Incision. The authors prefer a single, long, anteromedial incision; a single incision should cause less damage to the quadriceps mechanism, thus facilitating the return of function. The incision should begin at the patellar tendon insertion and extend proximally 2 to 3 inches into the quadriceps tendon, well lateral to the vastus medialis, which should be spared. The parapatellar portion of the incision should be made close to the patella. If this portion of the incision goes through the medial parapatellar retinaculum, excessive scar tissue overlying the medial femoral condyle can prejudice the return of function. The incision through skin, subcutaneous tissue, capsule, and synovium should be uniform, entering the synovial cavity directly in line with the skin incision with no undermining of skin or capsule. This will permit an immediate emptying of the joint and facilitate the synovial dissection.

Synovial Dissection (Five Distinct Steps). The dissection of the synovial membrane should not be a haphazard procedure but, rather, a well planned ablation of the diseased tissue (Fig. 3-1).

The superopatellar femoral pouches should be dissected first. The diseased synovium in the anteromedial femoral recess is excised in continuity with similar tissue behind and beyond the medial collateral ligament. The thickened synovial membrane in the lateral femoral recess is then similarly excised: the patella is dislocated laterally and the knee is acutely flexed; it is then possible to dissect underneath and beyond the lateral collateral ligament. Throughout this dissection, care should be taken to spare the subperiosteal blood vessels, which are prominent underneath the diseased synovial membrane.

If the synovial tissue is thickened and diseased underneath the quadriceps tendon, one should not hesitate to include it in the resected tissue. It is sometimes thin and almost normal in this area, in which case it need not be dissected.

The third phase of the synovial dissection ought to include the partial removal of the thickened and hypertrophied infrapatellar fat pad, which can by its sheer volume inhibit the extensor mechanism and interfere with full flexion. The removal of this tissue, which often appears normal, permits an easier and more complete visualization of the joint structures and allows a more complete synovectomy during the subsequent phases of the operation.

The fourth stage is a meticulous and complete removal of the perichondral pannus at the periphery of patellar and femoral articular cartilages. This tissue is usually thin and friable but very adherent to the underlying cartilage. It is best removed with a rongeur; abnormal cartilage is always exposed.

The final step is achieved by acutely flexing the knee while the patella is dislocated laterally. This exposes the inner surfaces of the intercondylar notch as well as the cruciate ligaments which must be denuded of their diseased synovial tissue. A pituitary rongeur facilitates this dissection and allows the surgeon to remove a good portion of the synovial tissue in the posterior compartment.

The Menisci and the Patella. Theoretically, a synovectomy does not include the surgical ablation of the menisci or the patella. However, the disease may so destroy these structures that they can be a cause of persistent pain and interfere with the postoperative rehabilitation, thus prejudicing the end result. Under such circumstances, they should be dealt with as part of the joint debridement. Similarly, peripheral femoral or tibial exostoses are removed with a rongeur.

The menisci should not be excised merely to do a more elaborate debridement; they should be left in place if they are grossly normal. If they are torn or fibrillated, one should not hesitate to remove them; it is then possible to remove the perichondral pannus around the tibial articular cartilage.

Every effort should be made to preserve the patella. The decision to save or remove the patella is sometimes difficult. If in doubt, it is better to postpone the patellectomy. Rheumatoid patients usually exhibit diffuse muscle wasting with poor muscle tone; quadriceps function is almost always weak, and flexion deformities are either obvious or imminent. Patellectomies should not be performed if passive knee extension is incomplete. However, a grossly degenerated patella may not be worth saving, particularly if passive knee extension is complete. If, after due consideration, the surgeon elects to excise the patella, a simple "shell-out" patellectomy is sufficient. There is no need to perform any type of patellar reconstruction or to modify the postoperative program.

Patellectomies were performed in association with synovectomies in 13 instances. If one considers that these joints were more seriously involved, the end results do not suggest that patellectomy prejudiced synovectomy. A few patients with residual flexion deformities complained of weak extensor power.

A synovectomy performed by a single anteromedial incision should remove approximately 90 per cent of the diseased tissue. This percentage will increase with the surgeon's experience, and no posterior incision is necessary unless the physician can palpate an obvious mass in the popliteal space. When the popliteal space is distended by a large cyst, there is no advantage in aspirating such lesions, since they are usually filled with fibrinoid tissue. Such lesions will obviously interfere with complete knee extension and should be removed through a separate posterior incision performed during the same anesthesia or as a separate procedure.

Table 3-2. Clinical Criteria for Assessment of Results

Rating	*Pain*	*Range of Motion*	*Functional Capacity*	*X-ray Evidence of Increased Joint Destruction*	*Patient's Assessment*
Excellent	None	Better or same as preop	Almost normal	Nil	Delighted
Good	Some but less than preop	Same	Improved	Nil or mild	Satisfied
Unsatis-factory	More than preop	Restricted	No permanent improvement	Obvious	Disappointed
Poor	Disabling	Limited with deformity	Gross restrictions	Advanced	Displeased

Postoperative Regimen. The postoperative regimen is planned before the operation and includes detailed instructions to the patient. Isometric quadriceps contractions are started *prior* to surgery under the surveillance of a physiotherapist who will visit him daily after the first postoperative day.

A Jones type of compressive dressing (with or without plaster shell) is applied without any wound drainage. The day following surgery the patient is allowed up on crutches but no weight bearing is permitted until quadriceps function is normal.

A postoperative joint manipulation is performed under anesthesia 1 week after synovectomy. If this is omitted and if patients are merely instructed to move the knee progressively, many will admittedly achieve a satisfactory range of motion. On the other hand, the identification of those patients who need a manipulation is not easy, and their need may be recognized too late to attain full motion. For these reasons, joint manipulation has been performed routinely; the resulting range of motion suggests that postoperative stiffness, once a dreaded complication, is no longer a problem (see Summary on page 22). The manipulation is extremely gentle; the hip joint is flexed and the weight of the leg is the only applied force to obtain at least 90° of knee flexion. The stitches are left in place and 1 cc. of intra-articular cortisone is injected after the joint has been aspirated. The procedure was repeated more than once on very few occasions.

POSTOPERATIVE RESULTS

The criteria of assessment and results obtained are summarized in Tables 3-2 and 3-3 and corroborate the findings of other similar series.

The poor results are most informative. The criteria of preoperative patient assessment are outlined in Table 3-4. The correlation of this assessment with the postoperative results (Table 3-5) clearly indicates that the operation can be successful in spite of mild cartilage lesions (Stage III). It also shows that a synovectomy can offer very little to a patient with far-advanced disease (Stage IV). The operation is primarily directed at the synovial membrane and cannot restore normal cartilage once it is destroyed. The importance of careful and

Table 3-3. Results in 52 Synovectomies

Result	*No. Patients*	*Per-centage*
Excellent	30	58
Good	10	19
Unsatisfactory	7	13
Poor	5	10

Table 3-4. Preoperative Assessment: Severity of Disease at Time of Surgery

	Stage I (4) Knees	*Stage II (22) Knees*	*Stage III (19) Knees*	*Stage IV (7) Knees*
Clinical signs and symptoms of rheumatoid arthritis	Mild	Obvious	Obvious, plus extra-articular signs	Gross Polyarticular involvement
Joint deformities	Mild	Obvious but not fixed	Obvious and fixed, but not gross	Gross and fixed
Function capacity	Almost complete but restricted	Adequate for every day activities only	Limited even for normal activities and self care	Largely or wholly dependent
x-Ray sign	Osteoporosis; joint line adequate	Slight diminution of joint line slight subchondral erosions	Obvious cartilage and bony lesions	Fibrous or bony ankylosis

Table 3-5. Relationship Between End Result of Synovectomy and Severity of Disease Process

Advancement of Disease (No. of knees)	*End Result*				*Percentage of Excellent and Good Results*
	Excellent	*Good*	*Unsatisfactory*	*Poor*	
Stage I (4)	4				100%
Stage II (22)	18	4			100%
Stage III (19)	8	6	2	3	75%
Stage IV (7)			5	2	0%
Total (52)	30	10	7	5	

judicious patient selection, as summarized above, is obvious. Poor results are the rule and not the exception if the operation is performed too late. On the other hand, the operation can rarely be performed too early; in no instance was the patient's condition aggravated locally or systemically by the operation.

Synovectomy is now well documented as sound therapeutic treatment of early rheumatoid disease. The more contentious question of its prophylactic value was discussed in a previous publication.[1] It was shown that the operation can arrest the local evolution of the disease and prevent cartilage destruction which would otherwise have been almost certain. The unpredictable course of the disease makes analysis of this aspect of the problem most difficult. Bilateral lesions are not necessarily symmetrical, but a comparison of their evolution, with and without surgery, has provided supportive information. Patients with early but irreversible synovial disease of both knees

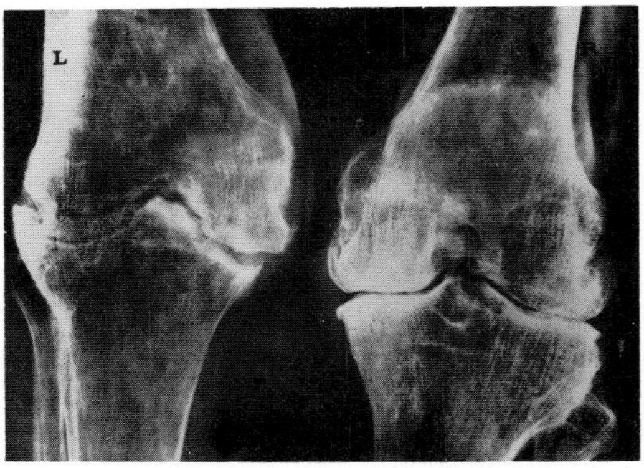

FIG. 3-2. Radiographs taken 10 years after unilateral synovectomy (right knee) for rheumatoid arthritis.

were usually submitted to bilateral synovectomies which were performed during different hospitalizations. On three occasions, contrary to instructions the patients did not return, as requested, for a synovectomy of the opposite knee. When they were examined later, it was obvious that the disease had progressed considerably in the "unoperated" side, whereas the "synovectomized" knee was less symptomatic and maintained superior function. In these three instances of bilateral knee involvement with a unilateral synovectomy, it appeared that surgery had protected the "operated" knee against further destruction; in that sense, the operation had achieved a prophylactic effect (Fig. 3-2).

Summary of 52 Knee Synovectomies

Postoperative ROM
- Decreased (maximum loss, 15°): 8
- Same: 36
- Increased: 8

Postoperative Knee Pain
- None: 20
- Less: 22
- Same: 6
- More: 4

Subjective Assessment
- Delighted: 30
- Satisfied: 18
- Hesitant: 4
- Would not repeat: 0

Table 3-6. Prophylactic Value of the Operation

	Local Improvement Persists	*Local Improvement Lost*
	(No. of patients)	
Systemic Deterioration	14	3
No Systemic Deterioration	1	0

The potential prophylactic effect of the operation may also be assessed by comparing the local progress of the disease in the "operated" knee with its systemic evolution in other "unoperated" joints (Table 3-6). There were seventeen patients whose records permitted such a comparison and whose disease obviously progressed systemically after surgery. In only three of these patients did knee joint function deteriorate significantly after synovectomy. The other 14 knees maintained their postoperative improvement, whereas the "unoperated" joints deteriorated considerably. It would appear that the synovectomy not only relieved the local symptoms but also protected those knees against further damage.

The therapeutic and possibly prophylactic effects of synovectomy may impress the surgeon, but it is usually the patient who is most gratified. Indeed, the subjective assessment of the operation was most encouraging; there were patients who were obviously disappointed with their long-term results, but none said that he would not repeat the experience. Every patient reported at least temporary relief of pain. Indeed, pain relief is the most striking effect of the operation (see Summary above). If this consideration is related to the fact that a synovectomy never aggravates the local condition, the surgeon can only err by operating too late. It is unlikely that he could ever operate too early.

REFERENCES

1. Gariépy, R., Demers, R., and Laurin, C. A.: Prophylactic effect of synovectomy of the knee in rheumatoid arthritis. Canad. Med. Ass., J., *94*:1349-1352, 1966.
2. Mignon, A.: Synovectomie du genou. Soc. Chir. Paris, *26*:1113-1115, 1900.
3. Speed, J. S.: Synovectomy of the knee joint. J.A.M.A., *83*:1814-1820, 1924.
4. Swett, P. O.: Synovectomy in chronic infectious arthritis. J. Bone Joint Surg., *6*: 800, 1924.

CHAPTER 4

The Surgical Management of Flexion Deformity in the Rheumatoid Knee

ROGER GARIÉPY, M.D.

Flexion contracture in the rheumatoid knee has many features. This clinical entity manifests a more or less permanent loss of full extension, while a relatively painless flexion motion is preserved. Whether unilateral or bilateral it is a formidable challenge to the rheumatologist, the physiotherapist and the orthopaedic surgeon. The treatment varies according to the stage of the disease, but it is aimed at restoring full use of the joint. In the advanced stage, conservative measures such as exercise, steroid injections, serial cast manipulations, and traction will fail to restore satisfactory function because of cartilage damage.

In all but the acute phase of arthritis the pain in flexion is usually mild. The position of flexion affords some relief of pain and the patient avoids extension beyond 15° to 20°. The inflamed synovium of the infrapatellar fat pad and the large volume of synovial fluid produce an extreme tension on the capsule when the knee is extended. Later the synovial pouches and the capsule become dilated. Full extension may still be recovered in spite of a persistent effusion. For various reasons, however, a certain number of cases will not recover. Large amounts of loose fibrinous bodies and villous synovium may interfere with the extension mechanism. A popliteal bursa may tense the flexor tendons and cause a permanent contracture. If the inflammatory process is allowed to persist the articular cartilage is destroyed and the articular surfaces become incongruous. As a result, dislocation in both planes may occur, since the flexion deformity is often associated with some degree of varus or valgus deformity. The latter is more common and often appears with external rotation of the leg. Severe deformities are more often bilateral. When they are limited to one knee only, the patient usually remains ambulatory. When the hips and ankles are also affected, ambulation may become so difficult that the patient stops walking. This usually happens when flexion exceeds 30°.

TREATMENT PROCEDURES

Preventive Treatment

Early and aggressive treatment of the disease as well as the synovitis may prevent deformity. Repeated aspirations of the joint and steroid injections, proper splinting and exercises are successful in the majority of cases. The deformity, however, often progresses insidiously, and the patient himself may fail to notice it.

Surgical Treatment

Joint Debridement, Capsulotomy and Tenotomy. A long term follow-up of synovectomies and bursectomies suggests that these procedures have a definite preventive effect on deformities. Synovectomy alone is still useful in the correction of flexion at an early stage. A total debridement of the joint should aim at recovering as much extension and internal rotation of the tibia as possible. This may include the excision or section of the cruciate ligaments, the lateral meniscus, the lateral ligament and the posterior capsule.

The following technique has been used when the cartilage had a relatively healthy appearance. The usual anteromedial knee incision is extended at the lower end, laterally and transversely, to reach the posterolateral aspect of the knee behind the bicipital tendon. The capsule is divided close to the medial aspect of the patella and the patellar tendon. A total synovectomy is carried out, after which the knee is tested for extension and rotation of the leg. If necessary, the capsule and lateral ligament are divided around the tibial plateau, and the lateral meniscus is excised if destruction is advanced. The iliotibial band is also divided when necessary. For further visualization of the joint structures the cruciate ligaments may be excised. The knee is immobilized in extension in a well-padded and bivalved plaster cylinder for 1 week. Exercises are resumed after a manipulation under anesthesia.

Osteotomies. The femoral osteotomy is usually described in textbooks as an accepted procedure. Our own experience with this operation has been disappointing. The supracondylar osteotomy attempts to align the leg by an angulation above the joint. We have found that this correction will not be satisfactory, unless some flexion is sacrificed and the motion thus limited to a very small weight-bearing surface represented by the posterior part of the femoral condyles.

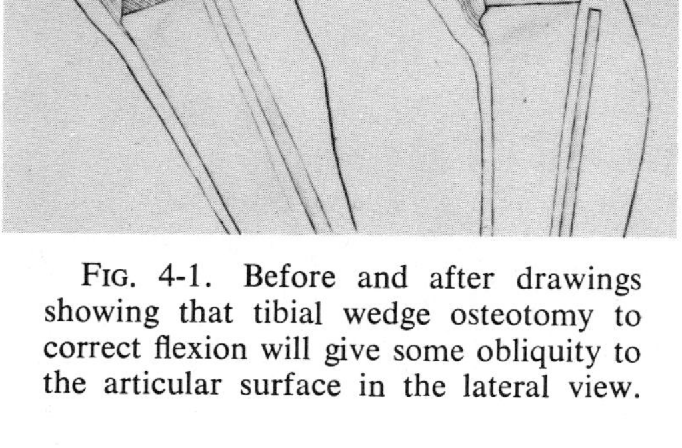

FIG. 4-1. Before and after drawings showing that tibial wedge osteotomy to correct flexion will give some obliquity to the articular surface in the lateral view.

The high tibial osteotomy, with or without excision of the fibular head, also has some theoretical mechanical drawbacks. The wedge osteotomy in the tibial epiphysis straightens the leg by an angulation below the joint. The weight-bearing surface is thus made oblique to an extent which depends on the degree of preoperative flexion (Fig. 4-1). In practice, however, this is well tolerated. The weight-bearing surface is wide, and the stress on the capsule is supported by strong elements anteriorly and posteriorly, provided the correction has not exceeded 15° to 20°. More important, distal to the joint, the tibial osteotomy does not interfere with knee function.

High Tibial Osteotomy. Following a total joint debridement, as described above, and provided the joint cartilage is still in fairly good condition, the knee is tested for extension. If more than 10° of flexion persists, the incision is extended transversely and posteriorly to the bicipital tendon. The peroneal nerve is identified and protected, and the head of the fibula is excised. A wedge is removed in the cortex of the tibial epiphysis just above the insertion of the patellar tendon, and the leg is manipulated into full extension, thus closing the space. (A valgus or varus deformity may also be corrected at this stage by the removal of appropriate wedges.) The wound is sutured anatomically, and the operative area is drained.

The knee alignment is maintained by a well padded and bivalved long-leg cast for 1 week. Exercises are then started after a gentle manipulation under anesthesia. A posterior slab splint protects the leg for 3 to 4 weeks more while progressive weight-bearing is permitted.

Following is a summary of results of tibial osteotomies in our patients.

Stage I: synovitis the only finding. None of our rheumatoid patients have had a tibial osteotomy at this early stage. Synovectomy has been the treatment of choice in these cases and it has been found that a few degrees of flexion deformity following a synovectomy is well tolerated by the patient.

Stage II: chronic synovitis with limited cartilage changes and a fixed but mild flexion contracture. Tibial osteotomies with synovectomies were carried out in eleven knees. Eight were performed in a single procedure, and three others were performed as a delayed correction (Fig. 4-2). This group has been followed for 6 years. The average flexion retained was 90° (Fig. 4-3). Pain is moderate, and all patients have resumed previous activities with minimal disability. There has been no recurrence of the flexion deformity, but most of the patients show an extensor lag when they attempt active extension.

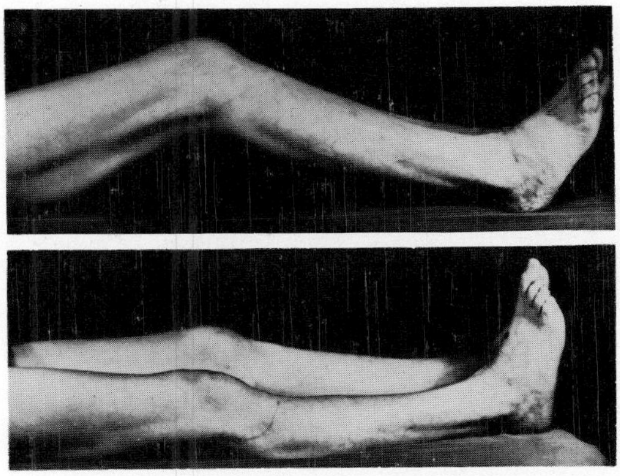

FIG. 4-2. Pre- and postoperative views of a knee in which osteotomy alone was performed for a flexion contracture.

Stage III (advanced chronic): small range of motion, severe pain in extension, a permanent flexion contracture, and narrowed knee joint space indicating significant cartilage destruction (Fig. 4-4). Twenty-three knees have been operated at this stage with an average follow-up of 6 years. Fifteen joints had tibial osteotomies only. Ten were improved and five were not. Those patients who improved are walking satisfactorily.

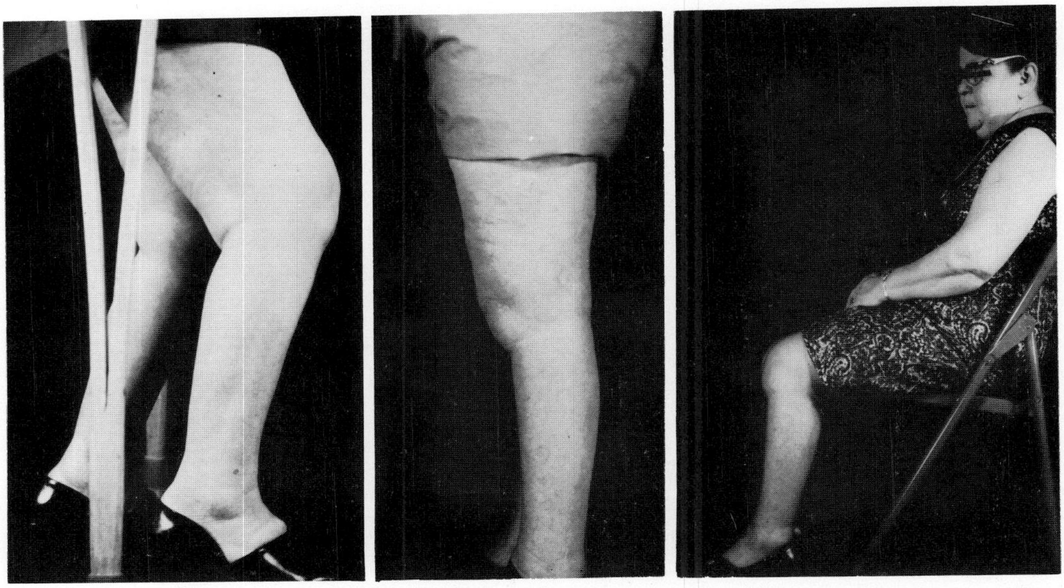

FIG. 4-3. (*Left*) A 45-year-old woman severely disabled by pain and flexion deformity. (*Center*) Ten years after synovectomy and osteotomy she walked independently without recurrence of flexion deformity. (*Right*) Active flexion approached 90°.

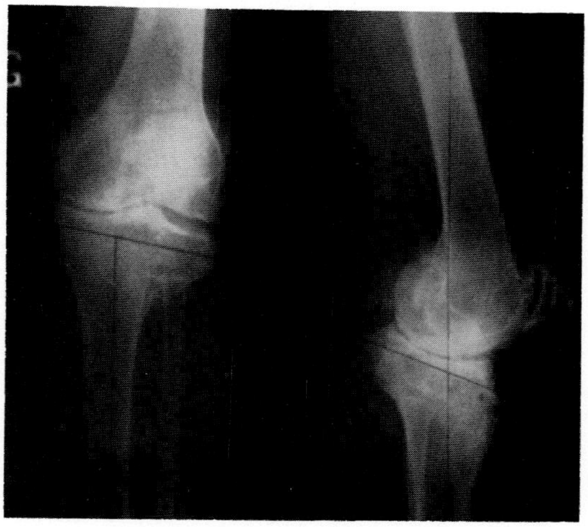

FIG. 4-4. X-rays of the knee of a 32-year-old woman 10 years after synovectomy and osteotomy for stage III disease. In spite of joint space narrowing and the obliquity of the articular surface, the pain had been relieved and function was good.

Eight knees had combined synovectomies and osteotomies; of these, two are improved and six are not.

Stage IV (late chronic): range of motion very limited, pain frequently slight, severe permanent flexion deformity in most cases. Five knees at this stage had tibial osteotomies only; none were improved.

COMMENTS

Flexion deformity in the rheumatoid knee is but one of many clinical features of the disease. The success of surgical treatment depends primarily on the progress of arthritis at the time of operation. Although some patients with minimal deformity will require only a synovectomy, the requirements for success with both tibial osteotomy and synovectomy are similar in regard to the joint. If most of the joint cartilage is preserved and the disease is not too severe, good and satisfactory results can be expected. The results of osteotomy in neglected cases with severe and often bilateral knee deformities are much less certain. Some of these severely deformed patients are so crippled as to be mainly sedentary. Because their flexion deformities do not prevent the limited ambulation that they can do, it may be preferable not to attempt any correction at all. Many such patients are, of course, candidates for arthroplasties, as are those patients with total destruction of the articular cartilage. Since many also have hip and distal joint involvement, the physician will have to decide which patients have the capacity to tolerate such extensive programs.

CHAPTER 5

Arthroplasty of the Knee in Rheumatoid Arthritis Using the Hemiarthroplasty Prosthesis

D. L. MacIntosh, M.D.

Because rheumatoid arthritis continues to be a disease of uncertain cause, uncertain duration, and uncertain control, many cases progress inexorably to a stage of severe and painful generalized disability. Of the many joints involved, the knee probably contributes more than any other to this disability picture because of its weight-bearing function, its frequency of involvement, and its proneness to unmanageable deformity.

Arthroplasty of the knee using the "hemiarthroplasty prosthesis" has been developed as a method of knee reconstruction. It is used in the late stages of rheumatoid involvement, when all articular cartilage on the weight-bearing surfaces has been destroyed and function is inhibited by pain and deformity.

We first used the hemiarthroplasty procedure in 1954 to correct the varus or valgus deformity that characterizes most cases of osteoarthritis of the knee. A prosthesis thick enough to correct the alignment was inserted on the wearing side of the joint. Initially it was felt that this procedure would not be applicable to the rheumatoid knee because of the more severe deformities and destructive changes, the softness of rheumatoid bone, and the general debility of the rheumatoid patient. Time has proved however that this type of arthroplasty has its most useful role in the rheumatoid patient.

Pathological Considerations

The Articular Cartilage. Rheumatoid arthritis begins as a synovial disease, but as it progresses, the cartilage on all articular surfaces of the joint is progressively destroyed, partly by pannus, but more by a direct chondrolytic process. In osteoarthritis usually only one tibiofemoral compartment is

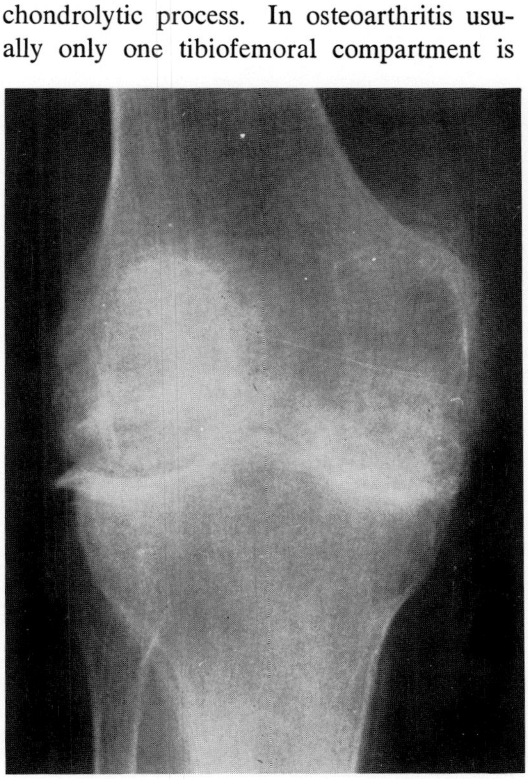

Fig. 5-1. Radiograph of a severely involved rheumatoid knee. The cartilage has been destroyed in both compartments.

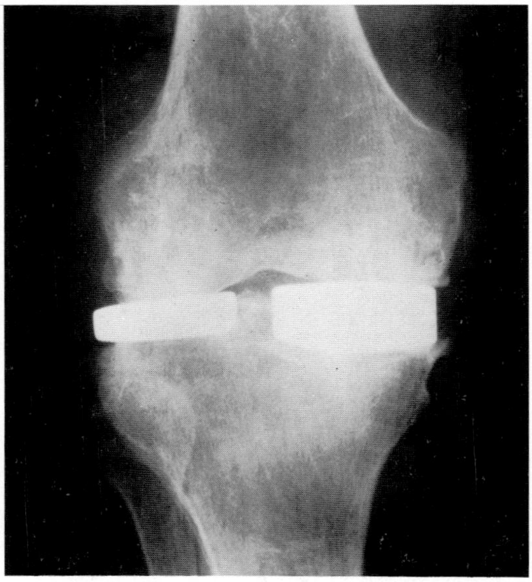

FIG. 5-2. Knee shown in Figure 5-1 following a double tibial hemiarthroplasty procedure.

severely involved, permitting correction of alignment and shift of the weight-bearing load onto the spared side of the joint by osteotomy or simple hemiarthroplasty. In the rheumatoid knee, however, the articular cartilage of both tibiofemoral compartments is being destroyed by the rheumatoid disease. By the time anthroplasty is undertaken, both compartments usually have worn down to bone-on-bone contact, so that two hemiarthroplasty units, one in each tibiofemoral compartment, are required (Figs. 5-1 and 5-2). If arthroplasty is done at a stage when cartilage in only one compartment has been completely destroyed, and alignment is corrected using only one tibial plateau prosthesis, then the cartilage of the other compartment is likely to wear even more rapidly. This cartilage is being attacked by the rheumatoid disease, and a second arthoplasty unit is likely to be required on that side later.

The Bone. Bone is involved too in rheumatoid disease, and it was felt at first that the soft or porotic bone of the rheumatoid patient would not provide adequate support for the hemiarthroplasty prosthesis. When the flat tibial bed is being prepared, the bone may be so soft that it can be cut with a knife. The prosthesis, however, distributes the weight load over its entire contact area with the tibia, and even the grossly porotic bone of the rheumatoid will provide stable support. The widest possible prosthesis is used to give the widest support area; no rim of bone is left, as best support is provided by the peripheral cortical area. A minimum amount of bone is removed in preparing the bed for the prosthesis, because the densest bone is at the articulating level.

The Ligaments. Hemiarthroplasty and double hemiarthroplasty procedures are dependent on intact collateral ligaments. At the stage of joint involvement at which arthroplasty is done the cruciate ligaments have frequently been destroyed completely by disease or by wearing, but in the limited function of the rheumatoid patient the cruciates are not essential for a successful arthroplasty. The collateral ligaments, fortunately, are rarely destroyed, even at a late stage of rheumatoid disease, and the arthroplasty procedure restores stability by building up the related tibial plateaus with prostheses thick enough to take up slack and restore tension in the adjacent collateral ligaments. Even cases with gross disalignment rarely exhibit collateral ligament insufficiency, but if a severe misalignment (usually a valgus deformity in the rheumatoid) has stretched the stressed collateral ligament, then tightening of that ligament will be required, as well as relief of tension on the ligament, by a little planned overcorrection. These are all procedures which add technical difficulties to the operation.

Operative Procedure

The Prosthesis. The hemiarthroplasty prosthesis is a simple D-shaped unit, usable in either compartment of either knee. Its upper surface, a low-friction surface for contact with the femoral condyle, is polished and slightly hollowed. Its lower surface, a high friction surface for contact with a prepared tibial bed, is rough and flat. The broad contact of this rough under-surface with a level tibial bed is all the friction that is required to provide a stable position.

The prostheses are made in three widths to fit joints of different sizes, and in five thicknesses to enable correction of varying degrees of misalignment. The first prostheses used were of acrylic, but the prostheses now used are of Vitallium.

Surgical Technique. The procedure is based on very simple and direct biomechanical principles, but accurate positioning of prostheses and attention to other details are demanded if the best result is to be obtained.

The approach must provide an adequate exposure for the preparation of level beds for the prostheses, for synovectomy, and for any reshaping of femoral condyles. An extended medial parapatellar incision has been found best in the average case. The vastus medialis is best detached from the upper medial border of the patella, and, above that, the quadriceps tendon is split in the line of its fibers. Below, the incision is carried to the patellar tendon insertion. The supermedial fibers of insertion can be detached until the patella can be completely everted, exposing the whole joint at the front.

A synovectomy is done if the synovium is still hypertrophic and "active." At the stage of disease at which arthroplasty is done, however, the synovium is often "burned out"; it is mainly thin, smooth and pale, and only remaining islands of active synovium need be removed. The synovium in the cruciate ligament area maintains an active rheumatoid appearance to a very late stage. The suprapatellar pouch in burned out cases is often sealed off and is then opened up by blunt or sharp dissection to promote movement.

The patellofemoral joint is invariably severely involved, but patellectomy at the time of arthroplasty is avoided if possible, because return to active function is slower and more difficult after patellectomy. The articular cartilage in the patellofemoral compartment has often been destroyed as well, but usually it is replaced by a thin, smooth, fibrous tissue covering which supplies satisfactory gliding surfaces for the limited function of the rheumatoid knee. The fibrous covering is carefully preserved. We have done a patellectomy only when the patellofemoral surfaces are faced with rough bone which locks or binds and does not glide. The patella may be grossly deformed, even saucer-shaped, with wide osteophytic margins. The projecting margins may be cut back, but the central articular area is left undisturbed.

In preparing beds for the prostheses, the intercondylar area of the tibia is left to serve as a buffer zone between the two prostheses and also to preserve cruciate ligament attachments, if they are still functioning. The first osteotomy cut on either side is thus a vertical cut defining the intercondylar zone. This cut is slightly inside the margin of the corresponding femoral condyle and parallel to it. The intercondylar area left should not be too wide and should not steal any of the weight-bearing articular area of the tibial plateau.

The beds for the prostheses are cut level, at right angles to both sagittal and coronal planes of the tibia. A right-angle instrument should be used to aid visual alignment. Any lateral slope of the prosthesis is avoided, because this may promote lateral shift of the tibia. Osteotomes are used to cut the bed, except at the back of the joint where the cut is completed with an oscillating osteotomy saw. Because the bone is soft, an osteotome may break off the posterior margin leaving the prosthesis without posterior support. No rim of bone is left at the back or at the sides. The prosthesis is introduced right to the posterior margin of the tibia, since in flexion of the knee the femoral condyles ride far back, and the prosthesis will tilt if the femur rides up on its posterior margin. As little bone as possible is sacrificed when the beds are prepared; just enough is removed to get to the bottom of the worn hollow of the tibial plateau. Below that level, very porotic bone is likely to be encountered, and support of the prosthesis may thus be jeopardized if the beds are cut too deeply.

The thickest prosthesis that can be inserted is used on either side. It may be inserted with the knee in flexion, or in extension, or in whatever position provides the best space for insertion. During insertion, the prosthesis is kept flat on the tibial bed so that the posterior margin of the prosthesis will not cut into the tibia.

The prostheses should be stable when the everted patella has been reduced and put through flexion to 90°. To be stable, the bed under each prosthesis must be flat; the femoral condyle must bear weight on the central part of each prosthesis and not at the margin. Shaping of the femoral condyle is often required to achieve this. If a long-standing varus or valgus deformity has been corrected, the femoral condyle may be worn unevenly, and when the tibia is brought back to a position of normal alignment, the high edge of the femoral condyle will bear weight eccentrically on the prosthesis. In that event, the prosthesis is likely to tilt, and the prominent margin of the condyle should be cut down around its whole circumference until the weight-bearing point is at the center of the condyle and at the center of the prosthesis.

Postoperative Management. A Jones compression bandage is applied, and the knee is kept in full extension for 4 or 5 days. If full correction of flexion deformity was difficult to achieve at operation, a Thomas splint to hold extension may be applied for the first day.

The wound is then inspected, and if it is healing well, assisted active movement is commenced with an objective of flexing to 90° within 2 weeks, (if that range was obtainable at time of operation). If this range is not being approached at 12 to 14 days, or if the recovery of flexion is slow and painful, gentle flexion of the knee to 90° is carried out under general anesthesia. This is repeated again 3 to 4 weeks after surgery if the range has not been maintained.

Flexion under anesthetic has been required in about 50 per cent of cases, chiefly in patients who have had a more extensive synovectomy. If flexion under anesthetic is to be used, it should not be delayed beyond 2 weeks, because only very gentle force can be applied with safety. Strong force to regain flexion will cause too much pressure on the prostheses and risks compressing them into the tibial beds.

Patients are allowed up with good walker support in 5 to 7 days and are permitted early moderate weight bearing. The first objective, however, is to gain flexion range, maintaining full active extension; weight bearing is increased carefully, well within pain tolerance. In a few weeks the patient progresses to crutches, and only to full weight bearing without support when this can be accomplished with complete confidence and without discomfort.

At the time of manipulation under anesthetic, a small dose of corticosteroid is often administered to facilitate the rehabilitation program. Postoperative joint effusion is rare. Quadriceps exercises are started within a few days of the operation. At first, only straight-leg lifting is done without added weight. After a few weeks, very light resistance is added, but no active extension exercises against resistance are performed because of the adverse effect of this activity on the patellofemoral compartment.

Results

The results of arthroplasty in the knee in the rheumatoid patient have to be related not only to the severity of destructive changes, deformity, and pain that existed in the particular knee, but also to involvement of other joints of the lower extremities, and to the general disability picture of the patient. Arthroplasty of a knee cannot be successful if its function continues to be limited by pain and deformity from other weight-bearing joints. In particular, correction of deformity of one knee by arthroplasty will not be maintained, and the knee will not function, if severe and painful deformity remains uncorrected in the other knee or in the hips. The program to rehabilitate the disabled rheumatoid patient must take all joints that are limiting function into consideration, and deal with them in appropriate sequence.

An independent review of the author's cases of arthroplasty of the knee, numbering more than 100, has been undertaken by Hunter.[1] The criteria on which results were assessed included relief of pain, the correction of deformity, range of movement, stability, and improvement of function and gait. His findings indicate that good results can be achieved by this form of arthroplasty in about 69 per cent of rheumatoid knees.

Causes of poor results or failures included infection (four cases), inadequate correction of deformity, lateral subluxation of the tibia, and failure of operative technique (including failure because of excessive bone destruction and prior ankylosis).

The availability of acrylic cement extends to some degree the application of the hemiarthroplasty procedure. Destruction of a femoral condyle to an extent that would prevent restoration of stability by a tibial plateau replacement remains a contraindication to a hemiarthroplasty procedure. It indicates, rather, hinge arthroplasty or a femoral condyle type replacement. Severe erosion of a tibial plateau that prevents full area support of the prosthesis can be filled in or built up with cement to provide a fully stable bed. We have not found it necessary to use cement to stabilize the prostheses when good bone beds can be formed.

Combined Procedures. Some more severe deformities, varus or valgus, are correctable if combined osteotomy and tibial plateau replacement procedures are used. These are done in separate stages, usually arthroplasty first in the rheumatoid because ligament stability is thereby restored. Osteotomy is then used to complete correction of a remaining alignment or flexion deformity.

Posterior Release. Some severe flexion deformities, including most deformities of more than 30°, have required a posterior release procedure to obain adequate correction. Up to 30° of flexion deformity is correctable at the time of arthroplasty by cutting away the ridge of bone on the femoral condyle that blocks extension, by cutting down to level bone beds for the prostheses, and by careful posterior capsular release, which is possible under good vision when the beds have been cut. Severe flexion deformities require division of all the limiting posterior structures, carried out through a posterior approach which permits one to visualize and protect the popliteal vessels and nerves.

Conclusion

Arthroplasty of the knee in rheumatoid arthritis using hemiarthroplasty prostheses permits correction of deformity, restoration of stability and function, and relief of pain. It is indicated only at a late stage of joint destruction, when all cartilage on the weight-bearing surfaces has been destroyed and "bone-on-bone" rub is demonstrable. Its use is limited by very advanced bone destruction, particularly of a femoral condyle. The use of arthroplasty can be extended if acrylic cement is used to stabilize the prosthesis when the lesion of the tibial plateau is too deep. Combined arthroplasty and osteotomy procedures may be used to correct some major deformities.

REFERENCES

1. MacIntosh, D. L., and Hunter, G. A.: The use of the hemiarthroplasty prosthesis in advanced osteoarthritis and rheumatoid arthritis of the knee. (Submitted for publication.)

CHAPTER 6

Mold Replacement in the Rheumatoid Knee

WILLIAM N. JONES, M.D.

In the past 20 years, more than 40 communications have been published concerning knee arthroplasty. A large variety of devices, applied to the femur, the tibia, or both, have been utilized. The results, with the exception of some small series and one reporting a method not now used, have generally resembled those reported for fascial arthroplasty.

In 1942, Dr. M. N. Smith-Petersen implanted free-moving Vitallium molds in both knees of a young woman who had bilateral rheumatoid ankylosis, and in 1950, a third mold of this same type was used. Dr. Smith-Petersen was disappointed in the results, and in 1952, we designed a mold to be applied to the femur.

After modifications of the intramedullary stem by Dr. Otto Aufranc and a lowering of the inner condyle walls by Dr. Smith-Petersen, a device has been produced commonly referred to as the M.G.H. knee mold. This chapter describes its use by the visiting and resident staff of the Massachusetts General Hospital and by Dr. William Kermond at the Lemuel Shattuck Hospital.

Materials and Methods

The Mold. The word *mold*, instead of *prosthesis*, is used to describe the joint implant in order to emphasize its intended function of opposing a new joint surface rather than replacing a joint or a portion of it. The structure of the mold at the time of its design was influenced by the intent to use it in knees affected by rheumatoid arthritis. It has been learned from fascia lata arthroplasties that the quality of bone in the distal femur was too poor to allow shaping to restore the contour of the distal femur.

In order to obtain motion beyond 90° in a reconstructed joint, it was felt that the height of the femoral condyles in the flexed knee position was important. In effect, a prominence is provided under which the tibial plateau may move posteriorly.

A hollow mold structure allows minimal sacrifice of bone, and when arthroplasty fails, joint fusion is easy to accomplish. The hollow structure, as it caps the distal femur, becomes somewhat fixed to it. A long (7½-inch) intramedullary stem, mounted at an angle of 15° valgus with the mold's joint surface (a little more than average valgus angle in the normal femur) provides additional fixation.

The internal surface of the hollow mold is flat, front and back. It slopes slightly outward proximally to allow easy fitting over the end of the femur (Fig. 6-1). The internal lateral walls are cut low to allow preserva-

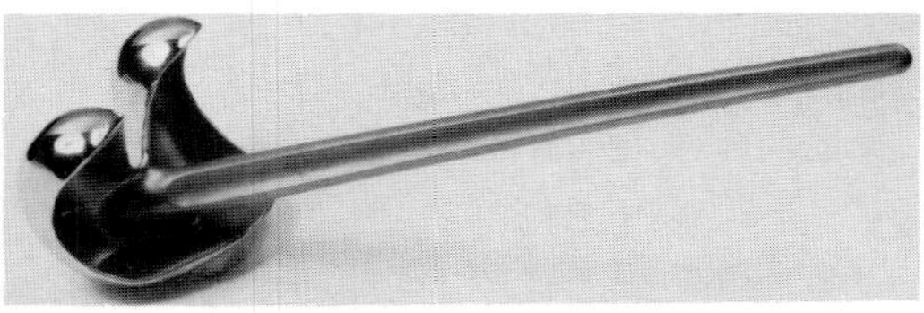

FIG. 6-1. A large left-knee mold. It is hollow, with a small posterior dome to provide the effect of the posterior portion of the femoral condyles when the knee flexes.

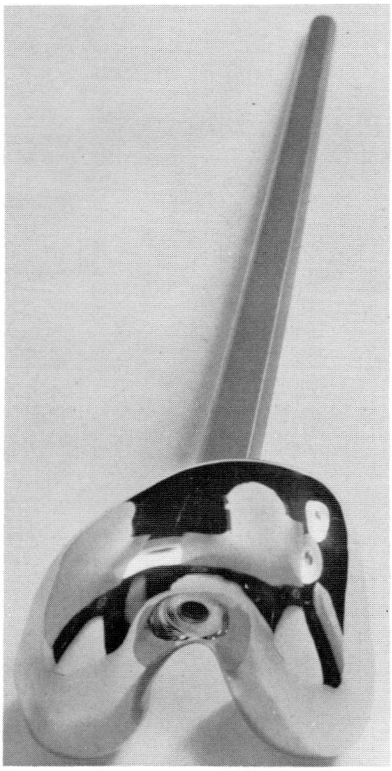

FIG. 6-2. A left-knee mold viewed from the articular surface. The central round depression is threaded for attachment of a Smith-Petersen nail driver.

tion of the cruciate ligaments when these are present, and the low outer walls allow preservation or reconstitution of the collateral ligaments.

The external contours of the intra-articular portion are a simplified approximation of those of a normal femur (Fig. 6-2). Three widths (66, 77 and 87 mm.) are available. Molds with perpendicular stems are used occasionally, when the knee is in severe valgus. A threaded socket for attachment of a Smith-Petersen nail driver is placed in a non-articulating area.

The mold is made of a chrome cobalt alloy (Vitallium), and none have broken to date. A patient who had molds implanted 2 years earlier fell a distance of 15 feet; he incurred bilateral os calcis fractures without damage to either mold or impairment of knee function.

Operative Technique. Three types of incisions are used: long para-patellar, transverse transpatellar, and long vertical incisions following the posterior border of vastus medialis (Fig. 6-3). The latter has been preferred by Dr. Aufranc. A deep U-shaped incision is not recommended. The choice of incision depends on the characteristics of the joint operated upon and on the surgeon's preference. It may influence the requirements of blood transfusion and early postoperative handling but probably does not affect the quality of joint function achieved. Special instruments are not necessary.

In most knees, only the anterior cortex of the patella has been left in the quadriceps tendon. In a few, the whole or a large mass of patella has been retained, and in some a

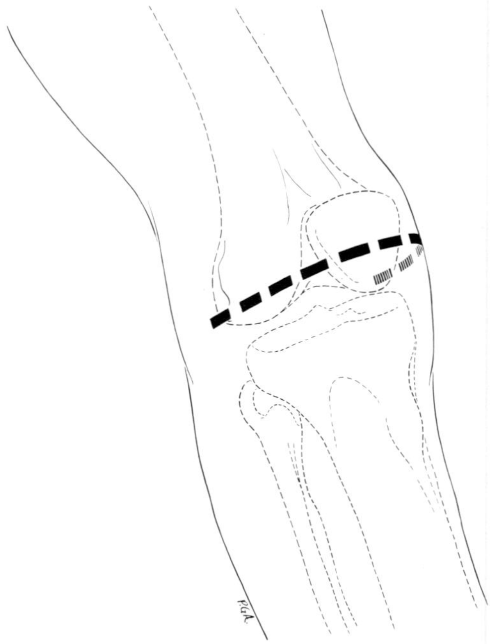

FIG. 6-3. The heavy broken line is the line of transverse incision for approach to the knee joint. It extends from beyond one collateral ligament to the other across the junction of the middle and lower thirds of the patella.

total patellectomy has been done. As with the incision, the management of the patella does not appear to be of importance in the results.

When a transpatellar incision is used, a portion of anterior patella just thick enough to allow a 21 gauge wire to be inserted within the substance of bone is preserved on both sides of the osteotomy cut. In fused joints, if the patella is ankylosed to the femur, it is detached and reflected with soft tissues (Fig. 6-4). Although disturbance of the collateral ligaments is usually unnecessary in mobile joints, detachment of their origins is often necessary in joints which are solidly ankylosed.

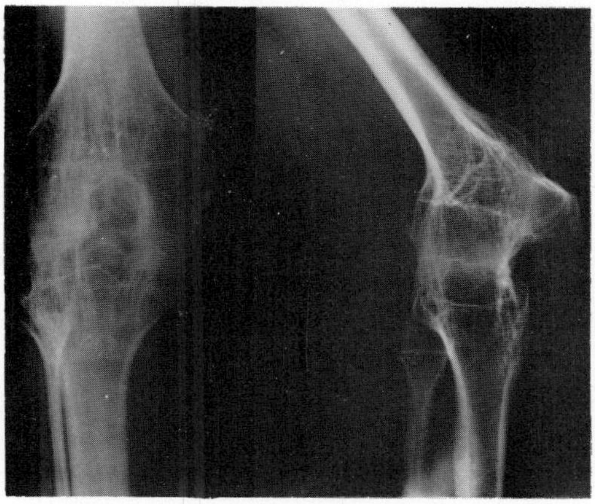

FIG. 6-4. Radiographs of solidly ankylosed right knee of a 23-year-old man with juvenile rheumatoid arthritis. He had had a free mold arthroplasty of the ankylosed left knee done by Dr. Smith-Petersen three years earlier.

Blunt subperiosteal dissection of the posterior tibiofemoral mass is done, protecting the posterior soft tissues. The tibia and femur are separated by gouges and osteotomes in line with the normal contours of the tibial plateaus.

The joint is flexed and the distal femur is shaped to conform to the inside contour of the hollow mold. Resection of the posterior portion of the femoral condyle facilitates exposure of the posterior capsule and cruciate ligaments. With long-standing bony ankylosis, the bone is likely to be soft in the cortex and mushy in the cancellous portions. A ronguer or scissors often cuts this bone more precisely than an osteotome.

With the knee in hyperflexion, a blunt instrument is passed carefully from both sides behind the posterior capsule, and a capsulotomy is done.

Shaping of the femur is continued, using a small gouge. A rounded hole is made well forward in the intercondylar area to conform to the size of the base of the intramedullary stem. Because of the valgus angle of its stem, the mold moves slightly from medial to lateral as it caps the femur, and more trimming of the medial than the lateral aspects of both condyles is needed to produce a snug fit.

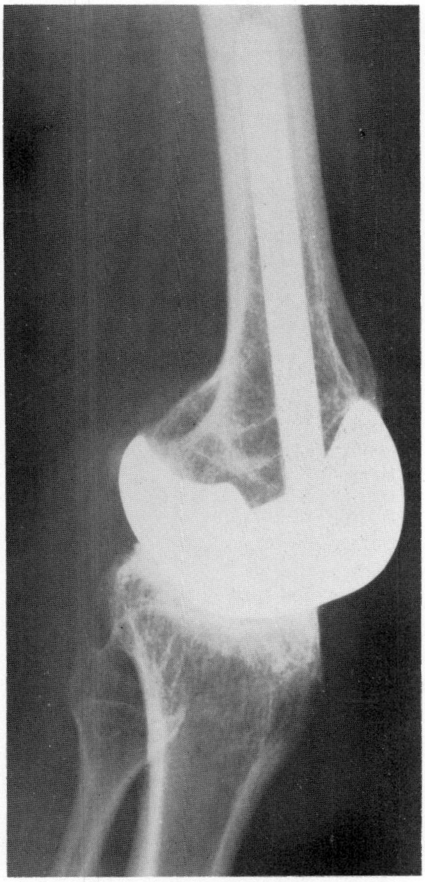

FIG. 6-5. Lateral postoperative view of right knee shown in Figure 6-4.

The amount of femur to be resected depends on the condition of the joint; with severe flexion deformity, shortening the femur may aid extension, while in a knee unstable in extension, little or no shortening should be done.

The shaft of the femur is palpated, and the introduction of the mold stem into the central portion of the medullary canal is carried out without difficulty. The long, tapered, blunt-edged, three-flanged stem is an aid in directing the mold. As the mold comes into contact with the femur, some additional trimming is usually needed. A Smith-Petersen nail driver is attached to the mold, which is then seated firmly over the femur. Ordinarily little force is required for this. If the medullary canal is very narrow, it may be drilled, or a portion of the stem may be cut off.

The proper plane of the femoral joint surface is established by placing the stem of the mold centrally in the medullary canal. Occasionally when a femoral shaft deformity exists, the stem is placed eccentrically to achieve the required correction (Figs. 6-8 to 6-10). This must be anticipated in shaping the distal femur; if the stem is pointed medially, the lateral condyle must be shortened more than the medial.

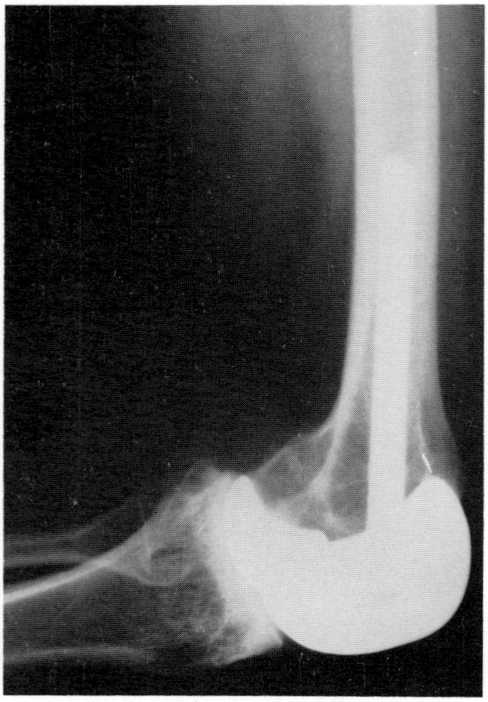

FIG. 6-6. Postoperative view of right knee shown in Figure 6-4 in flexion.

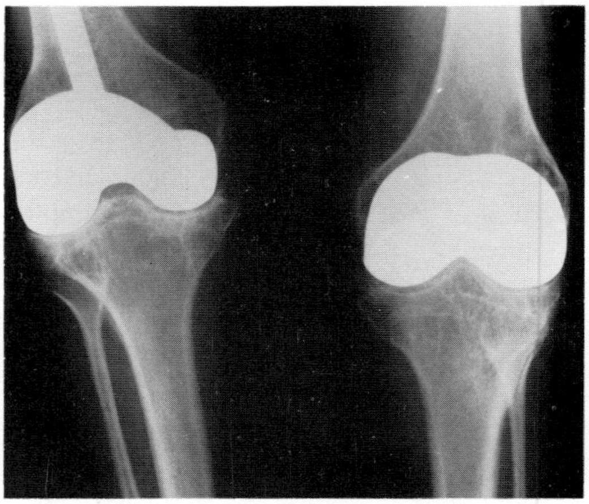

FIG. 6-7. Radiographs 16 years after a left arthroplasty and 13½ years after a right arthroplasty. Some mild impression of the tibia by the mold is evident in each, but function is unimpaired.

The articular surfaces of the tibia are shaped to allow secure seating of the mold; one plateau or the other may be trimmed to diminish varus or valgus deformity. The least resection of tibia which allows good alignment with the mold is desirable. The mold and tibia are brought into articulation, and after a trial of motion, further adjustments may be carried out. With fibrous ankylosis or in mobile deformed knees, the same sort of procedure is carried out. The cortex is usually better-defined and harder. Basic cuts in shaping the femur are through the posterior portions of both condyles, sloping slightly outward proximally. The anterior shield of femoral joint surface, which articulates with the patella, is resected (Fig. 6-11). The direction of these cuts in the coronal plane will determine the position of rotation in which the mold is seated and can be varied to compensate for rotation deformities.

When rotation deformity of the tibia on the femur exists (usually external in rheumatoid patients), new plateau facets may have developed. The edges must be cut away so that the natural contours of the two plateaus are restored. The tibia then aligns properly with the condyles of the mold.

A complete synovectomy is done in patients with active rheumatoid disease. In knees with substantial flexion deformity and subluxation, resection of the scarred cruciate ligaments may be necessary to allow restoration of joint alignment. The cruciates can be preserved in joints which extend well; they are debrided of abnormal synovium and left intact (Fig. 6-12). In knees affected by active rheumatoid disease, no loss of anteroposterior stability has resulted after cruciate resection. In joints affected by tumor, trauma, or other non-rheumatoid conditions, a "drawer-sign" and some sense of instability on descending stairs may be noted when the cruciates are resected.

Before closure, the position of the stem within the femur may be determined by x-ray examination; this should be done if heavy force was required to seat the mold or if varus or valgus deformity remains after the mold is in place.

Repair of the capsule and soft tissues with restoration of collateral ligament origins to bone is done. When a transpatellar incision is used, a 20-gauge wire suture is placed within the bone fragments. In some of the patients in whom transpatellar incisions were repaired with silk or catgut bone sutures, the patellar fragments separated considerably. Suprisingly enough, the patients were able to extend the knees completely as long as the lateral expansions were intact (Fig. 6-15). Various templates designed to guide shaping of the distal femur have not been of real value.

Although many more women than men have been operated on, more of the large molds have been used, the small size being reserved primarily for small juvenile rheumatoid patients. For average or large men the extra-large size is required.

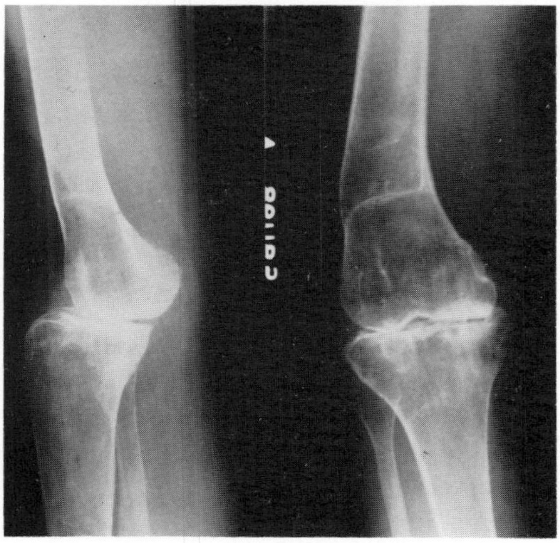

FIG. 6-8. The right knee of a 49-year-old woman with rheumatoid arthritis who had had a femoral osteotomy and fascial arthroplasty 25 years earlier. Severe varus deformity, instability and pain disabled her. Recent muscle transfers had not improved the joint. Motion was 10° to 80°.

Postoperative Care. Postoperative care varies, depending on the preoperative condition of the knee, the stability of the joint at the conclusion of operation, the incision used, and, to some extent, the surgeon's preference for immediate postoperative or delayed motion in inflammatory joint disease.

After arthroplasty has been done in a knee with solid fusion of soft bone (the operation having required detachment of ligaments), the use of a cast for about 3 weeks would be usual. This is followed with brace support for 4 months and crutches for partial weight bearing for 6 months or more. However, after the arthroplasty of a knee in which ligaments are not disturbed and tibial subchondral bone is firm, early exercise and early walking with crutches and without braces is the customary course.

If progressive gain of flexion is not evident by 3 weeks after mobilization of the joint has begun, manipulation under anesthesia should be considered. About one-third of the knees have been manipulated after operation, with substantial improvement.

Results

Of 98 patients (21 had bilateral operations), 53 had adult and 15 juvenile rheumatoid arthritis. Other preoperative diagnoses were degenerative arthritis in 15, effects of trauma in six, old septic arthritis in six, giant cell tumor in two and a form of dysplasia in one. Many had had earlier operations, some complicated by infection.

Of 110 knees in 89 patients who had had operations done a year or more before these figures were collected, 12 had bony ankylosis with deformity, nine had fibrous ankylosis with deformity; the large majority, 87, had pain, deformity, and instability combined.

Sex Incidence and Age. Seventeen patients were male, 72 were female. The patients' ages ranged from 14 to 76 years; the average age was 57½.

Complications. Complications were numerous; the most troublesome was infection in 12 knees. This required mold removal in five cases. Of the knees from which molds were not removed after infection, treatment resulted in fair to good function in six and poor in one. The last known infections occurred 53 and 45 months ago. Nearly 50 arthroplasties have been done since without this complication.

No correlation with operating time, tourniquet time, or the use of antibiotics could be established. Many of the early patients had severe active rheumatoid disease and were generally unwell. Subluxation occurred in three knees; all had flexion deformities greater than 35° and required massive freeing of soft tissues. Two patients had temporary peroneal nerve palsies; one had postoperative subluxation, one bled when anticoagulation went out of control while the leg was in a cast.

Three patients developed thrombophlebitis. Except in those patients who have had hip arthroplasties before knee arthroplasties, prophylactic anticoagulation is not routine, since early mobilization of the patient is ordinarily anticipated. Skin defects developed in four patients in whom long U-shaped incisions were used. Two had significant extension defects, one after skin slough and one after thrombophlebitis and partial wound disruptions. One patient developed cricoarytenoid arthritis, and one developed aplastic anemia after operation; both had rheumatoid arthritis.

Re-operations. Thirty-four re-operations were done. Eighteen molds were removed, five because of infection. Two molds were removed from one patient because of limited motion. These were replaced by hinged prostheses, and both knees became ankylosed. Ten molds were removed because of instability or pain. Many of these had not been considered wholly suitable for arthroplasty, but, in an effort to preserve motion, they had been done with the anticipation that fusion might later be required.

One amputation was done; the patient's knee had had four earlier operations, and the patient had complained of pain after surgical fusion. Instability and continuing pain followed arthroplasty. Small vessel disease was noted in the surgical specimen.

Twelve revisions were done, including two in one patient and three in another. Usually, these led to little improvement.

Follow-up. The times of follow-up ranged from 1 to 18 years, with an average of 4 years and 9 months. Of 110 knees operated upon, one was lost before a year after operation, and molds were removed from 18. Ninety-one knees were available for assessment of results. Seventeen knees had been followed for 10 or more years, 22 from 5 to 10 years, and 32 from 3 to 5 years.

Range of Motion. Forty-seven knees developed a wide range of motion from 85° to 120°, with an average of 97°. Thirty-two knees had a moderate range of 25° to 80°, with an average of 44° Twelve knees had very limited motion of 25° or less; when painless, even a little motion was useful in walking and superior to a fused knee.

Assessment of Results. It is especially difficult to grade the functional result of operation in a single joint when most others are abnormal. In none was a normal, wholly insensitive joint produced. Criteria for rating were range of motion, stability, and degree of discomfort.

Stable knees with 85° or more of motion and little or infrequent discomfort were considered very good; those with similar qualities but requiring use of bannisters or a cane were rated good. With motion range between 25° to 80° and the ability to walk or approach normal activity, the knee rated fair. Poor results included those knees with less than 25° motion; those which were painful, or had lateral instability or defective extension; and those from which molds were removed.

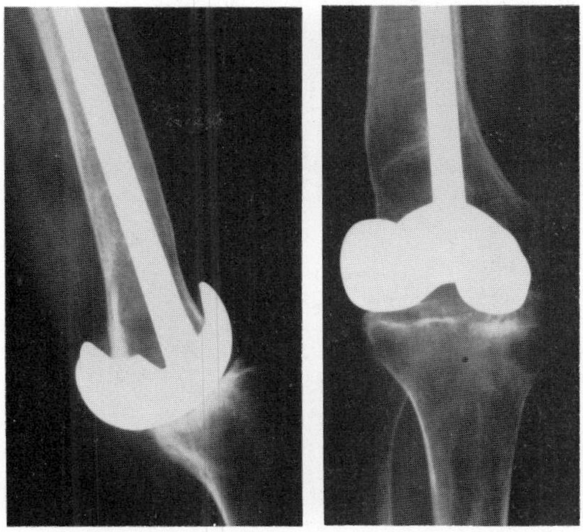

FIG. 6-9. Radiographs of patient in Figure 6-8 after arthroplasty in which a mold was used to reduce femoral varus. The substance of the mold over an unshortened femur tightened the joint. One year later motion was from 5° to 95° of flexion. She walks unsupported most of the time indoors but uses a cane outdoors.

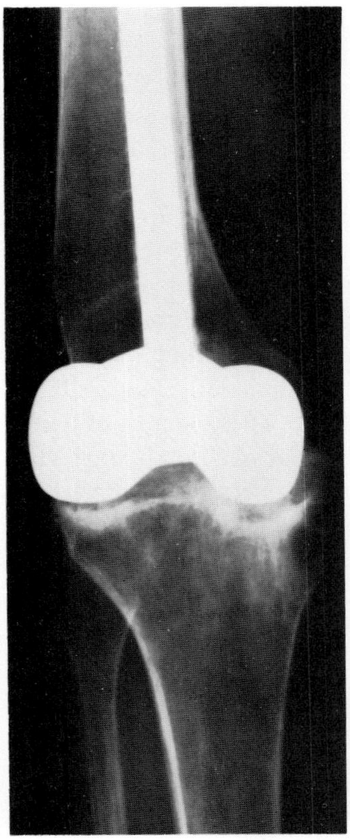

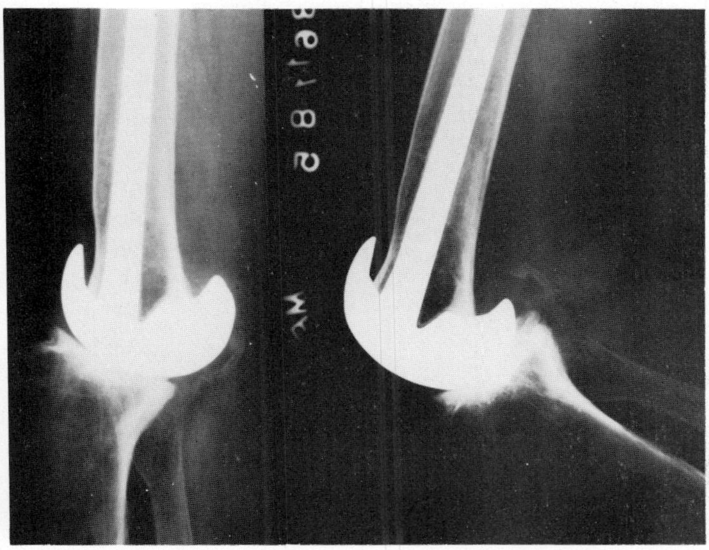

FIG. 6-10. (*Left*) Patient shown in Figure 6-8, 5 years after arthroplasty. The mold has impressed the tibial plateaus with some increase in lateral instability but no significant change in function. (*Center, right*) Lateral x-rays 5 years after operation.

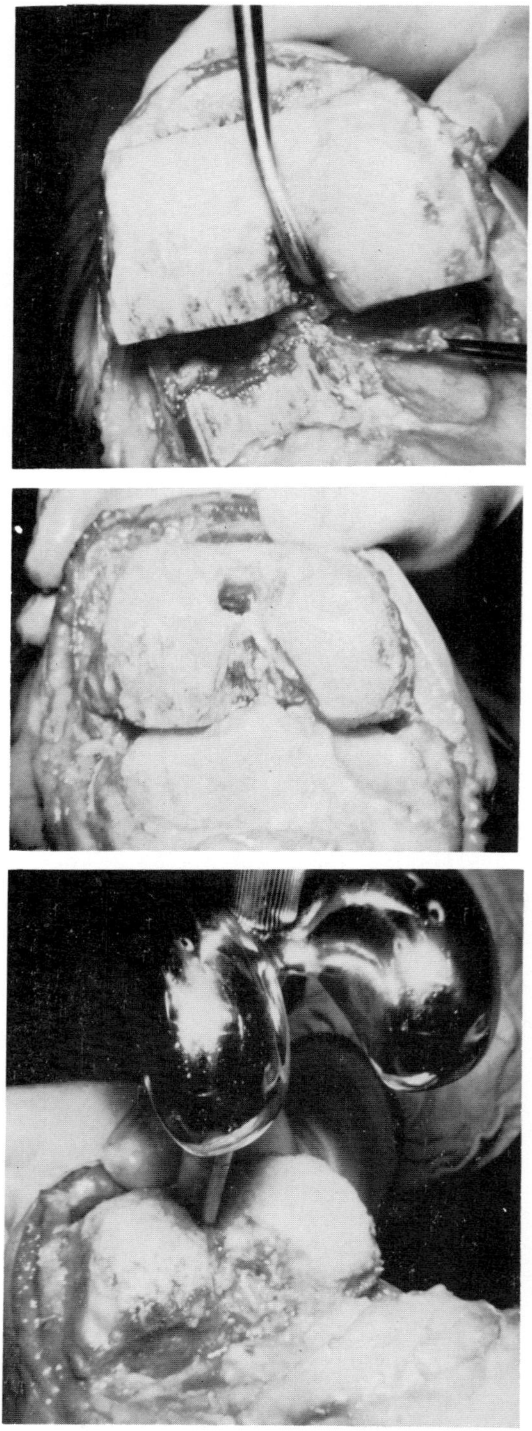

FIG. 6-11. (*Top*) Initial cuts in shaping the distal femur. (*Center*) The edges of the condyle are rounded. (*Bottom*) The mold is applied to the femur.

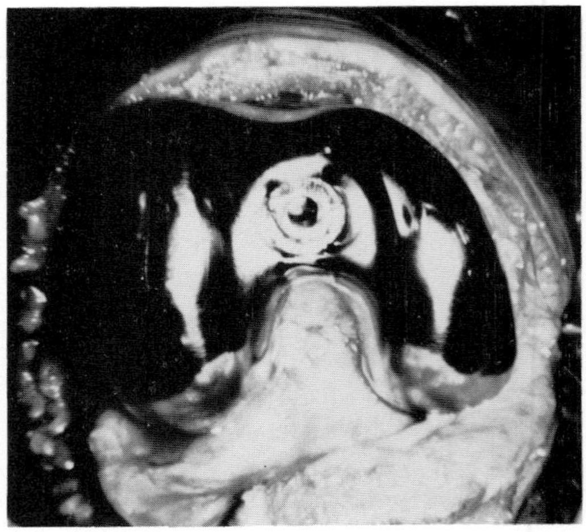

FIG. 6-12. A mold in place on the femur; the anterior cruciate ligament is intact.

Thirty-three were rated as very good and 13, good; these comprised 42 per cent of the whole group. Twenty-eight or 26 per cent were rated fair. Thirty-five or 32 per cent were poor. In general, the assessment of a knee 1 year after arthroplasty tends to be durable.

In all, some impression, or molding, of the tibial plateaus by the femoral mold was noted. This became apparent after 3 to 5 years in knees in which the tibial subchondral cortex was not disturbed, but much earlier when considerable remodelling of tibia had been done. These joints felt a little looser, but except for severe sinking when infection was present, significant deterioration in function was not found. In some of the older patients in whom arthroplasties had been done when they were in the sixth decade, the operated knees appeared to fail less than the rest of their joints. Loosening of the prosthesis in the femur has not been a problem.

Results in Various Conditions. Sixty-one arthroplasties were done to treat adult rheumatoid arthritis. In this group, results were good or very good in 30, fair in 14, and poor in 17 knees. A large portion of the complications listed earlier occurred in the

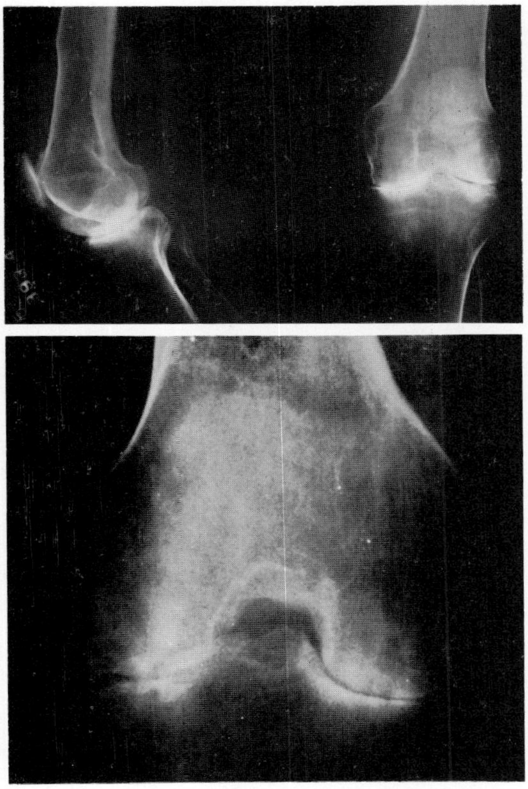

FIG. 6-13. (*Top*) The knee of a 63-year-old woman with rheumatoid arthritis who was disabled by pain. There was intense synovial thickening and a large effusion with the appearance of pressure remodelling of the anterior femur under the quadriceps pouch. A large ganglion was present in the popliteal space. (*Bottom*) Tunnel view showing beginning destruction of the lateral femur.

latter "poor" classification, and except for these, satisfactory improvement was fairly regular.

To generalize: in a knee affected by adult rheumatoid disease in which a wide range of motion is preserved but with pain, deformity, and instability, one may expect an arthroplasty result of satisfactory stability, improvement of pain and deformity and maintenance of a wide range of motion.

In this group seven patients had two hip and two knee arthroplasties; seven, two hip and one knee arthroplasty; and two, two knee and one hip arthroplasty. The patient with multiple severe lower extremity disabilities is a prime candidate for this procedure. (Fig. 6-16).

Of 20 knees affected by juvenile arthritis, only four were good or very good, seven were fair, and nine were poor. These patients had had very limited motion for many years and were often emotionally difficult. Though improvement of pain and deformity may be satisfactory enough to greatly improve the patient's ability to walk, a wide range of motion is not anticipated. Limited motion is the usual cause for poor rating in this group.

There were three fair and three poor results of arthroplasty in knees affected by old septic arthritis, the preoperative qualities of the joints being much like juvenile rheumatoid.

In knees operated on for degenerative joint disease there were good or very good

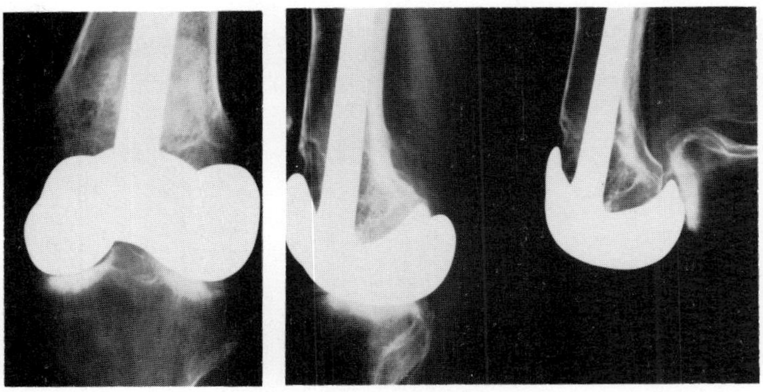

FIG. 6-14. Knee of patient in Figure 6-13 8 months after arthroplasty. (*Left*) Anteroposterior view. (*Center, right*) The patellar suture has disrupted. The tibia moves beyond a right angle over the condyle.

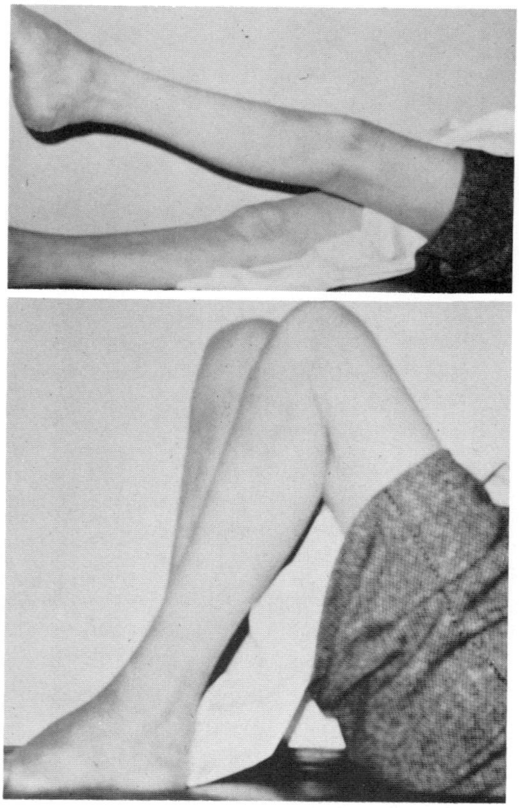

FIG. 6-15. The patient shown in Figure 6-13 demonstrates extension (top) and flexion (bottom). She has full active extension despite patellar separation. A wide range of motion developed early after operation.

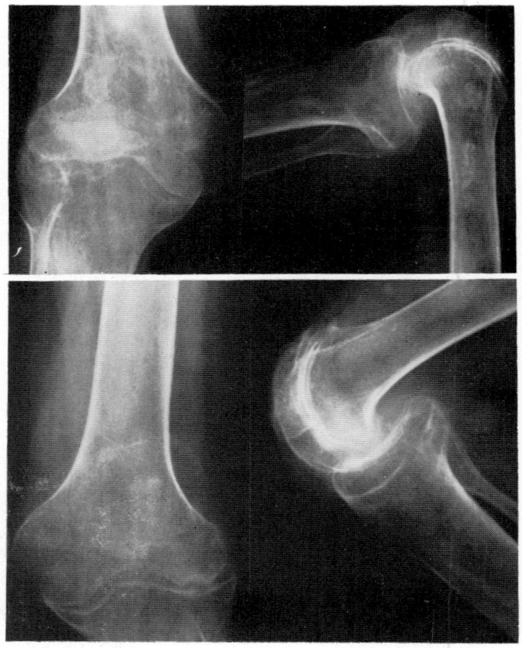

FIG. 6-16. (*Top*) Right knee of a 31-year-old woman with long-standing rheumatoid arthritis. She had been unable to be out of bed or without narcotics for 6 months. The principal disability resulted from knee pain, although the hips, too, were limited and painful. The right knee moved from 30° flexion deformity to 115° and was unstable. (*Bottom*) The left knee was unstable, moving from 20° flexion deformity to 100° of flexion.

results in ten, fair in two and poor in two. Improvement in function appears to be slower and to continue longer than in other conditions.

While the poor results in juvenile rheumatoid arthritis seem to be related to the disease, the poor results (two fair and four

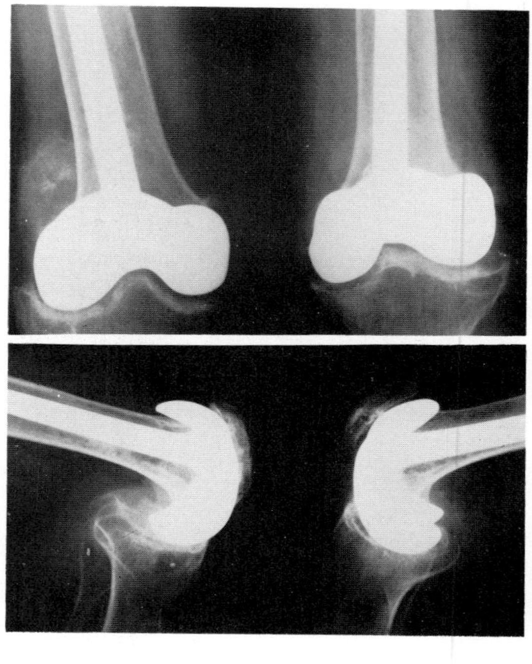

FIG. 6-17. (*Top*) Knees of patient shown in Figure 6-16 one year after right knee arthroplasty and 8 months after left knee arthroplasty. Impression of the tibial plateaus existed before the operations. (*Bottom*) The patient had full extension in both knees with 100° of flexion on the right and 75° on the left. Except for getting out of a chair of ordinary height, she was independent on crutches and needed a bannister on stairs.

poor) in the small group of knees affected by trauma may be artificial. One had had seven, one five, and one four earlier operations of the knee; two were considered addicted to narcotics; and in one an undersize mold was used.

In summary, the femoral mold arthroplasty is a useful procedure in the management of rheumatoid knees in which there has been severe destruction of femoral cartilage. Varus and valgus deformities may be corrected by appropriate placement of the prosthesis. The most frequent significant complication has been infection, though with increased experience, the incidence of sepsis has markedly diminished. The most gratifying results have been in those patients with multiple severe lower extremity disabilities.

CHAPTER 7

The Use of Hinged Joints in Rheumatoid Arthritis of the Knee

BORJE WALLDIUS, M.D.

In 1951, when this study began, the standard method of reconstruction of the knee joint consisted of the interposition of a flap of fascia lata between the articular surfaces. The result was a movable joint but hardly a stable and functional joint, because the stabilizing ligaments had to be sacrificed in the operation. An endoprosthesis of the hinged joint type could combine mobility with stability, provided that it could be firmly anchored in the bone. The conditions necessary for this seemed to be present, since the knee joints present bone surfaces which are large—twice as large as those of the hip joint. If the arthroplasty fails, it should still be possible to perform an arthrodesis after extracting the artificial joint.

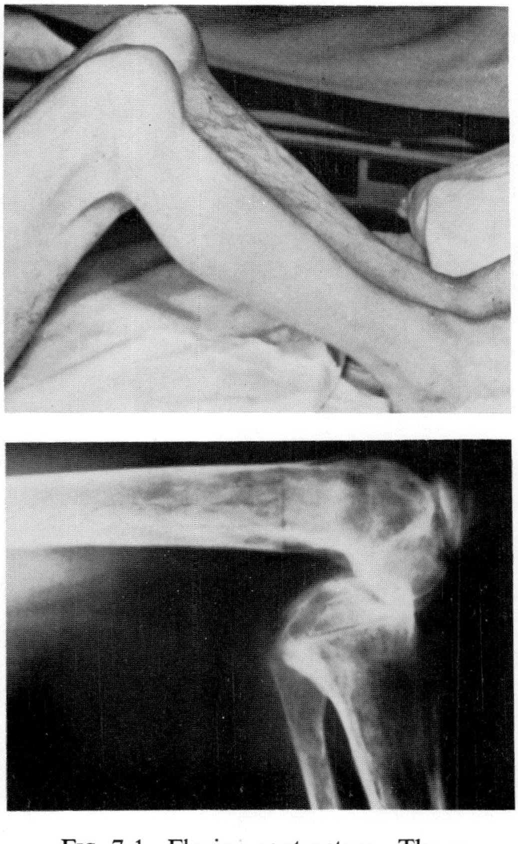

FIG. 7-1. Flexion contracture. The patient was unable to walk for 10 years.

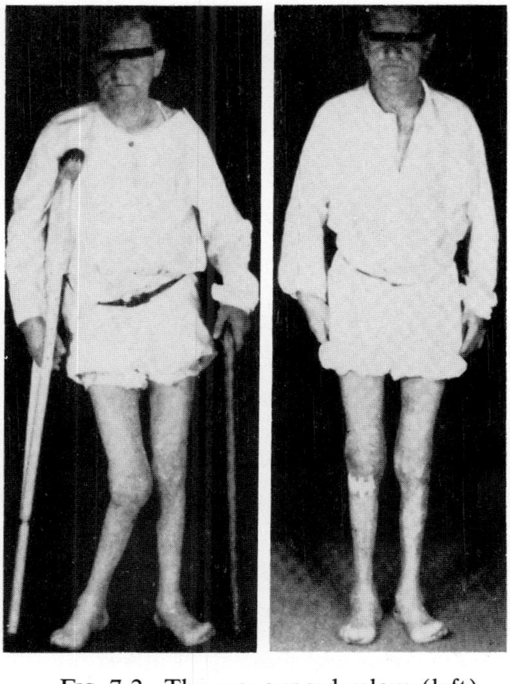

FIG. 7-2. The pronounced valgus (left) has been corrected by the operation.

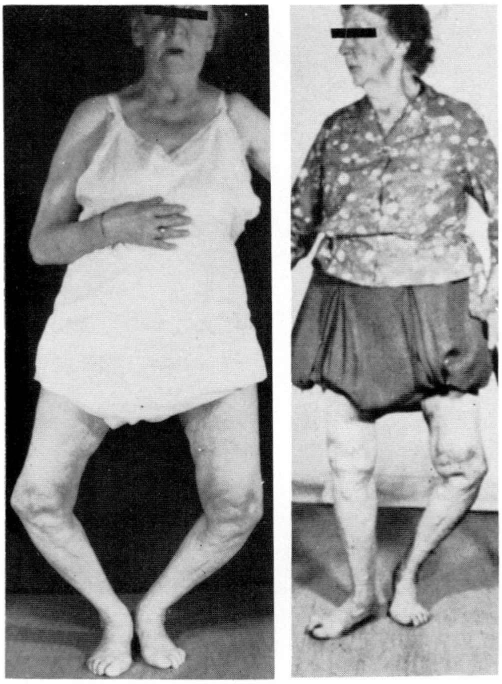

FIG. 7-3. A severe varus deformity (right knee) can be reversed.

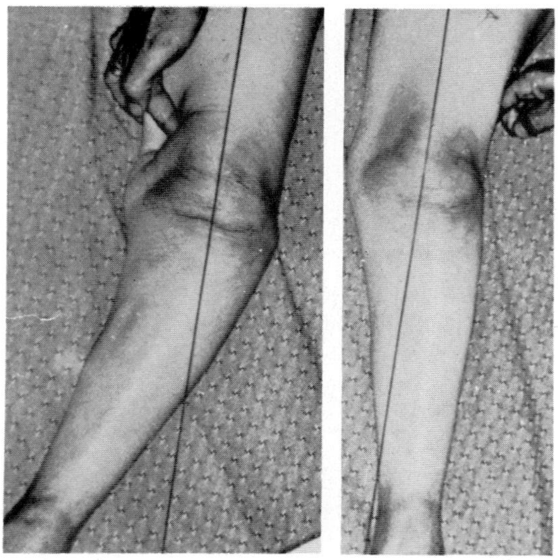

FIG. 7-4. The procedure may restore stability to the joint.

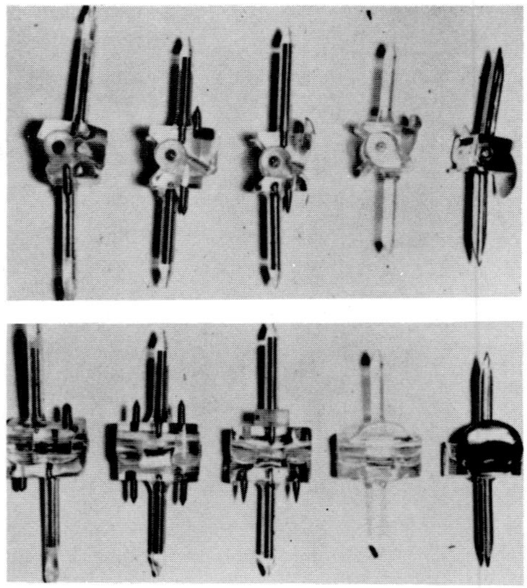

FIG. 7-5. The evolution of the design of the prosthesis.

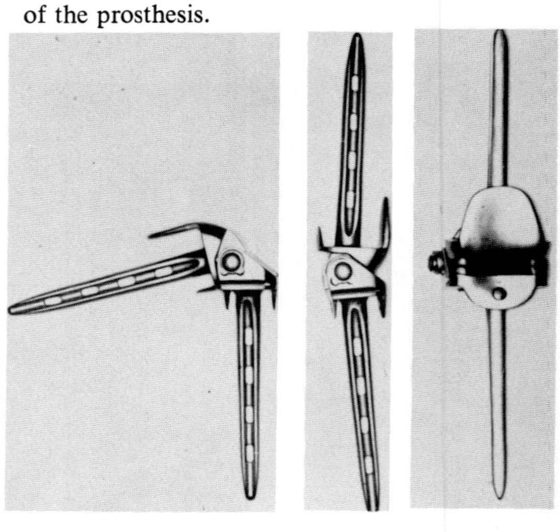

FIG. 7-6. The latest Vitallium model of the prosthesis.

Indications and Contraindications. The indications were the four common conditions and their combinations seen in the rheumatoid knee: (1) flexion contracture, (2) valgus deformity, (3) varus deformity, (4) instability (Figs. 7-1 to 7-4). Even the highest degree of deformity and instability can be treated. The requisite qualification is a properly functioning quadriceps muscle. The function in the other joints of the lower extremities must be sufficient to allow the patient to walk again.

Bedridden or wheel chair-bound patients who have had long-term treatment with cortisone followed by a high degree of osteoporosis are a group of patients in whom the

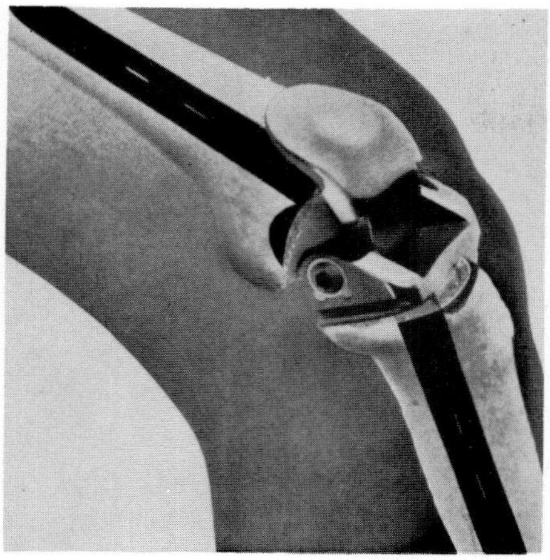

FIG. 7-7. The prosthesis in situ.

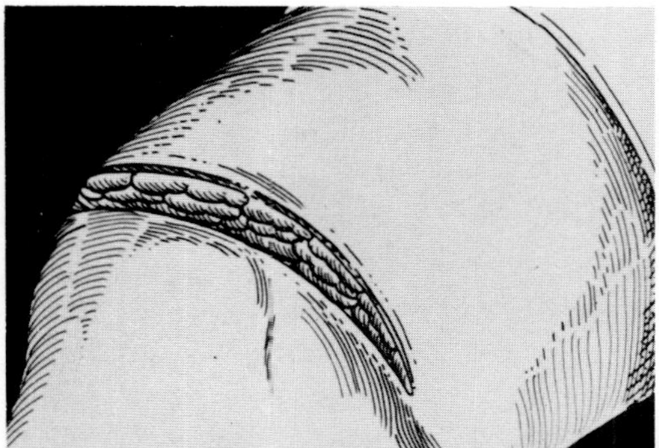

FIG. 7-8. A transverse incision across the middle of the patella.

operation may be contraindicated. The skin over the joint must be in good condition. Most of the rheumatoid patients were operated on at a relatively late stage of the disease, when the inflammation had become quiescent. A raised sedimentation rate, however, has not been regarded as a contraindication. The operation has not been performed in cases where one knee was intact and the other ankylosed but functioning well.

The Prosthesis. From 1951 to 1958 an acrylic prosthesis was used in 60 operations (Fig. 7-5). Since 1958, Vitallium prostheses have been used in 84 procedures. The design of the prosthesis has changed gradu-

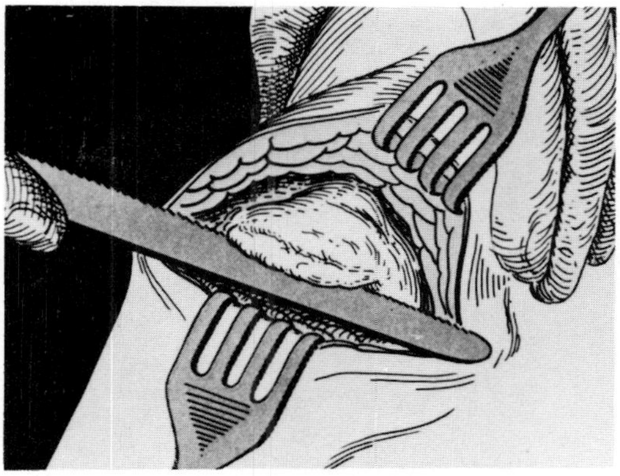

FIG. 7-9. Dividing the patella.

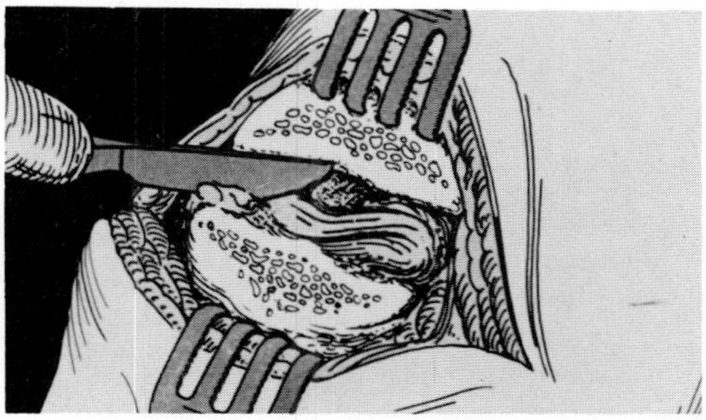

FIG. 7-10. Incision of the capsule.

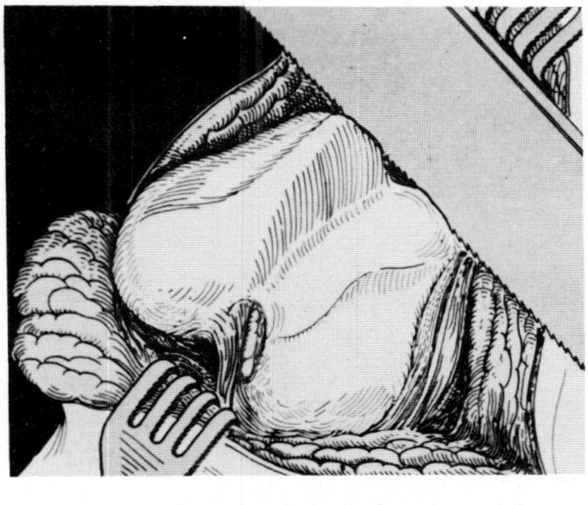

FIG. 7-11. Sawing off the femoral condyles.

ally during the years as a result of the experience gained. The present prosthesis has broad surfaces in contact with the bone, and frontal lips which extend over the anterior cortex (Figs. 7-6 and 7-7). Posterior lips insert into the cancellous bone

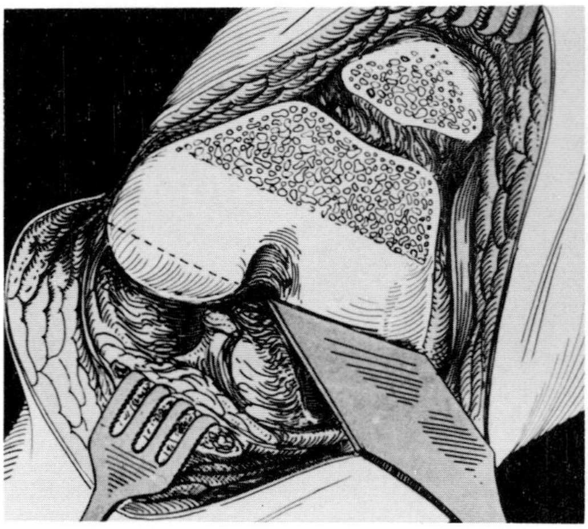

FIG. 7-12. Chiselling off the posterior portions of the femoral condyles.

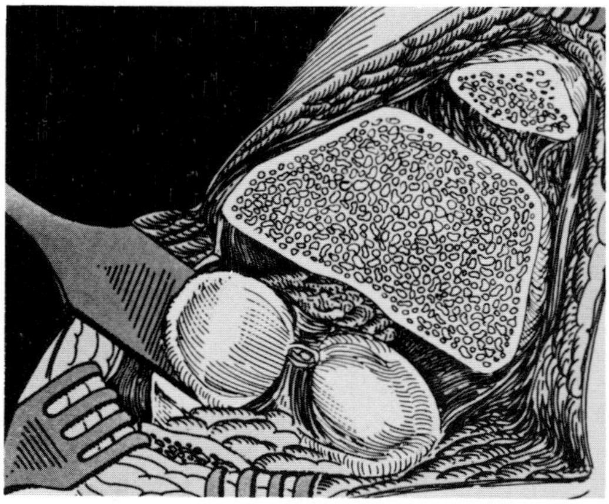

FIG. 7-13. Chiselling off the tibial surface.

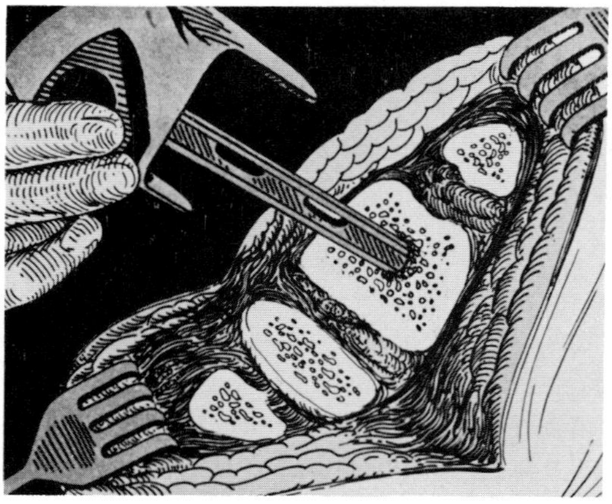

FIG. 7-14. Driving in the femoral member.

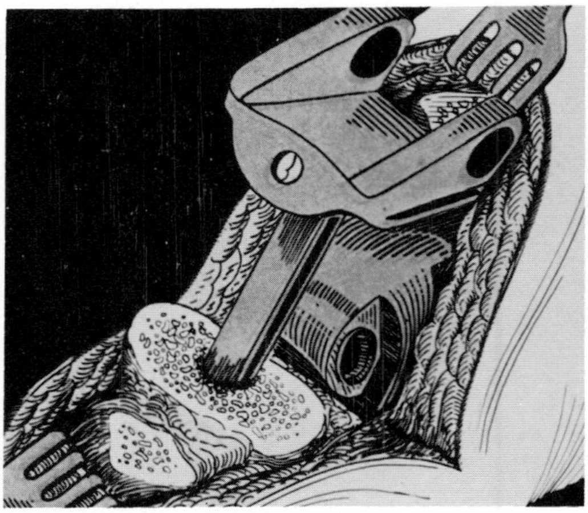

FIG. 7-15. Driving in the tibial member.

posteriorly. The medullary stems and the lips are perforated in an attempt to follow the self-locking principle. By these arrangements the prosthesis can be solidly anchored in the bone. Acrylic cement is not used.

Operative Procedure. The operation is performed under general or spinal anesthesia in a bloodless field. A transverse incision centered directly over the midpoint of the patella is used (Fig. 7-8). The patella is divided in the frontal plane with a saw in an oblique direction from the apex to the base (Fig. 7-9). The capsule is incised transversely on both sides of the patella (Fig. 7-10). The collateral ligaments are freed from the femoral epicondyles, and the suprapatellar recesses, which are often filled with adherent material, are opened by blunt dissection. The knee is bent to 90°, and the femoral condyles are sawed off, taking a slice measuring about 3 cm. in height (Fig. 7-11). The resected surface should be at right angles to the mechanical axis of the thigh. The posterior parts of the femoral condyles must be removed with an osteotome; otherwise, they will constitute an impediment to flexion (Fig. 7-12). The articular surface of the tibia is levelled off perpendicular to the long axis of the leg (Fig. 7-13). In cases with a varus or valgus deformity, the medial

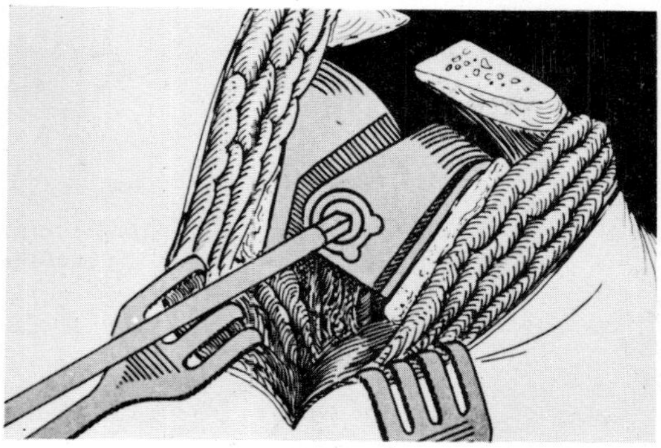

FIG. 7-16. Connecting the two members with a bolt.

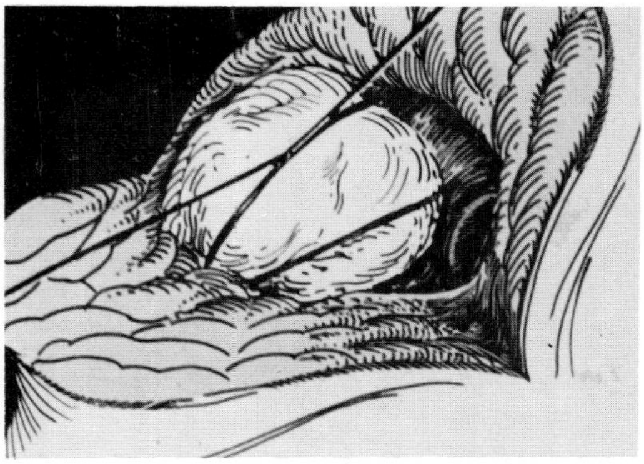

FIG. 7-17. Suturing the two parts of the patella.

and lateral parts of the articular surface, respectively, are more or less depressed. In these cases, only the undepressed part of the surface is removed.

Before the parts of the prosthesis are driven in, a probe of the same length as that of the medullary stems of the prosthesis is inserted into the medullary cavity to make sure that the stem will not impinge on the cortical bone. The femoral member of the prosthesis is inserted first (Fig. 7-14). The tibial member is then inserted with the lower leg in the position of 20° external rotation (Fig. 7-15). The two parts of the prosthesis are connected by a bolt. The bolt is locked with a washer and a screw (Fig. 7-16). Both stability and mobility are tested. If any impediment to flexion remains, the posterior parts of the resected surfaces are further chiselled away. The two parts of the patella are placed in an overlapping position with the apex as far as possible proximal and the base as far as possible distal. In this position they are sutured with strong nylon; first with a circular type of suture and then with a figure-8 suture (Fig. 7-17). In this manner the extensor apparatus is shortened and the axis

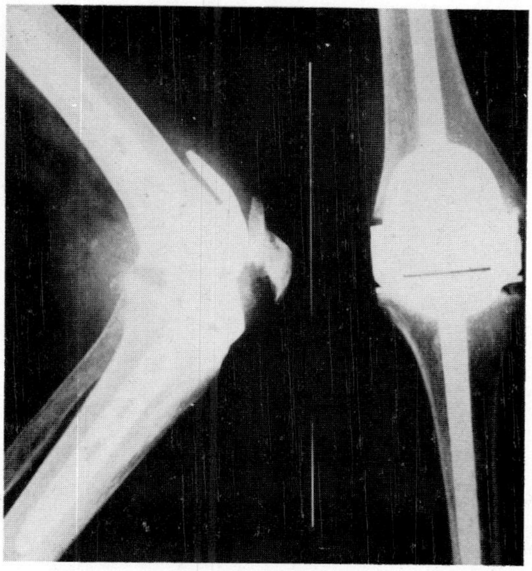

FIG. 7-18. The two parts of the patella have healed in an overlapping position. The patellar thickness has been increased and the reaction point moved further forward.

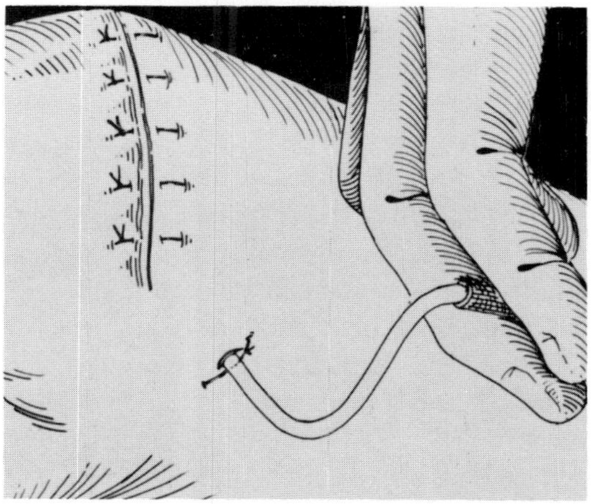

FIG. 7-19. Application of suction drainage.

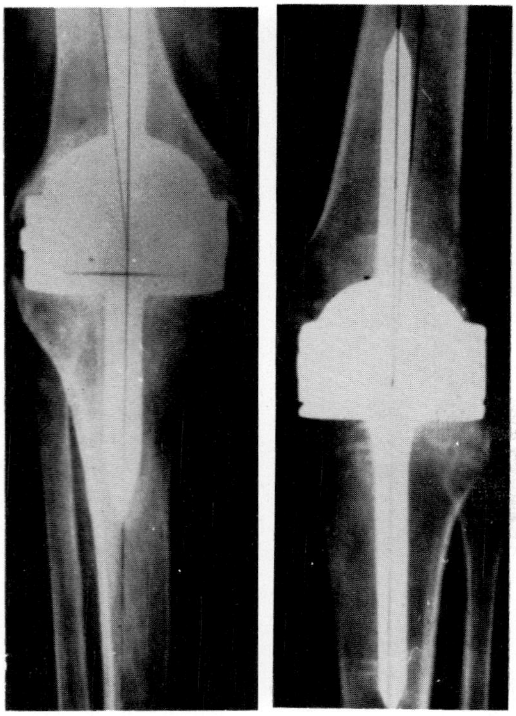

FIG. 7-20. X-rays with prosthesis in good alignment.

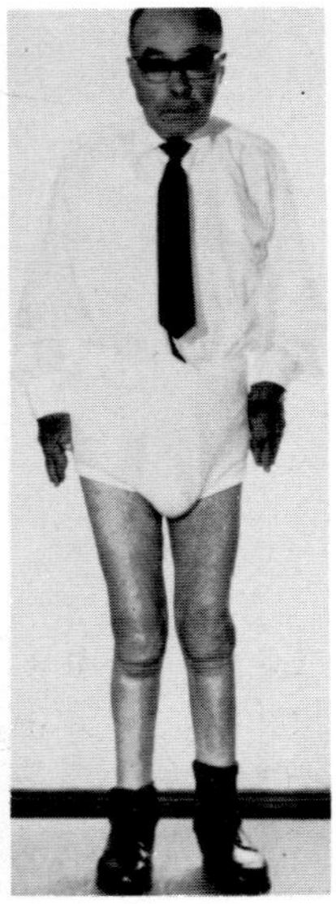

FIG. 7-21. This patient has been able to walk with properly functioning knee joints for a period of 12 years after operation.

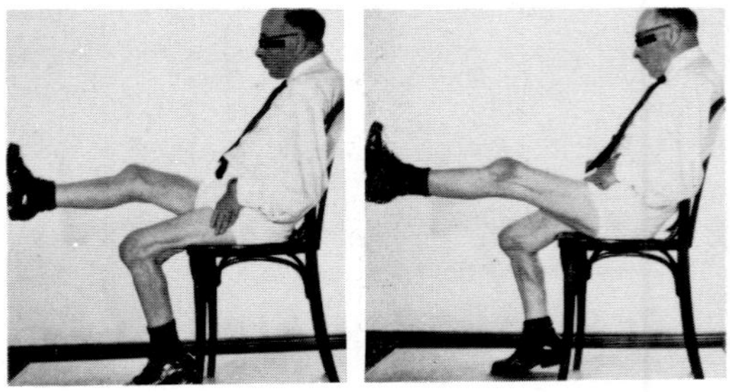

FIG. 7-22. Flexion and extension range in both knees is demonstrated.

of the lever for extension is lengthened, thereby helping to reinforce the quadriceps function (Fig. 7-18). A drainage tube is inserted into the posterior part of the joint (Fig. 7-19), and an amply padded cast is applied with the joint in full extension.

On the first postoperative day, the cast, the bandage, and the drainage tube are removed, and a new cast is applied. At this time 300 ml. to 400 ml. of blood is usually collected in the drain. After 3 weeks, the cast is taken off, sutures are removed, and exercises are started. When the patient can do a straight-leg raise, walking is begun and full weight bearing is permitted. This occurs after an additional 1 to 2 weeks and can usually be done without any pain or instability.

Results

During the period from 1951 to 1970, a total of 144 arthroplasties have been performed on 117 patients. Twenty-seven patients underwent operations on both knees. The ages of the patients range from 29 to 79 years. In 90 patients the primary disease was rheumatoid arthritis; in the remaining 27 it was degenerative arthritis. Since 1958, when the use of the Vitallium prosthesis began, good results have been obtained in 68 out of 84 joints (84 per cent). A good result is one in which the joint endures weight bearing on walking and is without pain. It must be fully stable and have a mobility of at least 60°. The best indication of the reliability of the operation is presented by those patients who underwent the procedure on both knees (Figs. 7-21 and 7-22).

Complicating Factors. The main complication has been infection, and for this reason arthrodesis has been performed in ten cases since 1958. During the same period, four patients underwent re-operation necessitated by loose prostheses. The prostheses were replaced by new ones with longer medullary stems; bone cement was used in order to obtain more stable fixation. Good results were obtained after these re-operations.

Peroneal nerve paralysis occurred in six cases, but recovery was progressive for up to 1 year after the operation, and there was no detrimental effect on the ability to walk. After trauma, two patients suffered almost identical fractures of their distal femurs. The fragments were not unduly displaced because of the medullary stems, and they healed in plaster without losing any motion in the joint.

The medullary stem of the prosthesis should be in alignment with the mechanical long axis. This suggests that the medullary stem in the femur should point to the medial side of the bone (Fig. 7-20). In three cases it has penetrated the cortical bone. The patients have complained of slight pain in this area during the first few months, but it then gradually disappeared.

The question of excision of the patella often arises, since congruence with the prosthesis cannot be obtained and a retained patella might cause pain. It is our experience that the joint between the patella and the prosthesis does not become a focal point for pain and that the patella is gradually transformed until full congruence with the prosthesis is obtained. One may wonder if the sensitivity of the joint is altered by the operation; that is, can the patient still sense the position of the joint with respect to the degree of flexion or extension? Patients have not found this to be any great problem. The main goal is that the muscular system of the joint should function well. In approximately half of the joints, the patellar reflex can be elicited. Structurally, the Vitallium prosthesis itself appears strong enough for the job. No prosthesis has ever fractured.

CHAPTER 8

Selection of the Surgical Procedure for the Rheumatoid Knee

NELSON MITCHELL, M.D., AND RICHARD L. CRUESS, M.D.

The surgical procedures available in the treatment of the rheumatoid knee can be divided into two main groups. Included in the first are those which at least temporarily eradicate the disease, relieve pain, and improve the function of the joint. These operations, then, are prophylactic as well as therapeutic and require a joint whose articular cartilage is more or less intact. Synovectomy, osteotomy, and posterior capsulectomies make up this group. When the disease has progressed beyond this point, salvage and reconstruction are the objectives, and these can be achieved by some form of arthroplasty or, in certain circumstances, by arthrodesis.

Synovectomy

This operation is frequently indicated when painful effusions have persisted for 6 weeks or more in spite of adequate medical therapy. Best results are obtained when little or no cartilage destruction is evident, as shown by a near normal joint space and absence of erosions on ordinary x-rays. A moderate degree of cartilage destruction, ligamentous instability, or a flexion contracture up to 15° prejudice the final result, but they are not contraindications. Clearly, the operation should not be performed in the presence of severe cartilage destruction, gross ligamentous instability, or a deformity of greater than 15° in any plane. Synovectomy may be carried out alone or in conjunction with any of the other surgical procedures advocated for this joint. In the presence of advanced patellofemoral disease a patellectomy may be performed at the time of synovectomy, but is better done later. Age is rarely a contraindication, nor is the general activity of the rheumatoid disease as a whole, providing the patient is well enough to tolerate surgery.

Osteotomy

The purpose of an osteotomy is to correct disabling deformities about the knee. These may be either valgus or varus but are most frequently due to a flexion contracture. An osteotomy to correct a flexion contracture is best suited for one between 15° and 30°. It may be done in conjunction with a synovectomy but should not be performed before or during arthroplasty or arthrodesis, because a correction of this magnitude can easily be obtained as a result of these procedures themselves. One may choose either a femoral or a high tibial osteotomy, although the rapid union and low morbidity with the latter make it the preferred method currently. Minor degrees of varus and valgus may be corrected simultaneously with the flexion deformity. The procedure relies for its success on the presence of adequate amounts of articular cartilage and should not be done in the presence of advanced disease or severe joint destruction. Age is not a contraindication to osteotomy, although deformities of the child and adolescent may often be correctable by more conservative means.

Capsulectomy and Tenotomy

This operation may be indicated for correction of flexion contractures of greater than 30°. It may also be used for lesser contractures which are not associated with various angular deformities necessitating osteotomy. The operation is frequently combined with lengthening of the hamstring tendon, and postoperatively multidirectional skeletal traction may be employed in an effort to lift the tibia forward and prevent hyperextension and subluxation. This can best be accomplished by a modified Russell type skeletal traction applied through the tibial tubercle and the os calcis, simultaneously. The correction of contractures of greater than 30° may be a hazard to neurovascular structures and should, possibly, be carried out in stages. A capsulectomy should not be carried out in the presence of severe joint destruction. Like the osteotomy, once the deformity is corrected the capsulectomy relies for its success on a relatively normal joint. In advanced stages of the disease, the obstruction to extension may be a mechanical block in the knee rather than a tight posterior capsule. The operation may be indicated as an adjunct to arthroplasty when flexion deformity is so severe that it cannot be corrected by the removal of bone during the arthroplasty procedure itself.

Arthroplasty

Current techniques of arthroplasty all involve the interposition of a foreign material, either plastic or metallic, between the femoral and tibial articular surfaces. In the last decade, most implants have been made of Vitallium, although recently there has been considerable interest in the use of plastics, either to cement a metal implant in place or to form half of a prosthesis articulating with a metallic member.

Tibial Replacement Arthroplasty. Indicated in the treatment of moderately advanced tibial disease, it may be used in cases where the destruction of articular cartilage is too advanced for synovectomy alone. Mild angular deformities may be corrected during the procedure, but severe deformities must be treated by other surgical procedures as noted above. Both medial and lateral plateaus should be replaced, and a synovectomy is usually considered a part of the operation. The contraindications to this procedure are severe deformity, extreme ligamentous instability, and advanced femoral articular disease with structural collapse. A general reluctance to perform the operation in younger patients prevails.

Femoral Mold Arthroplasty. As the tibial replacement arthroplasty is indicated for advanced disease affecting primarily the tibia, so the femoral mold arthroplasty should be used for advanced disease localized in the femur with collapse of the bony architecture. A synovectomy should also be carried out in conjunction with this operation, and a patellectomy may be performed, although it is not a prerequisite for a good result. Femoral mold arthroplasty should not be done in the presence of severe angular deformity or in the presence of marked tibial plateau destruction. This procedure is avoided in younger patients and those with monarticular disease.

Total Knee Joint Replacement Arthroplasty. Total knee joint replacement is reserved for the extremes of articular joint destruction. It has been used primarily in patients severely crippled by disease who, in many instances, were unable to walk at all. Angular deformities of up to 30° may be corrected at the time of surgery, but greater deformities should be dealt with by other means. Synovectomy is usually considered part of the operation and, if possible, the patella should be retained to give optimum extensor function. It may be used as a salvage procedure for a failed femoral or tibial arthroplasty. Mild or monarticular disease and youth are the main contraindications.

Arthrodesis

It has been axiomatic that arthrodesis should not be carried out in a progressive, unpredictable, multi-articular, and symmetrical disease such as rheumatoid arthritis. There are probably two main indications, however, for arthrodesis. The first is in a patient who has had a total joint arthroplasty which has failed. Secondly, it may have a place in a young vigorous patient in whom the arthritis has been limited to one joint for a sufficiently long period of time to suggest that the disease will remain monarticular.

CHAPTER 9

Synovectomy of the Hip in Rheumatoid Arthritis

RICHARD L. CRUESS, M.D.

Although there are references in the literature to synovectomy of the hip in conditions other than rheumatoid arthritis, only one report refers to this procedure in the rheumatoid hip.[2] This is noteworthy because it is now generally accepted that synovectomy arrests the local progress of the disease, at least temporarily, and in many instances may prevent further disintegration of the involved joint. This paradox may be explained by the fact that the hip is a deep ball and socket joint, and surgeons have been reluctant to carry out procedures early in the course of rheumatoid disease because of a fear of worsening the patient's condition. They have, therefore, waited until the indications for synovectomy are no longer present and a reconstructive procedure is necessary to give the patient the best possible functioning joint. Our experience, while not extensive, does suggest that synovectomy of the hip should be considered early in the course of the disease, as it is in other joints.

Indications for Synovectomy

The indications for synovectomy of the hip in rheumatoid arthritis are, theoretically, fairly straightforward. The procedure should be considered in the presence of known rheumatoid disease when there is persistent pain in the hip associated with evidence of failure to respond to an adequate medical regimen. This failure to respond should be manifested by either early destructive changes in the cartilage or the development of fixed deformities about the hip (usually a flexion deformity). The operative procedure can also be carried out in hips that are being biopsied and in which a tentative diagnosis of rheumatoid arthritis can be made at the time of surgery. Not infrequently, such biopsies reveal a proliferative synovitis with evidence of pannus growing across the cartilage. Usually the pathological diagnosis is "chronic synovitis compatible with rheumatoid arthritis." In our experience these patients benefit from an early synovectomy, and many will later be shown to have generalized rheumatoid disease.

The contraindications include excessive narrowing of the joint line, excessive erosion of the bone on either side of the joint, or joints in which there is very little motion remaining.

Technique

It is possible to do an adequate synovectomy through a single excision. It has been our practice to do this through a classical anterolateral Watson-Jones incision (Fig. 9-1). The standard skin incision is made beginning at the antero-superior spine, curving posteriorly to the greater trochanter and continuing distally for 2 to 3 inches. The interval between the tensor fascia lata and the gluteus medius is developed, and the neck is approached from its anterior aspect. The capsule and synovium are opened with a single H-shaped incision and are opened outwards like the pages of a

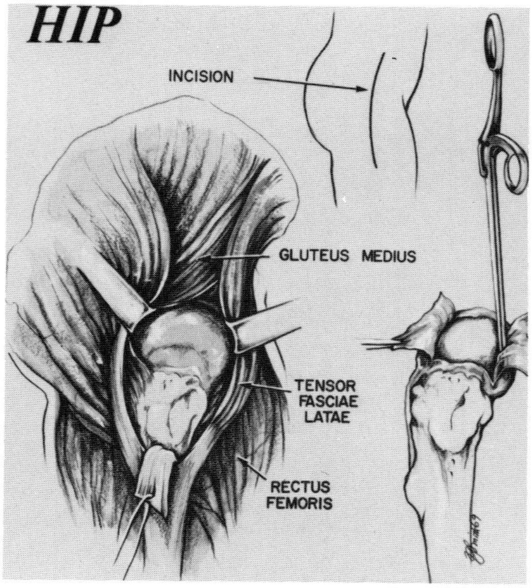

FIG. 9-1. Drawing illustrating the anterolateral Watson-Jones approach recommended for synovectomy of the hip.

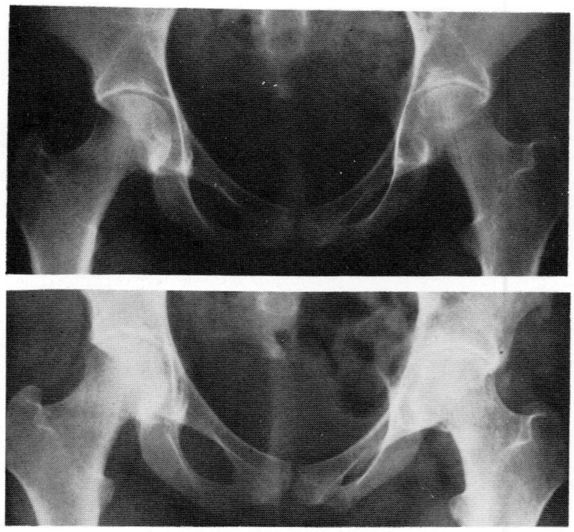

FIG. 9-2. (*Top*) Preoperative view of the hip in a 19-year-old woman subsequently shown to have rheumatoid arthritis involving multiple joints. There is narrowing of the joint space with regional demineralization prior to synovectomy. (*Bottom*) X-rays taken 2½ years after synovectomy. There has been no further loss of joint space or remineralization of the bones around the hip. The patient has no pain with a flexion contracture of 20°.

book. It is essential that the parallel arms of the H be carried as far superiorly and posteriorly as is possible on both the acetabulum and at the base of the neck, in order that access to the joint be adequate. A synovectomy and capsulectomy is next carried out, removing the tissue as far medially as can be done under direct vision. This is facilitated by first flexing and externally rotating the hip while working on the inferior and medial aspects of the neck and then internally rotating the hip while working on the superior and posterior neck. When all visible synovium has been removed, that portion of the posterior synovium which cannot be visualized directly is removed by means of straight and curved pituitary rongeurs. Over 90 per cent of the synovium can be removed through this single incision. No attempt is made to close the remaining capsule. The tight structures restricting motion are sectioned. Suction drainage is used only if hemostasis is difficult, and standard wound closure is utilized. The patient starts active exercises immediately, and partial weight bearing is commenced at 4 weeks. A manipulation under anesthesia at 10 days is carried out if there is excessive stiffness.

The Watson-Jones incision is preferred, because it does not detach muscles and rehabilitation is rapid. If, however, the surgeons feel that it is essential to reach both the anterior and posterior aspects of the joint, the lateral approach described by Harris[1] would be preferable, because both anterior and posterior portions of the joint could be reached after removing the greater trochanter. We do not believe that the hip should be dislocated because of the danger —in theory at least—of avascular necrosis.

Results

Four synovectomies of adult hips have been followed for between 1 and 3 years. One was for Marie-Strümpell arthritis, and three were for rheumatoid arthritis. In all, pain relief has been complete during the period of follow-up. One patient with rheumatoid arthritis now has complete range of motion (Fig. 9-2). The other two have flexion contractures of 15° and 20°, respectively. Both have approximately 20 per cent limitation of rotation, but flexion is full and abduction is normal. The patient with Marie-Strümpell arthritis has essentially fibrous ankylosis of the joint. While he is satisfied with the pain relief, we feel that the operative procedure has not been successful.

No complications have followed this operation, and, it should be noted, no avascular changes have been noted in the hips. The results of synovectomy in children's hips are also satisfactory (see Chap. 10).

Conclusions

Theoretically, synovectomy for rheumatoid arthritis should work as well in the hip as it does in other joints if it can be carried out before extensive destructive changes affect the hip joint. In extremely ill patients with multiple joint involvement it offers the advantage of being a much simpler procedure than reconstructive procedures in this region. In addition, synovectomy does not introduce foreign materials into the body, and if these hips remain satisfactory over many years, the end results should make it preferable to other operative procedures. However, it is apparently difficult to obtain suitable patients. We recognize that the sample reported here is not large enough to form the basis for strong recommendations. In theory, the operation should arrest the progress of the disease with very little risk to the patient. It is to be hoped that more information will be available soon in order that the true value of synovectomy in the surgery of the rheumatoid hip can be more accurately assessed.

REFERENCES

1. Harris, W. H.: A new lateral approach to the hip joint. J. Bone Joint Surg., *49*:891-898, 1967.
2. Law, W. A.: Reconstruction of the hip joint in rheumatoid arthritis. International Society of Orthopaedic Surgery and Traumatologies. International Congress of Orthopaedic Surgery, 9th. Symposium and Special Communications, p. 158. Brussels, A. Bailleux, 1964.

CHAPTER 10

Results of Surgical Management of the Hip in Patients with Rheumatoid Arthritis or Rheumatoid Spondylitis

RICHARD S. BRYAN, M.D., WYLIE T. SCOTT, JR., M.D., AND WILLIAM H. BICKEL, M.D.

Arthroplasty of the hip, as a treatment for the painful hip or the stiff hip, has interested surgeons since the beginning of the 19th century. Early in the development of arthroplasty, the concept of an interposition membrane was common. Almost every known substance was tried, but the vast majority proved unsatisfactory. To Dr. M. N. Smith-Petersen belongs the credit for the interposition of materials that would allow the reformation of a smooth articular surface suitable for weight bearing. He first used glass in 1923, and in 1925 he tried viscaloid. In 1933, he returned to Pyrex glass, and in 1937 he used a Bakelite interposition mold.[10] In 1938, after the work of Venable,[12] Vitallium was utilized for the first time as interposition material. This solved the problem of breakage, which had occurred with the other materials, and changed the original two-stage operation to a one-stage operation with revision only in those cases in which it was necessary.

Smith-Petersen used an anterior iliofemoral approach on 26 patients with rheumatoid arthritis. The cases of these patients were reported by Law in 1948.[7] Twenty-two of the 26 patients were satisfied with the result obtained, although the duration of follow-up was short. Moreover, 13 of the 22 patients required further surgical attention.

In 1950, Gibson described posterolateral exposure of the hip joint, with removal of the gluteus medius and minimus from their insertion on the trochanter.[5] This procedure was so widely accepted that Denham and Law, in 1957, although they still preferred the anterior approach, were ready to accept the Gibson approach as almost equally beneficial.[3] They condemned the lateral trochanteric displacement, which has since been widely accepted because of Harris's common use of it in his lateral approach to the hip joint.[6]

At first, orthopaedic surgeons were enthusiastic about the use of the Vitallium mold arthroplasty in patients with rheumatoid arthritis (Fig. 10-1), but according to Friberg, by 1948 or 1949 most surgeons had abandoned the method.[4] He stated that orthopaedic surgeons at that time generally

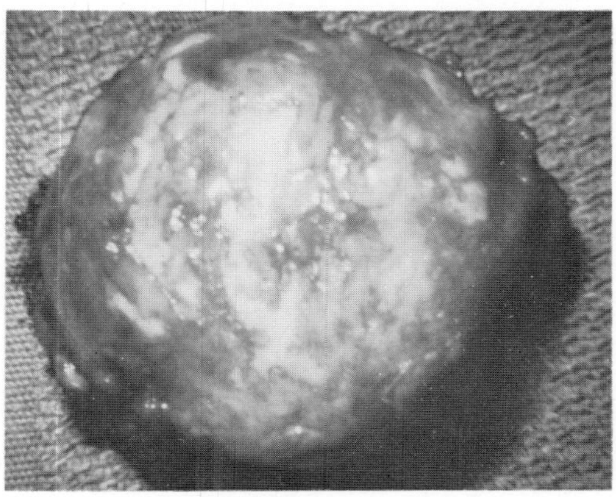

FIG. 10-1. Appearance of femoral head in active rheumatoid arthritis.

preferred arthrodesis, although the patients preferred arthroplasty, because they imagined their joints would regain almost normal mobility and good muscular strength. This, of course, was not always the result. In 1957, Aufranc stated that not infrequently a result rated unsatisfactory by the surgeon was good or excellent in the patient's evaluation. In particular, bedridden patients with bilateral bony ankylosis who had been mobilized to a sitting position by one or more procedures tended to give high evaluations.[1] Schwartzmann, in 1959, reported the cases of 48 patients with rheumatoid arthritis in whom 53 hips had been treated by Vitallium mold arthroplasty and 15 by prostheses.[8] Satisfactory results were obtained in 73 per cent of the selected cases.

In 1962, Solomon and Aufranc were able to obtain follow-up data on 90 of 297 patients with rheumatoid disease. Of the 90 patients, 54 had rheumatoid spondylitis and 36 had rheumatoid arthritis.[11] In 57 of the 90, both hips were involved. Fifty-one per cent of these patients had periarticular ossification after operation. The 18 patients who were on steroids responded much better than expected. Supplementary surgical procedures were needed by 51 patients. Thirty-five of them required further operations because of stiffness; only eight underwent re-operation because of pain. Of the 51 patients, 15 had rheumatoid arthritis and 36 had rheumatoid spondylitis. In 87 per cent relief of pain was achieved and maintained. The range of motion was satisfactory in 56 per cent, but the functional result was good in 73 per cent of the entire operated group. Although 67 per cent of the entire group continued to use crutches, 67 per cent of all patients were satisfied with their result. The final overall rating of Solomon and Aufranc was as follows: excellent, 8 per cent; good, 47 per cent; unsatisfactory, 12 per cent; and failed, primarily because of poor mobility, 33 per cent. They concluded that better results were obtained with Vitallium mold arthroplasty in older patients than in younger patients and in rheumatoid arthritic patients than in those with rheumatoid spondylitis.

In 1967 Schwartzmann wrote that reconstructive operations, especially the mobilizing surgical reconstructions, of the hip in a patient with rheumatoid arthritis are, for the most part, palliative rather than permanently definitive.[9] He defined the objectives of such surgical procedures as: (1) relief of pain, (2) correction or prevention of deformity, (3) maintenance or restoration of mobility, (4) maintenance of ability to walk, (5) improvement of status of related joints, (6) facilitation of self-care, and (7) occupational rehabilitation. His preoperative requirements were: (1) failure of conservative treatment, (2) control of the patient's physiologic status, (3) voluntary control by the patient of his musculature, and (4) life expectancy and mental attitude justifying the operative procedure.

We have reported the results of Vitallium mold arthroplasty in rheumatoid spondylitis and rheumatoid arthritis at the Mayo Clinic over the period 1939 to 1954.[2] Forty-five patients with rheumatoid spondylitis, 43 with rheumatoid arthritis, one with psoriatic arthritis, and one with scleroderma and rheumatoid arthritis underwent one or more hip operations at the Mayo Clinic. Every patient had involvement of at least one hip joint. Sixty-two were men and 28 were women. Final follow-up information was obtained by examination in 31 cases and by correspondence in 59. The 59 patients had been examined on several occasions subsequent to operation, but the final decision was based partially on correspondence.

Our criteria for evaluating results were as follows: very good, 90° or more of flexion and extension with little or no pain after the first operation; good, flexion and extension of 30° to 90° with little or no pain; fair, flexion and extension of 10° to 30° with little or no pain; poor, motion of less than 10° to 15° or pain that was more than slight. For 71 patients whose condition was followed for 2 or more years our results were very good in nine cases, good in 22, fair in nine, and poor in 31.

We have now reevaluated all hip operations performed on rheumatoid arthritics and rheumatoid spondylitics at the Mayo Clinic from 1939 through 1968 except total hip arthroplasties. The number is now 150 rheumatoid arthritics, 11 of whom have been under follow-up for less than 1 year, and 60 rheumatoid spondylitics, five of whom have been under follow-up for less than 1 year. Of the 139 rheumatoid arthritics whose condition has been followed for a year or longer, 103 have undergone 143 Vitallium mold and eight Lucite arthroplasties. Rheumatoid arthritics have received 26 Austin Moore, ten Matchett-Brown, and two Vitallium Judet prostheses. Two patients had a cup in one hip and a prosthesis in the other. Five hips in three patients were treated by Girdlestone's method. One patient underwent osteotomy on both hips, and one patient had a Voss procedure. In the rheumatoid spondylitics who have been followed for more than a year 69 mold arthroplasties were performed on 50 patients, and 11 prostheses were placed in seven patients. Two patients underwent osteotomy and one, Jones' pseudarthrosis.

RESULTS

The results of Vitallium mold arthroplasty in rheumatoid arthritic patients with follow-up of more than 1 year are presented in Table 10-1 and are compared with results of follow-up for 5 years or longer and for 10 years or longer. It is apparent from the figures that the joints slowly deteriorated; this was manifest primarily as reduced motion rather than as recurrence of pain. Long-term results of Vitallium mold arthroplasties performed since 1950, when the technique had been standardized, are considerably better (see Table 10-2). The initial result was good or very good in 73 per cent of the patients, and even after 10 years, 50 per cent continued to have a good or very good result. Table 10-3 shows that age was a significant factor. Sixty-two per cent of patients under 50 years of age experienced a good or very good initial result; of patients 50 years and older, 83 per cent had a good or very good initial result. Table 10-3 also shows that little difference was noted between patients with bilateral hip involvement and those with unilateral

Table 10-1. Results of Vitallium Mold Arthroplasties in Rheumatoid Arthritis

Duration, years	*Number of Hips* *Total*	*Very good*	*Good*	*Fair*	*Poor*	*Percentage of good and very good hips*
1 to 5	143	23	58	21	41	57
5 to 10	78	12	33	14	19	58
10 or longer (average 16)	43	1	16	11	15	40

Table 10-2. Results of Vitallium Mold Arthroplasties Performed Since 1950

Duration, years	*Number of Hips* *Total*	*Very good*	*Good*	*Fair*	*Poor*	*Percentage of good and very good hips*
1 to 5	100	22	51	15	12	73
5 to 10	52	12	28	10	2	77
10 or longer	16	1	7	7	1	50

Table 10-3. Results of Vitallium Mold Arthroplasties Performed Since 1950 and Followed for More than 1 Year

		Number of Hips				*Percentage of good and very good hips*
	Total	*Very good*	*Good*	*Fair*	*Poor*	
Age, years						
Less than 50	53	11	22	13	7	62
50 or more	47	10	29	3	5	83
Involvement						
Bilateral	64	10	35	14	5	70
Unilateral	36	11	17	2	6	78

Table 10-4. Results of Vitallium Mold Arthroplasties in Rheumatoid Spondylitis

		Number of Hips				*Percentage of good and very good hips*
Time of operation; years follow-up	*Total*	*Very good*	*Good*	*Fair*	*Poor*	
Performed before 1950						
1 to 5	59	3	16	7	33	32
5 or longer	39	2	10	4	23	31
Performed since 1950						
1 to 5	23	3	7	1	12	43
5 or longer	15	2	5	1	7	47

Table 10-5. Results with Austin Moore or Matchett-Brown Prostheses in Rheumatoid Arthritis

		Number of Hips				*Percentage of good and very good hips*
Years duration	*Total*	*Very good*	*Good*	*Fair*	*Poor*	
1 to 5	36	5	15	4	12	56
5 or longer	17	0	4	3	10	24

involvement. The results of Vitallium mold arthroplasty in patients with rheumatoid spondylitis were not as good as the results in the arthritics (see Table 10-4). Again, when the cases in which the surgical procedure was done before 1950 are excluded, the results are improved.

Table 10-5 shows the results with Austin Moore or Matchett-Brown prostheses, which are reasonably comparable; cases followed for 1 to 5 years are compared to those followed 5 years or longer. It is notable that 56 per cent initially achieved a good result, whereas after 5 years results in only 24 per cent remained good. We operated on only six hips in rheumatoid spondylitics; the Austin Moore prosthesis was used in every case. The condition of all patients was followed for 5 years or longer. One hip showed a fair result and two hips, a poor result. Surprisingly, a good result obtained in three of the six.

Our results demonstrate that any operation on the rheumatoid patient is a palliative procedure, but that more lasting satisfaction is achieved by mold arthroplasty

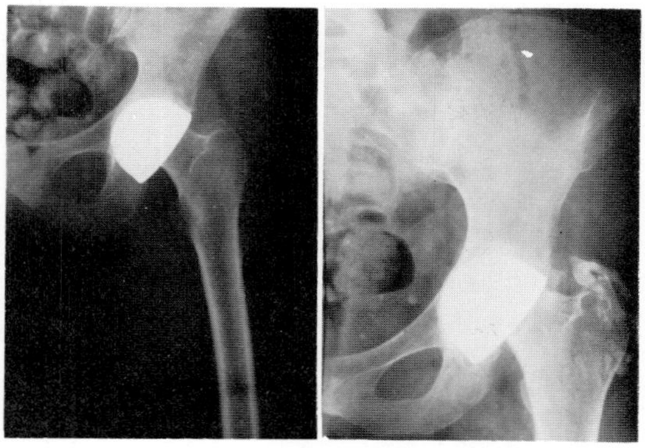

FIG. 10-2. (*Left*) Appearance of left hip of 49-year-old rheumatoid arthritic 2 weeks after operation. (*Right*) Appearance of same hip 1 year later. Note settling of cup and reaction around trochanter. At the time of this photograph, the patient was walking with a cane with a range of motion of 0° to 90° and little pain.

than by metal prostheses. We did not have enough patients undergoing the other procedures to permit comparison. There was no question that the rheumatoid arthritics did better than the rheumatoid spondylitics and that the older rheumatoid arthritics achieved better end results than the younger, possibly because of retarded progress of the disease.

Our technique varied somewhat. In most patients a Gibson posterolateral approach was used, but a lateral approach with transplantation of the trochanter was used in a number of instances. In a few cases the iliopsoas tendon was transplanted to the anterior capsule. In all cases total excision of the capsule and synovium (with reaming of the acetabulum and head to bleeding cancellous bone) was performed and reshaping of the acetabulum (doming it at least ¼ inch) was attempted. In recent years, a suction drain of one type or another has been used for 24 to 48 hours in most patients.

Postoperative treatment also has varied. When postoperative treatment of total hip arthroplasty does not include muscle-building exercises, one wonders to what extent postoperative care is based on factual knowledge. In general, we have preferred to use

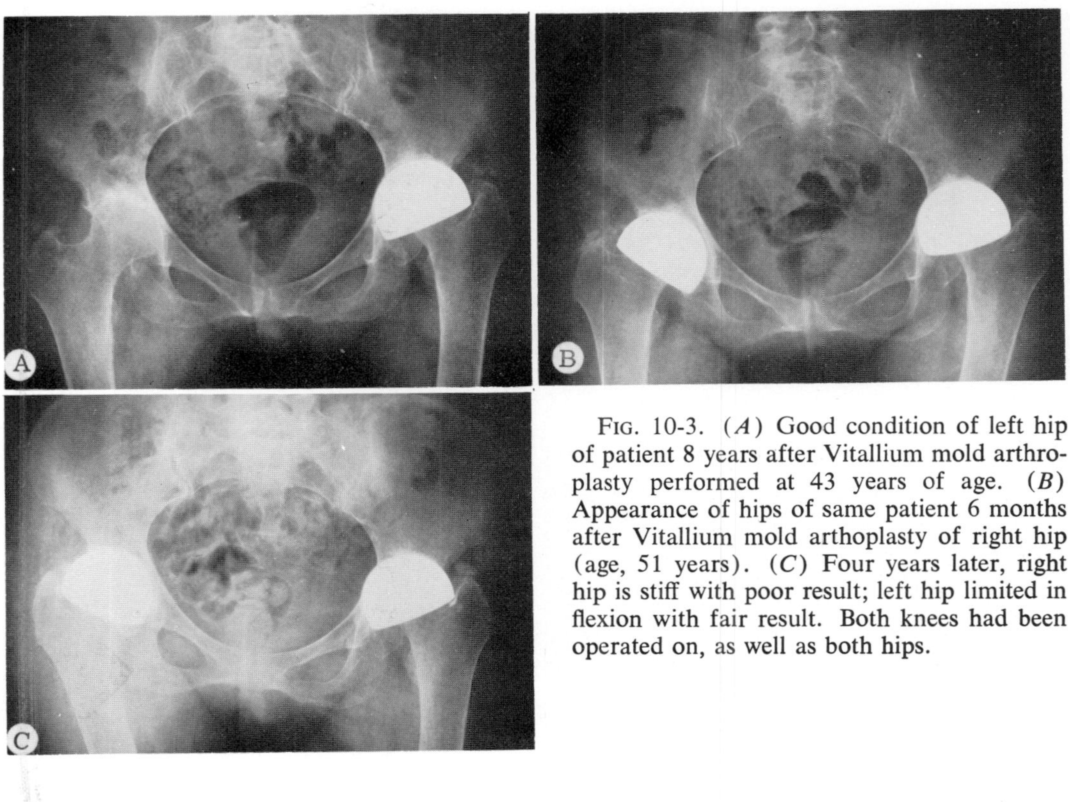

FIG. 10-3. (*A*) Good condition of left hip of patient 8 years after Vitallium mold arthroplasty performed at 43 years of age. (*B*) Appearance of hips of same patient 6 months after Vitallium mold arthoplasty of right hip (age, 51 years). (*C*) Four years later, right hip is stiff with poor result; left hip limited in flexion with fair result. Both knees had been operated on, as well as both hips.

the Hodgen splint for 8 to 10 days, followed with active motion and exercises on a skateboard. The use of the powderboard in exercising is begun at 2½ to 3 weeks, and the patient is usually hospitalized for 4 to 5 weeks. Crutches are used for at least 3 months, preferably for 6 months.

We have found that, in general, the condition of patients who have undergone mold arthroplasty tends to improve with time and exercise. (Improvement is greater in osteoarthritics than in rheumatoid arthritics.) In rheumatoid arthritics we have observed a tendency toward further erosion of bone both of the neck and of the acetabulum over time. This subsequently limits the motion of the hip joint (see Fig. 10-2). Recognizing as we do that the results will slowly deteriorate, it nevertheless remains our opinion that Vitallium mold arthroplasty is the treatment of choice in young rheumatoid arthritics (see Fig. 10-3). This procedure relieves pain, permits patients to live active lives for varying periods, and makes subsequent conversion to total hip arthroplasty easier, if and when this procedure becomes necessary.

REFERENCES

1. Aufranc, O. E.: Constructive hip surgery with the Vitallium mold: A report on 1,000 cases of arthroplasty of the hip over a fifteen-year period. J. Bone Joint Surg., *39*: 237-248, 1957.
2. Bickel, W. H., and Bryan, R. S.: Results of cup arthroplasty of the hip in patients with rheumatoid arthritis and rheumatoid spondylitis. Surg. Gynec. Obstet., *123*:243-250, 1966.
3. Denham, R. A., and Law, W. A.: Arthroplasty of the hip. J. Bone Joint Surg. [Brit.], *39*:614-622, 1957.
4. Friberg, S.: On arthrodesis and arthroplasty. Acta Med. Scand. Suppl., *341*:169-172, 1958.
5. Gibson, A.: Posterior exposure of the hip joint. J. Bone Joint Surg. [Brit.], *32*:183-186, 1950.
6. Harris, W. H.: A new lateral approach to the hip joint. J. Bone Joint Surg., *49*:891-898, 1967.
7. Law, W. A.: Post-operative study of Vitallium mould arthroplasty of the hip joint. J. Bone Joint Surg. [Brit.], *30*:76-83, 1948.
8. Schwartzmann, J. R.: Arthroplasty of the hip in rheumatoid arthritis: a follow-up study of sixty-eight hips. J. Bone Joint Surg., *41*:705-721, 1959.
9. ———: Reconstruction of the hip in rheumatoid arthritis. J. Bone Joint Surg., *49*: 398-410, 1967.
10. Smith-Petersen, M. N.: Arthroplasty of the hip: a new method. J. Bone Joint Surg., *21*:269-288, 1939.
11. Solomon, L., and Aufranc, O. E.: Vitallium mold arthroplasty of the hip in rheumatoid arthritis. Arthritis Rheum., *5*:37-54, 1962.
12. Venable, C. S.: Osteosynthesis in the presence of metals: Studies on electrolysis. Southern Med. J., *31*:501-508, 1938.

CHAPTER 11

Total Hip Replacement in Rheumatoid Arthritis and Marie-Strümpell Arthritis of the Hip

J. WATSON-FARRAR, F.R.C.S. (ENG.)

In the past the results of the surgical treatment of rheumatoid arthritis have been more disappointing than those obtained in the treatment of osteoarthritis, and even in that condition there has been room for improvement. The same surgical procedures used in the treatment of osteoarthritis, namely osteotomy, arthrodesis, arthroplasty or Girdlestone pseudarthrosis, were performed on the rheumatoid hip. The underlying pathological changes in the two conditions are so different that perhaps it is not surprising that the results of surgery differed. Osteoarthritis is a progressive condition, involving the articular surfaces initially and, subsequently, the underlying bone. Soft tissue changes occur at a relatively late stage in the disease. In rheumatoid arthritis the initial changes develop in the soft tissues; only later do the articular surfaces become involved. The bone of a rheumatoid hip is softer than a normal bone, whereas the bone in an osteoarthritic hip is always appreciably harder than normal. Admittedly this is a rather simplified description of the basic differences.

Because the two conditions are so dissimilar, it seems unreasonable to suppose that an operation which works in one must of necessity give satisfaction in the other. To have this expectation of osteotomies and arthroplasties is especially unwarranted. The only procedure that could be expected to give similar results is an arthrodesis, which is not intended to preserve or restore function. The multiplicity of affected joints in a rheumatoid patient precludes the consideration of an arthrodesis, because the additional handicap this causes would lessen rather than increase the patient's mobility.

Ignoring for the moment any form of total joint replacement, all other forms of arthroplasty depend for their success upon the integrity of the patient's bones. For example, a femoral prosthesis relies upon the ability of the acetabulum to accept the stresses imposed upon it by an artificial femoral head. In the rheumatoid hip the prosthesis too often tends to migrate inwards and upwards. When this occurs the quality of the end result is usually reduced.

A cup arthroplasty presents the same risks. Not infrequently, absorption of bone, both of the femoral head and of the acetabulum, occurs with consequent deterioration in the quality of the result. In favor of an arthroplasty is the fact that a capsulectomy must be performed, since the joint is exposed. The capsulectomy can overcome some disabilities which result from soft tissue involvement. An osteotomy, being a totally extracapsular procedure, does nothing to overcome any soft tissue factors, and, like an arthroplasty, depends for its result upon the physical properties of the joint, both articular and bony. Often the state of the joint is such that little benefit results from this procedure.

The technique of total joint replacement demands an almost total capsulectomy. By virtue of the fact that the two components of the artificial joint are anchored to the recipient bones by means of an acrylic resin, the forces acting across the patient's acetabulum are spread over a wide area. Thus no single area of the acetabulum is exposed to a high load per unit area factor and bony absorption due to this high load factor is avoided. Furthermore, the bony pelvis is not exposed to any moving part, and therefore wear from friction and consequent absorption of bone should not occur. Despite the softness of the bones in a rheumatoid hip, we have never had a case where the cup and its surrounding plastic have migrated into the bony pelvis.

If the answer to the problem of the arthritic hip, irrespective of etiology, lies in the hands of the surgeon, then that answer must be some form of operation performed early in the course of the disease which will arrest the condition and, if possible, reverse the changes that have already occurred. It appears that synovectomy is beneficial (at least initially) in the more accessible joints, if performed early. Whether good results will be permanent remains to be seen. In the light of present surgical knowledge, therefore, it would seem logical to perform a synovectomy of this kind in the very early stages of the disease. Nevertheless, it takes a brave surgeon to embark upon a fairly major procedure when symptoms are minimal until such a procedure has proved its worth. Most surgery of the rheumatoid hip is undertaken when the symptoms have reached such proportions that something must be done to help the patient. By this time some form of arthroplasty is usually required.

Indications and Choice of Operative Procedure

Until recently a mold arthroplasty has been the operation of choice. It would appear, however, that a total hip replacement is now generally preferable once the stage has been reached where some form of arthroplasty is required. Finally, if all else fails, and this includes the insertion of a complete hip, the surgeon can resort to a Girdlestone pseudarthrosis by removing a failed total hip replacement. In fact, an excision arthroplasty probably gives better results if performed after previous surgery. This is because the scar tissue resulting from previous major hip surgery tends to give a more stable pseudarthrosis than is obtained when the operation is performed as a primary procedure.

By choosing total hip replacement one is, in effect, acknowledging that the joint is beyond redemption, just as when an excision arthroplasty is decided upon. However, having reached this conclusion, the surgeon takes positive steps to offer a satisfactory alternative in the form of a stable, mobile and painless artificial joint.

The advantages of artificial joints in the treatment of rheumatoid hips are several. First, the operative procedure removes most of the involved tissue around the joint. Secondly, the technique employed ensures that the subsequent load is spread across a wide area of the patient's osteoporotic bone, so that there is a relatively low load per unit area factor, which prevents bone absorption. Thirdly, the patient recovers from the operation rapidly and equally rapidly reaps the benefit of this procedure. Postoperatively there is no waiting for bone to unite as in an osteotomy, and no period of traction followed by weeks or months on crutches, as is often required after a mold arthroplasty. If the correct technique is used, one does not even have to wait for muscles to heal. Because of this, the patient can be allowed out of bed 4 days after the operation and can bear full weight on his hip using two canes. Total hip replacement can be used to stabilize an unsatisfactory pseudarthrosis or to salvage a failed mold arthroplasty, an arthrodesis, or a failed osteotomy.

Materials

The four essentials for a successful artificial joint are: (1) the use of inert materials, (2) a satisfactory design, (3) correct operative technique, and (4) secure and permanent fixation of the components to the bone. At present three basic types of total hip replacement are in common use. The McKee-Farrar utilizes metal upon metal and relies upon the acrylic resin, methylmethacrylate, as a fixing agent. Charnley's, which is metal upon plastic, also relies upon methylmethacrylate fixative. The joint devised by Ring relies on mechanical fixation.

Metal upon metal was chosen because plastics have an unhappy history as a bearing surface in orthopaedics. McKee, who started work in this field in 1951 when he inserted his first artificial joint, always used metal upon metal. Nothing has occurred to suggest that this was a mistake. Obviously it is vital that the metal used be inert, and chrome-cobalt alloy meets this condition. Previous models had failed because of one or the other component working loose. When Charnley published his paper in 1960 on the use of methylmethacrylate as a fixing agent[1] the present McKee-Farrar was designed. A prime requisite for successful joint replacement surgery is that the fixation of the component parts of the joint be secure and permanent. Methylmethacrylate seems to fulfill these requirements. After 10 years of use in our work and some 12 to 13 years in Charnley's, there is still no evidence of any adverse reaction in the body due to its presence.[2]

In Ring's joint everything depends upon a screw maintaining its anchorage in the pelvis. Because it is a technically difficult operation, the screw is not always inserted correctly. There is a danger that the screw will gradually work loose, especially in the relatively soft bone of a rheumatoid patient, and there is a possibility of fatigue fracture of the junction of the cup and the threaded stem. At the present time the Charnley and McKee-Farrar procedures appear to give equivalent results.

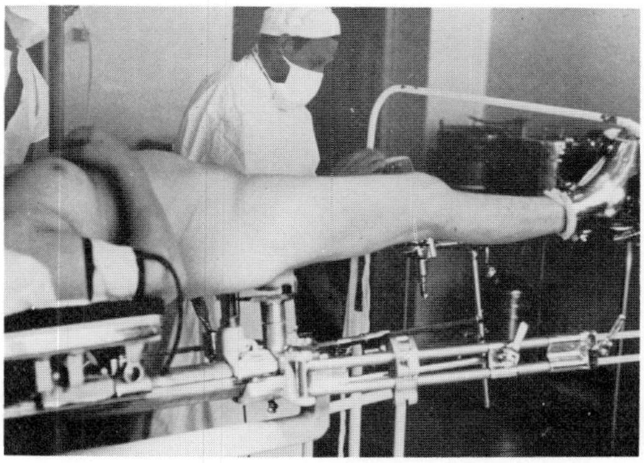

FIG. 11-1. Patient on the orthopaedic table prior to surgery.

Surgical Technique

The antero-lateral approach is used. This does not cause any muscle damage and gives the surgeon the best possible view of the acetabulum, the adequate preparation of which is the most vital step in the operation. Although the operation can be performed satisfactorily on an ordinary operating table, an orthopædic table allows freer manipulation of the leg (Fig. 11-1). The patient may be tilted towards the opposite side so that the hip being operated upon is inclined upwards towards the surgeon, thus improving his view of the acetabulum.

The incision commences one inch posterior to the anterior superior iliac spine, skirts in front of the greater trochanter and extends down the shaft of the femur for an inch or two (Fig. 11-2). The incision is deepened down to the deep fascia which is then incised opposite the interval between the tensor fascia lata, anteriorly, and the gluteii medius and minimus posteriorly. This interval is found most easily immediately proximal to the level of the greater trochanter. Very often it is marked by a change from muscle fibers of the tensor fascia lata to fascial fibers overlying the gluteii. If this sudden transition is present, it marks the line in which the incision is

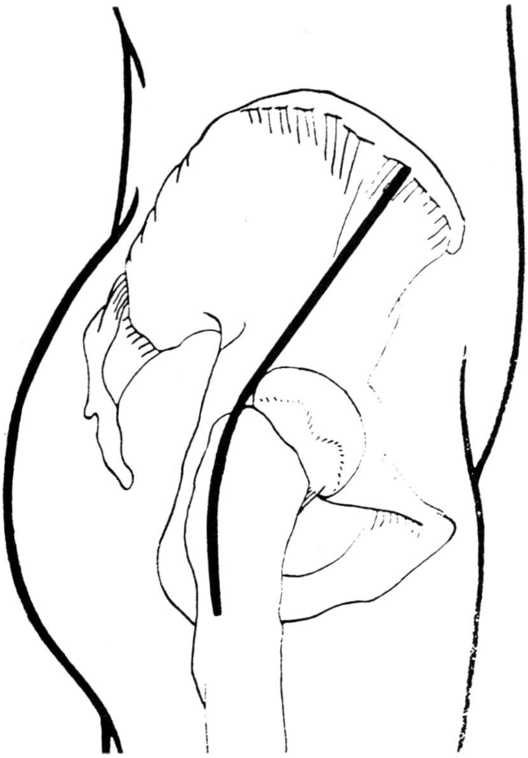

FIG. 11-2. Diagram of the skin incision for prosthetic replacement.

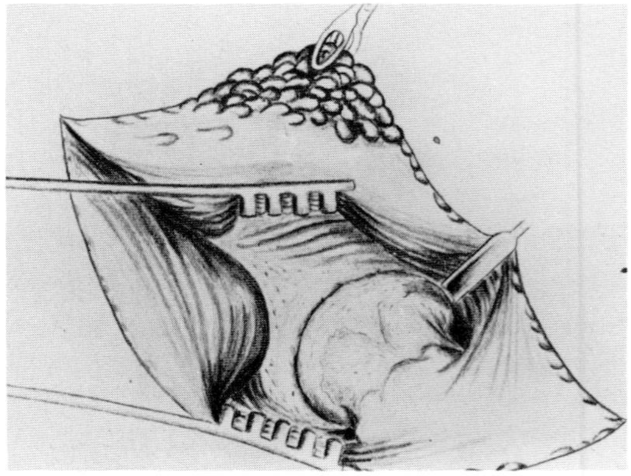

FIG. 11-3. Drawing of the exposed hip following capsulectomy.

made to develop the interval between these muscle groups. If not, the deep fascia immediately anterior to the greater trochanter is incised and a finger inserted through this incision to find the interval between the muscles. This is a vital step, for once this plane has been found the rest of the approach is extremely easy. The gap between these muscles is developed proximally, requiring sharp dissection, because the muscles become blended near the anterior superior spine.

Retractors are now inserted and the gap is opened. A leash of blood vessels is always found in this gap and will require controlling. When the gap is opened the nerve to the tensor fascia lata is invariably divided; this in no way affects the functional result. A finger in the gap will readily palpate the femoral neck. The anterior capsule is then excised distally to the level of the trochanteric line and superiorly to the mouth of the acetabulum. The hip joint is now clearly displayed (Fig. 11-3).

Next the femoral head is dislocated. Any osteophytes at the mouth of the acetabulum are removed to facilitate dislocation of the joint. In rheumatoid cases, care should be taken in this maneuver. Dislocation can be very difficult if the head is misshapen or if there is an element of protrusio acetabuli. Naturally an ankylosed hip cannot be dislocated. If the hip will not readily dislocate, a safer procedure is to divide the femoral neck high up using an osteotome; this avoids the risk of fracturing the femoral shaft if too much rotational force is applied in an effort to dislocate the hip. Obviously in a case of ankylosing spondylitis, dislocation is impossible, and it is essential to osteotomise the neck.

Once this is done it is often impossible to rotate the femoral shaft externally, and a further section of neck needs to be removed in order to gain access to the side wall of the pelvis so that the ankylosed femoral head can be removed piecemeal. The object is to recreate an acetabulum large enough to accommodate a cup. Frequently there is a plane of cleavage, between the head and acetabulum, which a curved gouge will find. If the head dislocates easily, it is removed with a Gigli saw, taking care that the line of section is just beneath the head. It is important not to remove too much neck, since this could result in a loose and consequently unstable reduction. It is always possible to remove more, if necessary.

Attention is now directed to the acetabulum (Fig. 11-4). If secure and permanent fixation is to be achieved, the preparation of the acetabulum is vital. All remnants of cartilage are removed. The fovea, which makes a very satisfactory keying point for the plastic, is cleaned of all soft tissue. A series of 1 cm. holes is drilled in the walls of the acetabulum; it is difficult to push the plastic into smaller ones. As many holes as possible are made, usually six. Finally, a large pit is gouged out towards the ischial spine to add yet another keying point (Fig. 11-5).

If the acetabulum loosens, it always does so at the junction between the plastic and the bone; the cup does not become loose in the plastic. The weakest point of fixation is between the bone and plastic, and it is for this reason that as many keying points as possible are made. Collapse from a weakened pelvis has not as yet occurred. Of the three cup sizes available the largest one that can be totally or almost totally contained within the acetabulum should be used (Fig. 11-6). If this dictum is followed, the cup is entirely supported within the acetabulum, so there is no need to insert screws above the acetabular mouth and build up plastic around them.

With the acetabulum prepared, the femoral shaft is cleared. The track down the neck, around the calcar and into the medullary canal is found with a template. It is at this point that the one drawback of the anterolateral approach is met. In a fat or muscular patient the bulk of soft tissue tends to throw the head of the template forwards so that the tip of the stem pierces the posterolateral aspect of the shaft. It is in such cases that the use of the orthopaedic table is advantageous. If the leg is dropped in full external rotation, the stump of the neck presents better in the wound and allows the

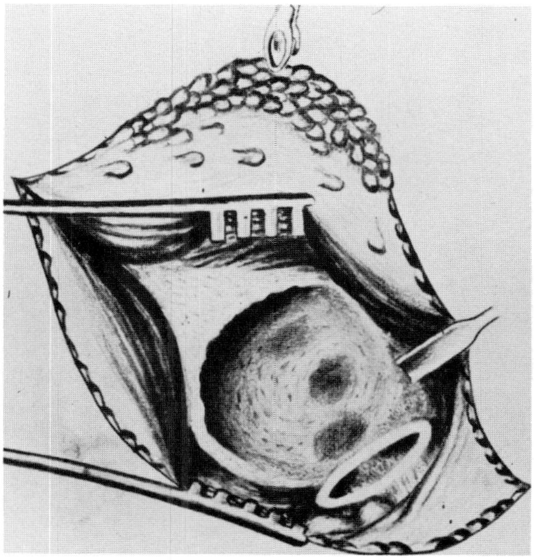

FIG. 11-4. The acetabulum prior to final preparation.

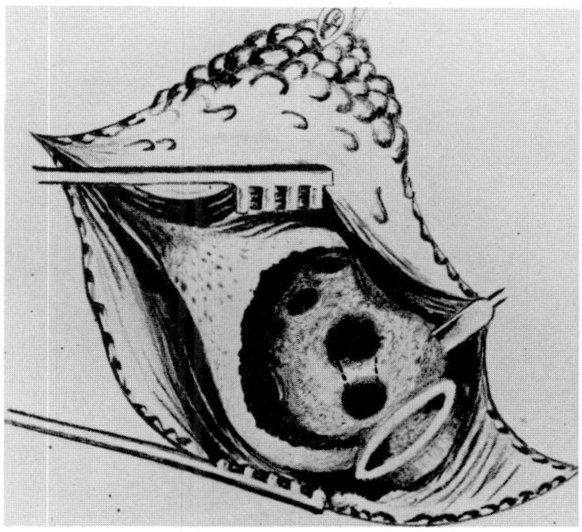

FIG. 11-5. The acetabulum after drill holes have been inserted.

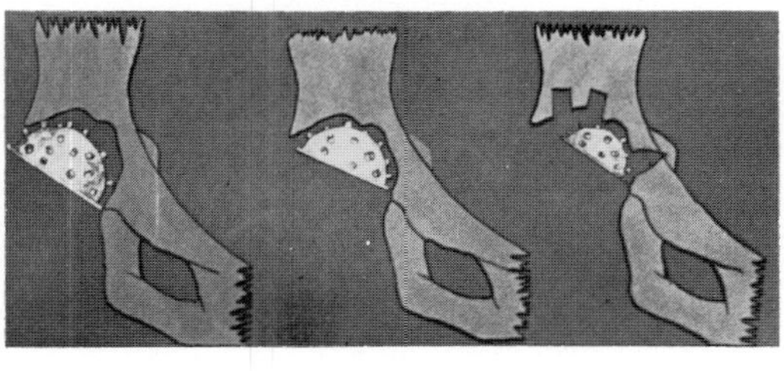

FIG. 11-6. The selection of the proper cup size for insertion into the hip is most important. (*Left*) Cup too large, (*Center*) correct size cup, (*Right*) cup too small.

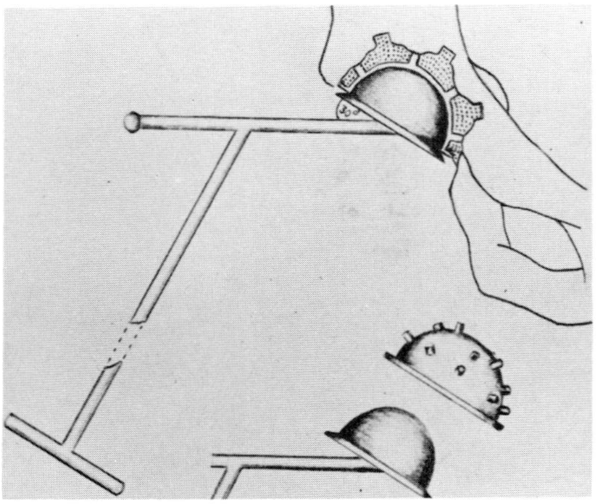

FIG. 11-7. Insertion of the acetabulum using the cup holder.

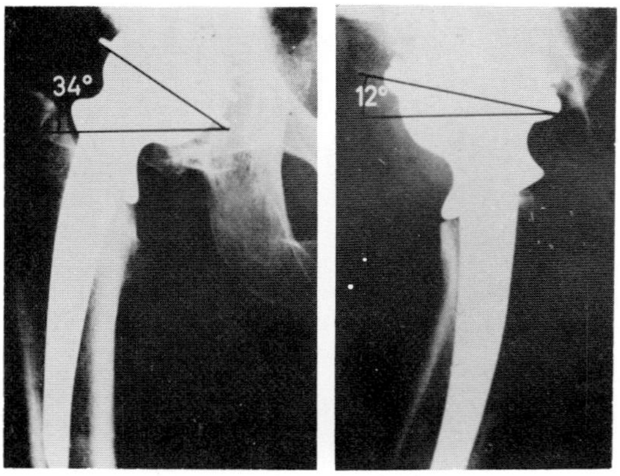

FIG. 11-8. Demonstration of the proper angle of the cup in the anteroposterior and lateral projections.

head of the template to be laid back. The risk of "coming out of the back" is avoided. Once the correct path is found, the track is widened with a rasp until the stem of the femoral component fits snugly in the femur. All cancellous bone is not removed, because it provides a firmer bond.

The cup is inserted next. The methylmethacrylate is mixed and when ready for use (when the plastic no longer sticks to the surgeon's gloves) it is inserted into the acetabulum. An effort must be exerted to push the plastic into the various holes that

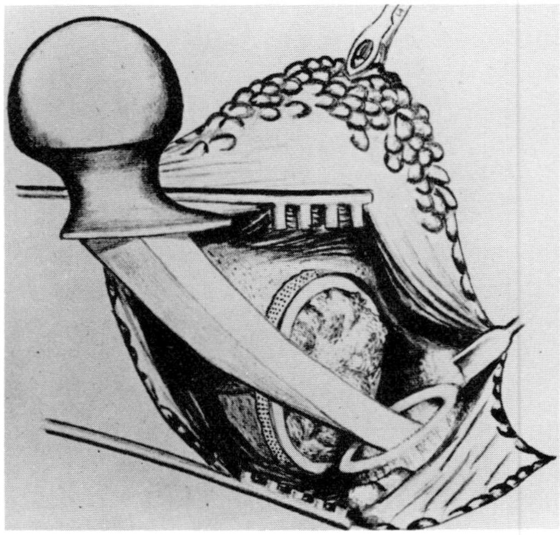

FIG. 11-9. The femoral head component is inserted into the shaft and a tibial reduction is carried out.

have been made in the acetabular walls; the plastic is not sufficiently fluid to find its own way into these keying points. The cup is then inserted into the plastic with the special introducer in order to achieve the correct position (Fig. 11-7).

The position of the cup is not as critical as was initially suggested. It was originally thought that it should lie at an angle of 30° to the horizontal and be anteverted by about 5° to 10° (Fig. 11-8). There is, however, an appreciable amount of latitude before stability is impaired. Just how much, can only be ascertained from experience and initially, at least, an effort should be made to insert the cup according to the figures given.

Once the plastic has set, the cup is securely anchored to the acetabulum. At this stage the cup should be examined and any plastic removed that may have been pushed into it with the introducer. It is also wise to run a finger round the edge of the cup to ensure that no plastic is protruding which might prevent the reduction of the femoral head. If any plastic is found, it is easily removed with a chisel or gouge.

The cup is then filled with swabs to prevent the actual reduction of the femoral head in the "trial reduction procedure" (Fig. 11-9). The femoral component is inserted into the femoral shaft. An effort is made to reduce the cup, but this effort stops short of actual reduction. The surgeon is simply making sure that reduction will be possible once the femoral portion has been cemented in. If it is apparent that reduction is *not* possible, more femoral neck is removed. Once it is evident that a reduction *is* possible, the plastic is mixed and forcefully rammed down the femoral shaft, and the femoral component is then inserted. When the plastic has set, but not before, the joint is reduced (Fig. 11-10).

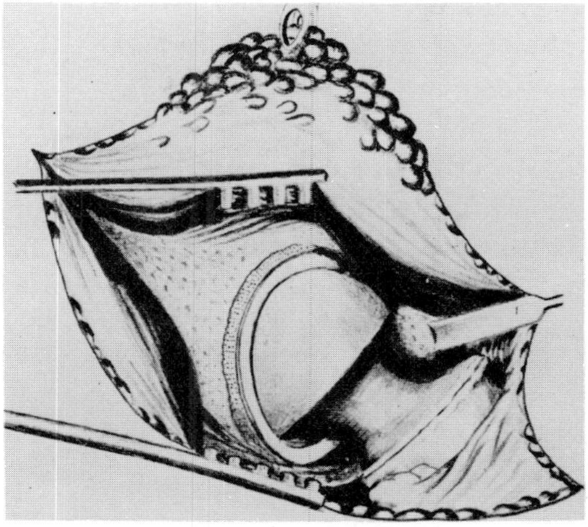

FIG. 11-10. The head has been reduced into the cup prior to closure.

Wound closure is simple, because once the retractors are removed the muscles fall together. Suction drainage is used to lessen the chances of hematoma formation and its accompanying risk of sepsis. Antibiotics in the preoperative and postoperative periods are also recommended.

Physiotherapy commences on the first postoperative day. If the physiotherapist has demonstrated the exercises to the patient before surgery, the patient will find them easier to do. Four or 5 days after the operation, the patient is allowed out of bed, and immediate weight-bearing is permitted with the aid of two canes. Thereafter, the rate of progress depends largely upon the determination of the patient and the degree of preoperative stiffness. Undoubtedly, the quality of the result is related to the preoperative condition. The range of movements present in the hip preoperatively is the starting point for the recovery of function. Obviously, recovery is quicker and more complete in a relatively mobile hip than in an ankylosed hip.

Results

In Norfolk and Norwich Hospital, a personal series of 50 rheumatoid hips on which this procedure was carried out had a success rate of 85 per cent. The follow-up period was 3 to 7 years. Osteoarthritic hips so treated had a 92 per cent success rate. These figures refer to the percentage of cases that fall into the good or excellent categories as described in the original report of this operation.[3] The complication rate has been low. The mortality rate is less than 1 per cent, with one death from cerebral hemorrhage and a second from peritonitis. The rapidity of postoperative mobilization has given a rate of pulmonary embolus of only 2 per cent, and no deaths have resulted from thromboembolic disease. The infection rate is 5 per cent, but only .5 per cent required removal of the prosthesis. (The criterion for infection is a discharge, other than blood, from the wound.) No late infections have developed. The rate of loosening is 3 per cent. Loosening is treated by reinserting whichever component is loose.

In ankylosing spondylitis the results are not as good as in other conditions for which this operation can be used. Nevertheless, it can increase the patient's mobility by restoring a useful range of movements. One patient who was unemployed before the operation obtained a job as a parking lot attendant after a total hip was inserted into his fused right hip. Only four such operations have been done, and they have not achieved more than 60° of flexion. Nevertheless this is a considerable improvement over the preoperative condition and makes the procedure worthwhile. So far, new bone formation has not developed, possibly because the procedures were done when the disease was burnt out.

REFERENCES

1. Charnley, J.: Anchorage of the femoral head prosthesis to the shaft of the femur. J. Bone Joint Surg. [Brit.], *42*:28-30, 1960.
2. ———: Acrylic cement in orthopaedic surgery. Edinburgh, E. and S. Livingston, 1970.
3. McKee, G. K., and Watson-Farrar, J.: Replacement of arthritic hips by the McKee-Farrar prosthesis. J. Bone Joint Surg. [Brit.], *48*:245-259, 1966.

CHAPTER 12

Excision Arthroplasty of the Hip (Girdlestone Pseudarthrosis) in Rheumatoid Arthritis and Ankylosing Spondylitis

T. K. F. TAYLOR, F.R.C.S., SIG T. HANSEN, JR., M.D., AND D. KAY CLAWSON, M.D.

The surgical treatment of the hip joint is still highly controversial, and the diversity of operations used in its management is evidence of the lack of a simple generally successful procedure. Only too frequently in the past have attempts been made to tailor the patient to fit the procedure rather than the more desirable reverse. Total hip replacement is gaining widespread popularity for a variety of hip disorders. We feel it is currently the procedure of choice for most patients with rheumatoid arthritis and ankylosing spondylitis who need reconstructive hip surgery. The permanence of the early excellent results is yet to be established.

Excision arthroplasty of the hip has never gained acceptance in the United States as a primary procedure for hip disease. It has, however, been employed in a number of centers in Great Britain, notably the Oxford School.[3,6,7,8,9] There the procedure is correctly regarded as an arthroplasty requiring the same meticulous attention to detail and operative techniques and postoperative care as any arthroplasty. In the United States the operation is considered a salvage procedure employed after all else has failed.[5] Although the role of the operation in hip surgery has changed because of the development of the total hip replacement, it remains the procedure of choice when the joint has been destroyed by infection. Because infections appear to be with us for the forseeable future, this procedure should be in the armamentarium of all surgeons who treat disorders of the hip. Between the years 1960 and 1969, excision arthroplasty was performed for a wide variety of conditions on 66 patients at the University of Washington hospitals. Six operations were carried out on patients with rheumatoid arthritis or ankylosing spondylitis.

Advantages and Disadvantages of Excision Arthroplasty

The principal advantage of the operation is that 90 per cent of the patients obtain complete and permanent relief of pain. This attribute is sadly lacking in most operations designed for reconstruction of the hip joint, except arthrodesis. The deformity is corrected, and a mobile hip allows the patient to sit in comfort. In ankylosing spondylitis a range of 60° to 70° of flexion can be obtained.

Stamina is reduced, since increased effort is involved in walking, and prolonged exercise may result in diffuse aching of the hip. The necessary shoe raise and the awkward gait are drawbacks, but when a cane is used, the patient with unilateral pseudarthrosis walks surprisingly well. Instability is produced but the joint is certainly not flail

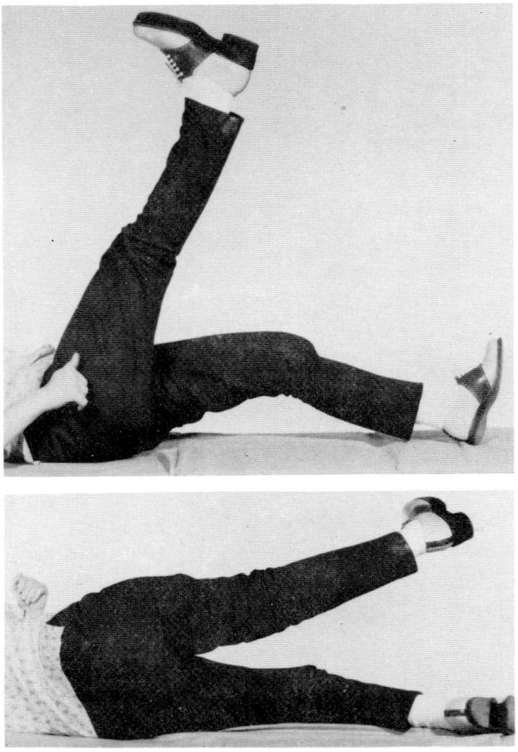

FIG. 12-1. Demonstration of the range of active flexion and abduction in the right hip of a 25-year-old female patient with severe rheumatoid arthritis on whom excision arthroplasty had been carried out previously.

(Fig. 12-1), and a remarkable degree of control can be obtained when the patient develops good strength in the hip musculature. This is directly dependent upon the enthusiasm of the patient for the postoperative exercise program, upon which the final result will depend. An obese or debilitated patient is at an obvious disadvantage.

Role of Excision Arthroplasty in Rheumatoid Arthritis and Ankylosing Spondylitis

In general terms it can be stated that excision arthroplasty should always be considered in patients for whom pain relief is absolutely necessary and when, for one reason or another, one operation only can be performed. The procedure has limited use in rheumatoid arthritis, primarily because of the need for external support, for which moderate strength in the upper limbs is required. The dipping of the pelvis on the operated side puts considerable strain on an arthritic valgus knee and may aggravate the knee symptoms. Similarly the telescoping of the pseudarthrosis forces the contralateral hip into adduction. This may increase symptoms from that joint.

Hip Joint Infection Complicating Previous Surgical Treatment. Here, excision arthroplasty is the procedure of choice. It is preferred to an approach of first attempting to eradicate the infection and later attempting reconstructive surgery. The functional result after sepsis is improved by scar tissue, which increases stability. Septic arthritis in the aged or debilitated patient carries a high mortality. When the wound is packed open, the mortality rate is over 25 per cent. With wound closure over a closed suction-irrigation system, mortality has been reduced to less than five per cent.

The Grossly Disabled Patient. The patient largely confined to bed or wheelchair who suffers hip pain can benefit considerably from unilateral or bilateral excision arthroplasty. Extensive involvement of joints in the upper or lower extremities leaves such persons little hope of walking. An excision arthroplasty ensures pain relief; wheelchair life is more tolerable; and all aspects of nursing are facilitated.

Failed Arthroplasty. The over-all results of treatment of the rheumatoid hip joint with either cup arthroplasty or prosthetic replacement have not been entirely satisfactory. While it is hoped that total hip replacement will solve many of the problems encountered in the past, its usefulness in patients with failed arthroplasty has yet to be determined. When conventional arthroplasties fail, excision arthroplasty is an ideal solution, because the intense fibrotic reaction that acompanies such failure will improve the stability and the end result.

Ankylosed Hips. Our experience with this condition is limited. R. G. Taylor[8] has reported the results of bilateral pseudarthrosis in nine patients, and the results were satisfactory with one exception, attributed to faulty technique. Most of the patients reported regained 50° to 60° of flexion at the hip joint and were able to sit with ease and to walk with support. The marked muscle wasting makes the after care extremely demanding. Until the advent of total hip replacement, bilateral pseudarthrosis was the procedure of choice in patients with bilateral fixed hips. It is still considered a useful approach in management, both primarily and when other attempts at reconstruction have failed.

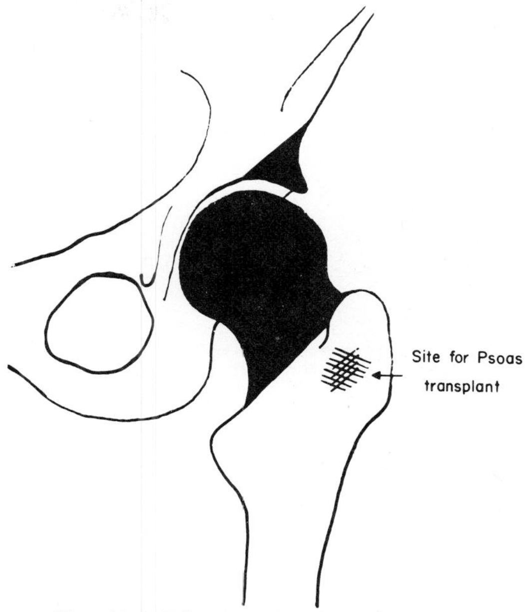

FIG. 12-2. Diagram showing the amount of bone to be resected in an excision arthroplasty. The line of bone division runs from the trochanteric fossa to the lesser trochanter. The acetabular rim, shown here in black, is removed together with all osteophytes. The psoas muscle is transferred anterolaterally below the intertrochanteric line.

Technique of Excision Arthroplasty

Preoperative Management. The patient must be aware of what is entailed in the postoperative treatment process and the function that can reasonably be expected. It is important that patients understand the problems associated with hip instability, for when pain is abolished they tend to become unduly concerned with this problem. Their memory for the intensity of preoperative discomfort is short. It is advisable to have a prospective candidate for this operation visit other patients who have had the procedure.

The overweight subject with an excision arthroplasty is at a disadvantage, since obesity reduces the overall physical capacities. The operative procedure is more difficult, postoperative complications more prevalent and rehabilitation time is prolonged. When possible, operative intervention is postponed until a satisfactory weight level has been achieved.

Preoperatively the patient is introduced to the therapist and a muscle-strengthening program. Pain usually limits an effective preoperative exercise program; however, when possible, it is useful to strengthen the gluteal and quadriceps musculature to shorten postoperative convalescence. A marked flexion contracture is reduced preoperatively with skeletal traction, which makes the operative procedure technically easier.

The Operative Procedure. The object of the operation is to create a pseudarthrosis (Fig. 12-2). Inadequate bone resection may lead to later bony contact and recurrence of pain, which would prejudice the functional result. We have used the anterior Smith-Petersen approach routinely, except in those instances where the surgical exposure is dictated by factors such as a sinus.

The patient is positioned with a small pillow under the buttocks. The standard Smith-Petersen approach provides a wide exposure. *Sharp dissection should be used at all stages of the operation*, avoiding periosteal elevation which can later lead to heterotopic bone formation.

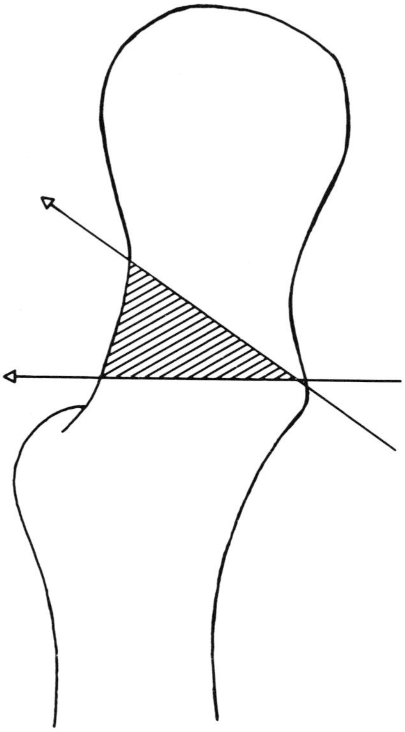

FIG. 12-3. Diagram showing how oblique division of the femoral neck from the intertrochanteric line anteriorly results in a sizeable posterior spur, which, by abutting against the pelvis, can cause pain.

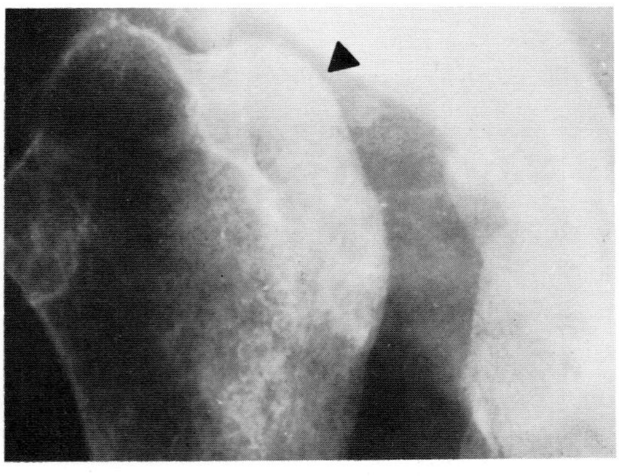

FIG. 12-4. An anteroposterior roentgenogram demonstrating the appearance of the posterior spur abutting against the pelvis.

An anterior capsular flap based on the intertrochanteric line is opened to expose the head and neck of the femur. This can be turned over the raw femoral surface and sutured to the posterior capsule at the close of the procedure to provide a cushion between the femur and the acetabulum.

Dislocation of the hip is often difficult, and forceful manipulation carries the risk of fracturing an osteoporotic femur. To avoid this complication, the acetabular margin is trimmed first, and the neck of the femur is osteotomized by taking an anteriorly based V wedge and then removing the femoral head.

The shaping of the femoral surface is carried out with rongeurs. This should be done with the limb in neutral to avoid leaving a buttress of calcar posteriorly (Figs. 12-3 and 12-4). The line of bone division must run smoothly from the trochanteric fossa to the base of the lesser trochanter. A residual calcar spur, such as that on which a Moore type prosthesis rests, exacerbates postoperative pain (Figs. 12-5 and 12-6).

The entire acetabular margin, particularly posterior-superior, should be removed. More needs to be taken away than appears on cur-

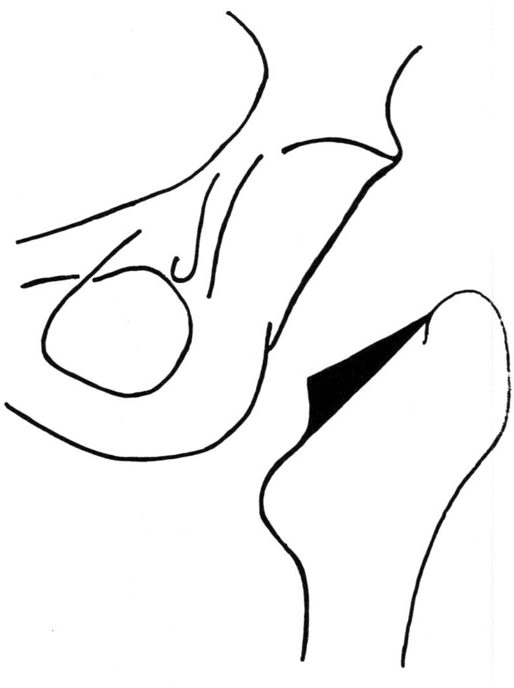

FIG. 12-5. Diagram showing the residual calcar which requires attention when a prosthesis of the Moore type is removed.

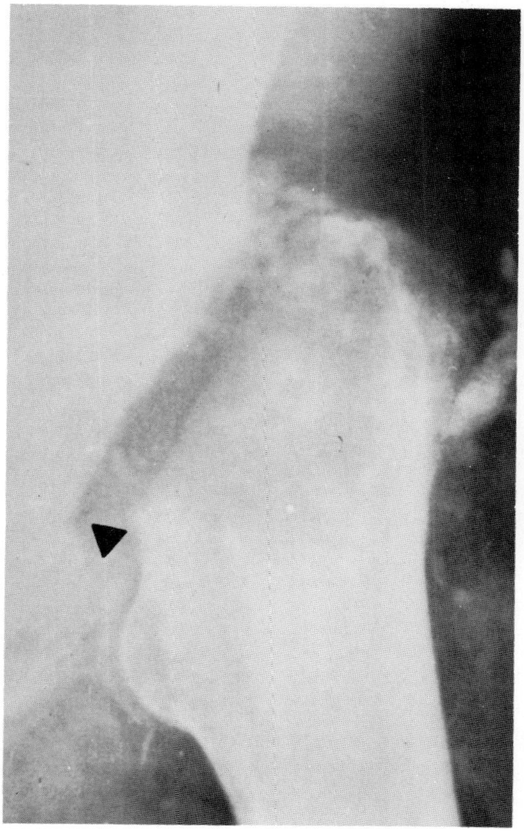

FIG. 12-6. Anteroposterior roentgenogram demonstrating residual calcar following removal of a Moore prosthesis.

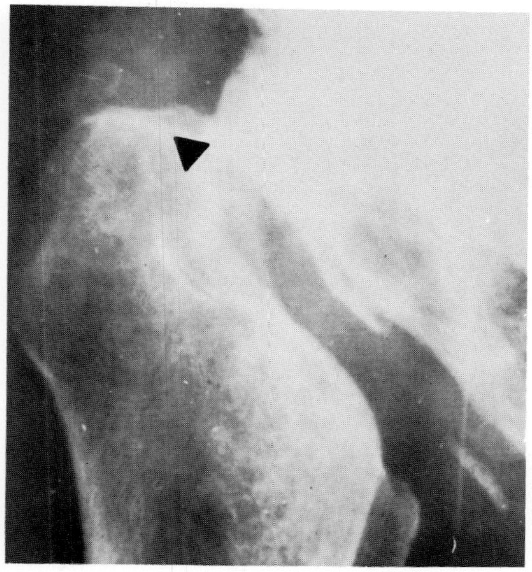

FIG. 12-7. Anteroposterior roentgenogram demonstrating insufficient removal of the posterosuperior acetabular margin.

sory examination (Fig. 12-7). A radiograph on the operating table is a valuable precaution. The sciatic nerve and the anastomosis between the obturator and medial circumflex arteries should be protected by a flat malleable retractor when the posterior-inferior margin of the acetabulum is trimmed.

After preparing the opposing surfaces, the surgeon observes the pseudarthrosis while the hip is telescoped by an assistant. All fragments of bone are carefully removed from the acetabulum, and the wound is irrigated with copious amounts of solution. Except in cases with significant sepsis, the iliopsoas muscle is transferred anterolaterally. The lesser trochanter is drilled at its base and divided with an osteotome. The tendon is mobilized proximally, preserving the iliacus component as much as possible. The femoral nerve must be protected at this stage. The trochanter is then attached to the previously denuded anterolateral surface of the femur just below the lateral extreme of the intertrochanteric line using two No. 22 stainless steel sutures passed through drill holes (see Fig. 12-2). The transplanted iliopsoas muscle acts as a stabilizing factor by exerting a sling effect under the wing of the ilium. Further, it controls the external rotation deformity which invariably appears if it is left in situ. Just before tendon transfer, the capsular flap is turned over the surface of the femur and sutured to the posterior tissues. The rectus femoris is reattached to the pelvis and the fascia lata closed carefully, because it aids in the stability of the hip in extension.

In cases without sepsis, the wound is closed without drains. A hemovac suction may be used for 24 hours. In the septic hip, closure is carried out for continuous suction-irrigation as described by Clawson and Dunn.[1]

A soft spica of alternating layers of cot-

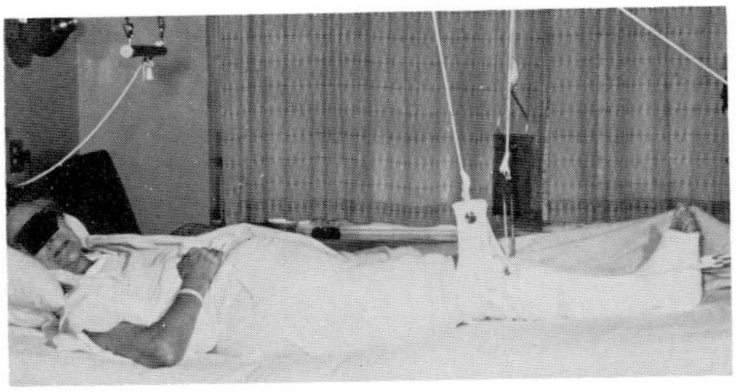

FIG. 12-8. A patient in the postoperative period showing the soft spica dressing about the hip and thigh. The leg is in a modified Hamilton-Russell traction incorporating a Steinmann pin through the tibial tubercle into a short-leg cast.

ton and stockinet is applied with the hip slightly flexed to insure firm pressure anteriorly when the limb is extended. A Steinmann pin is passed through the tibial tubercle and incorporated in a below-knee cast with the foot at a right angle. Hamilton-Russell traction is used (Fig. 12-8). The pin-cast technique avoids many of the complications which can attend skin traction. A pulley and weight system (2 to 3 lb.) is attached to the lateral side of the tibial pin to control external rotation and to protect both the iliopsoas transfer and the plicated capsule. An alternative to this is the use of a horizontal bar attached to the plaster cast, which will also prevent external rotation.

Excision Arthroplasty in the Presence of Infection

Experience in the last decade has clearly indicated the advantages of closed suction-irrigation treatment of osteomyelitis and septic arthritis when this is coupled with meticulous excision of all infected bone and soft tissue.[1,2] The dense scar tissue is a potential source of organisms and must be removed to avoid failure, even in the presence of adequate antibiotic coverage, since these substances diffuse poorly into relatively avascular fibrous tissue.

Operative Procedure. After debridement, two ¼-inch diameter siliconized perforated tubes are inserted into the dead space, one anteriorly and the second posterolaterally. Their ends should be overlapped and in close approximation throughout the perforated length. It may be advisable to tie them loosely together with catgut, for if these tubes drift apart they may plug with blood clots and debris and become ineffectual. The suction and irrigation, using large quantities of fluid, must be commenced as soon as the tubes are inserted and maintained continuously throughout wound closure. If the dead space is large, a second parallel system may be used.

In case of infection a one and one half plaster spica is used instead of the soft spica. The spica cast immobilization has many advantages in addition to any potential benefit in early wound healing. The immobility that results lessens postoperative hemorrhage, which can cause clotting of the tubes and loss of the suction-irrigation system. In addition, it provides a method of securely anchoring the tubes so that they are not inadvertently moved or removed.

The suction-irrigation system and immobilization are continued until a sinogram shows obliteration of the dead space. Appropriate systemic antibiotics are administered preoperatively and maintained postoperatively until there is complete wound healing.

Postoperative Management. The dressings are retained for one week. A check anterior-posterior radiograph is taken to insure that there is adequate separation between the femur and the pelvis (Fig. 12-9). Isometric gluteal and quadriceps exercises are begun as soon as pain will permit. Skeletal traction is continued for 4 weeks, after which skin traction is used so that the patient can have pool therapy.

Postoperatively, the patient lies flat, except at meal times, for the first 4 weeks to avoid a flexion contracture of the hip. Strengthening exercises for the adductors, abductors and internal rotators are commenced by the second week. These exercises can be facilitated by the use of a skateboard or powderboard. The upper limbs are exercised in order to prepare the patient for walking with crutches.

Our experience has led us to dispense with the previously used ischial caliper in most instances. A brace is cumbersome and handicaps the already disabled patient. The patients are allowed to toe-touch in crutch walking as soon as there is reasonable muscle control, usually at 7 to 8 weeks. Once good muscle control has been achieved, patients are allowed to walk with a cane. Full weight bearing is discouraged; however, many patients will gradually discard the cane, particularly for indoor walking. A sole and heel raise is provided of about 1 to 1½ inches. Because of the telescoping that occurs on weight bearing, measured shortening does not reflect the actual shortening that occurs during walking. The shoe lift should not compensate fully for leg length disparity to allow the patient to clear the ground in the swing phase of gait and to ascend stairs. The postoperative management after excision arthroplasty for infection does not differ from that in the uncomplicated case once the wound is healed, though progress is usually slower.

A feature of an excision arthroplasty is the steady improvement which usually takes place postoperatively for up to three years. When patients apply themselves vigorously to the exercise program, the functional result is improved considerably. If an excision arthroplasty is painful, the most likely cause is bone contact between the femur and the pelvis due to inadequate removal.[7]

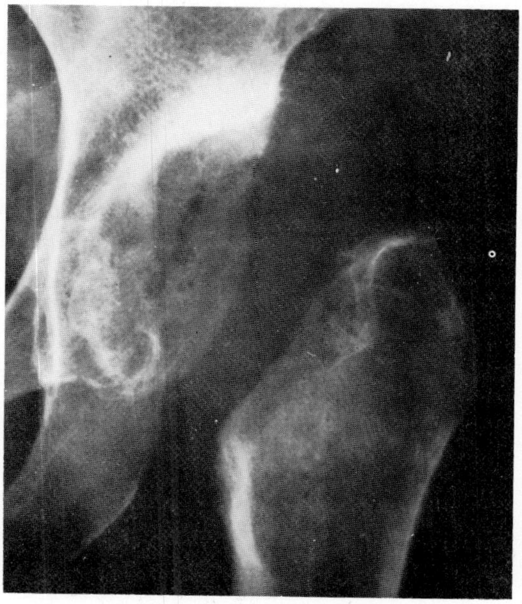

FIG. 12-9. Anteroposterior radiograph made in the immediate postoperative period, which demonstrates an "ideal" excision arthroplasty. The femur is held well away from the pelvis by skeletal traction, creating the optimum conditions for the development of a pseudarthrosis. The line of bone division on the femur is approximately parallel to the slope of the pelvis. All osteophytes have been removed as well as most of the acetabular margin.

Summary

1. Excision arthroplasty as a technique in rheumatoid arthritis and ankylosing spondylitis should probably be reserved for complications of sepsis, failure of conventional arthroplasty, or total hip replacement. The possible exception to this is the severely handicapped patient who is confined to bed or wheelchair. In such cases the procedure is unusually predictable in providing relief of pain while maintaining motion.

2. The operative technique is demanding; meticulous attention must be paid to details in both operative technique and postoperative management if the patient is to obtain optimum result.

3. Although an objective evaluation of the benefits of iliopsoas transplant is possible, it is felt that this transfer, originally described by J. Trueta, is a valuable stabilizing factor, acting as a dynamic sling under the wing of the pelvis as well as providing effective control of external rotation.

4. The advantages of excision arthroplasty are: (a) it is the most reliable procedure for pain relief, (b) correction of

even severe deformities can be achieved, (c) results are usually permanent, and the arthroplasty tends to improve with time, and (d) an adequate range of hip motion is assured.

5. Disadvantages of excision arthroplasty are: (a) limb shortening, and (b) instability which produces a pronounced limp, weakness of the extremity and fatigability.

6. Even though the scope of reconstructive surgery has been widened by the recent advent of total joint replacement, it is the authors' opinion that excision arthroplasty should be in the armamentarium of all surgeons who treat disorders of the hip joint.

REFERENCES

1. Clawson, D. K., and Dunn, A. W.: Management of common bacterial infections of bones and joints. J. Bone Joint Surg., *49*: 164-182, 1967.
2. Clawson, D. K., and Stevenson, J. K.: Treatment of chronic osteomyelitis. Surg. Gyn. Obst., *120*:59-69, 1965.
3. Girdlestone, G. R., Watson-Jones, R., Stamm, T. T., and Pride, K. H.: Discussion on treatment of unilateral osteoarthrosis of the hip joint. Proc. Roy. Soc. Med., *38*: 363-368, 1945.
4. Lee, M. L. H.: Pain following pseudarthrosis of the hip joint. Proc. Roy. Soc. Med., *55*:1062, 1962.
5. Murray, W. R., Lucas, D. B., and Inman, V. T.: Femoral head and neck resection. J. Bone Joint Surg., *46*:1184-1197, 1964.
6. Scott, J. C.: Pseudarthrosis of the hip. Clin. Orthop. Related Res., *31*:31-38, 1963.
7. Taylor, R. G.: Pseudarthrosis of the hip joint. J. Bone Joint Surg. [Brit.], *32*:161-165, 1950.
8. ———: Girdlestone pseudarthrosis of the hip joint in patients suffering from rheumatoid arthritis and ankylosing spondylitis. Proc. Ninth Congress Soc. Internat. Chir. Traumatol., pp. 152-157, 1963.
9. ———: Pseudarthrosis of the hip joint. Proc. Roy. Soc. Med., *49*:963-964, 1965 (Section of Orthopaedics).

CHAPTER 13

The Selection of the Operative Procedure for the Rheumatoid Hip

RICHARD L. CRUESS, M.D., AND NELSON MITCHELL, M.D.

The selection of the operative procedure to best treat rheumatoid arthritis of the hip depends, as it does in other joints, on many factors. The amount of destruction in the hip reflects the local progress of the disease and is of paramount importance. However, the number of other joints affected, the patient's occupation, his personality, and his ability to use crutches or canes to achieve the necessary early ambulation are other factors which must always influence the choice. Of these factors, the amount of local destruction in the region of the hip joint determines whether a so-called prophylactic or a reconstructive procedure may be utilized.

Minimal Local Destruction

It is axiomatic that there must be a stage in the evolution of rheumatoid arthritis of the hip in which articular cartilage is still adequate and erosion of bone is minimal. At this point, it is reasonable to assume that synovectomy will arrest the course of the disease, even if only for several years, and, therefore, it is recommended that a synovectomy be attempted at this stage. However, if the joint space is extremely narrow or irregular, if large erosions of bone are seen, or if there is essentially no motion of the hip, it is felt that too much joint destruction has occurred and reconstructive procedures are therefore indicated.

Indications for Synovectomy. (a) At the time of biopsy in apparent rheumatoid arthritis, (b) adequate cartilage interval visible radiologically, (c) adequate range of motion (60° flexion), and (d) minimal bone erosion.

Contraindications to Synovectomy. (a) Extensive cartilage destruction (observed roentgenographically or at the time of surgery), (b) very little motion of the hip (less than 60° flexion), or (c) extensive bone destruction.

Extensive Local Destruction

In a relatively young patient whose lower extremities are not so severely involved as to interfere with ambulation and who can walk with a crutch, it seems best to use a mold arthroplasty in the rheumatoid hip. Such an operation does not preclude other surgical procedures later and in many instances it will produce a permanently useful hip. There are many difficulties associated with this operation when several joints are involved, primarily because of the prolonged period of rehabilitation without weight bearing which is required. The early weight bearing and shortened period of rehabilitation associated with total hip replacement make this procedure attractive in the treatment of rheumatoid arthritis. At present it is not possible to recommend total hip replacement in the younger patient because of uncertainty about the life expectancy of the material used.

Prosthetic replacement of the femoral head without acetabular replacement has very little place in the treatment of rheumatoid disease, because in almost every instance the acetabulum is as severely involved as the femoral head. Because of the generalized osteoporosis, settling of the prostheses in the femoral shaft as well as protrusion into the pelvis frequently lead to early deterioration. It is also felt that primary resection of the femoral head, with or without osteotomy, is contraindicated in the treatment of rheumatoid arthritis because of the instability which results and because of the severe stress placed on the knee following a so-called Girdlestone procedure. Because the rheumatoid knee is osteoporotic and frequently affected by arthritis, it is particularly susceptible to valgus deformity due to altered stresses.

Indications for Mold Arthroplasty for the Rheumatoid Hip. (a) Too much destruction for a synovectomy, (b) relatively young patient (less than 50 years old), (c) other joints not so severely involved as to preclude eventual ambulation, (d) relatively stable patient who is able to participate actively in a prolonged rehabilitation program, and (e) failed cup arthroplasty in a young patient.

Indications for Total Replacement. (a) Total hip replacement may benefit those patients whose hips have been destroyed to such an extent that a synovectomy cannot be considered. (b) Rheumatoid patients above age 50 could be considered for this procedure if other factors also favor its use. When the hips are primarily involved and there is very little involvement of the other joints, it seems logical to raise the minimum age to 60 years. On the other hand, severe involvement of the upper extremities or of other joints of the lower extremities, which would make rehabilitation after cup arthroplasty extremely difficult, lowers the minimum age. (c) Total replacement is recommended in any condition which makes immediate ambulation more desirable than usual in the rheumatoid patient. (d) The surgeon is wise to consider total hip replacement, rather than a revision, in a patient over the age of 45 with failed cup arthroplasty. (e) Any accompanying medical conditions which limit life expectancy lower the minimum age at which total hip replacement should be contemplated.

Indications for Resection in the Treatment of Rheumatoid Arthritis. This procedure should be utilized only to salvage hips on which previous operations have failed. It is probable that an infected cup or total hip replacement are the only instances in which resection is indicated.

The Selection of the Operative Procedures in Marie-Strümpell Arthritis of the Hip

This particularly distressing condition is one of the most difficult types of arthritis to treat. No procedure available at the present time is entirely satisfactory. Synovectomy has been given an inadequate trial, but the nature of the disease does not offer much hope that synovectomy will arrest the course of the disease, as it may well do in rheumatoid arthritis. The results of mold arthroplasty in Marie-Strümpell arthritis of the hip are also disappointing. Total hip replacement probably offers patients the greatest hope of some useful motion with little or no pain and good stability, although it does not restore as great a range of motion as it does in other conditions. Resection or resection-angulation osteotomy is offered as a second choice and would also be utilized to salvage a failed total hip replacement. It must be emphasized that these recommendations are based on an analysis of many small series. There is no report of any single center's experience with this condition that is extensive enough to support firm conclusions.

CHAPTER 14

Treatment of Rheumatoid Arthritis of the Foot and Ankle

WILLIAM N. JONES, M.D.

Non-Operative Treatment

The majority of patients complaining of painful feet affected by rheumatoid arthritis will never have real indications for operation. Though conservative treatment may fail in many because of advanced joint disease, some may have relief of pain when joints ankylose. In adults spontaneous ankylosis often occurs in subastragalar joints, occasionally in midtarsal, and rarely in metatarsophalangeal and ankle joints. Ankylosis is much more common in juvenile rheumatoid patients.

Remissions may occur, and mechanical devices can have a very valuable part to play in protecting the foot during periods of activity. A great variety of soft pads, metal plates and plastic molds are available, and other devices, such as Jones bars may be useful. Simple stretching of ordinary shoes over local prominences is very effective, if done well. If foot distortion is considerable, SPACE shoes can be used. A skillful shoemaker can produce footwear to reduce pressure or stress even in feet severely deformed by arthritis.

If active disease affects the subastragalar joint, varus or (more commonly in adults) valgus deformity is likely to develop (Fig. 14-1). It produces stress on the hind-foot and fore-foot. In that phase, when deformity is the effect of muscle spasm and not fixed, a combination of Whitman plates and a wedged inflare or outflare heel is extremely helpful. The plate will "fix" the foot to the shoe and prevent broken counters, allowing the corrective force of the heel wedge to tilt the hind-foot. (A simple wedge on an ordinary heel is much less effective and tends to wear down rapidly.) This sort of support often seems to cause diminution of joint inflammation. A caliper brace is much less satisfactory.

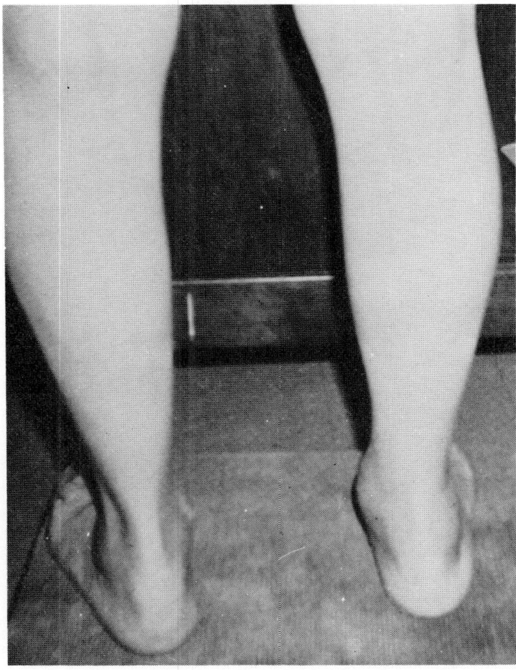

FIG. 14-1. Right foot has active subastragalar rheumatoid arthritis, peroneal spasm, and valgus deformity.

This method of heel positioning also tends to relieve the stress from an inflamed ankle. Light elastic supports or bandages

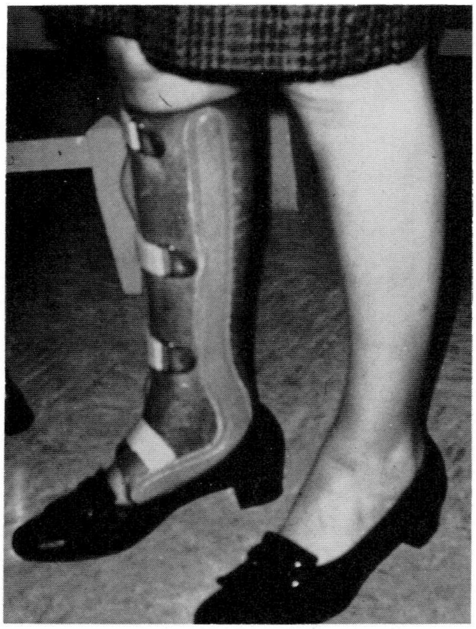

FIG. 14-2. A leather boot for ankle immobilization.

will afford some comfort in mild or temporary bouts of active disease. In the long-term, severely affected, and painful ankle, a leather boot can be used, with satisfactory relief of pain (Fig. 14-2). These will fit into unaltered shoes, including women's pumps; they are lighter, less cumbersome, and more comforting than calipers.

All such measures and devices cause some inconvenience; some are unsightly, and some, used over the years, entail substantial cost. All, of course, may fail to achieve the desired effect. It is estimated that about one out of 30 patients with rheumatoid foot complaints presenting to an orthopedic surgeon receives operative treatment.[1]

Operative Treatment

The Fore-foot. Metatarsophalangeal joints are involved about ten times as frequently by rheumatoid arthritis as any other joint in the foot, and the same ratio probably applies to the frequency of operation. The relative regularity of satisfactory results from the classic Fowler-Keller operation, when compared with other joint reconstructions in rheumatoid arthritis, contributes to this frequency.

Limited procedures such as simple bunionectomy and operations for clavus are indicated occasionally, and in patients with moderate fore-foot deformity and "burned-out" disease, metatarsal neck osteotomy or head recession may be adequate to relieve pain. The basis of deformity, however, is intra-articular disease, and joint operations are usually preferable.

Synovectomy of the metatarsophalangeal joints has been done in a limited number of feet. In the state of our present knowledge of synovectomy, this appears to be a logical procedure when synovial inflammation rather than joint distortion is the cause of symptoms. Unfortunately, patients usually present after joint destruction and deformity have occurred, and then bone procedures—either metatarsal head or full metatarsophalangeal joint resection—are necessary.

The foot should be free of ulcers and other infected lesions before surgery; this may require a period of abstention from weight bearing or protection by temporary foot coverings and adaptive soles to relieve pressure points. Supramalleolar Esmarch tourniquet is used unless circulation is precarious; skin edges should be carefully protected from over-retraction.

The transverse dorsal incision described

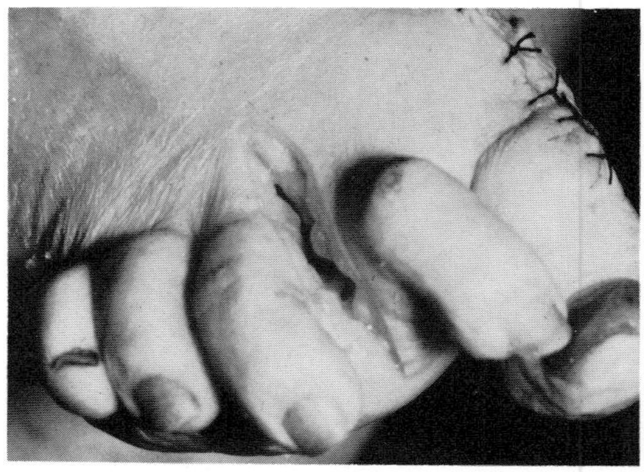

FIG. 14-3. A longitudinal dorsointerdigital incision.

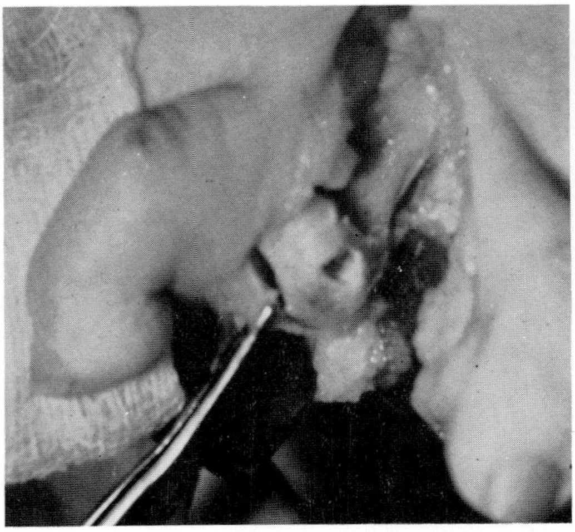

FIG. 14-4. Exposure of the metatarsal.

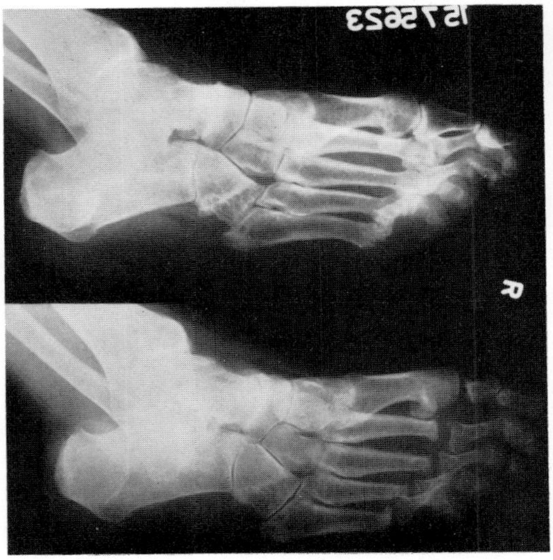

FIG. 14-5. X-ray appearance of the foot after a Keller operation with metatarsal head resections for a moderately deformed forefoot.

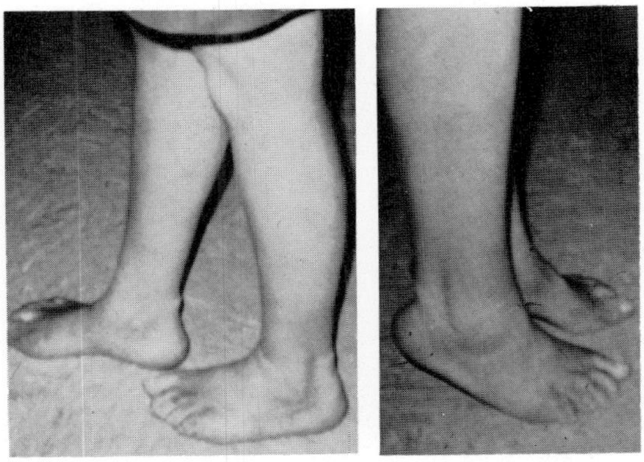

FIG. 14-6. A and B. Appearance of a foot after a Keller operation with resection of other metatarsal heads.

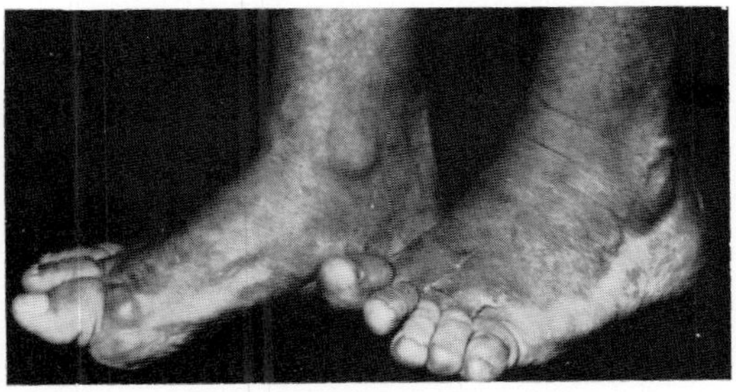

FIG. 14-7. The appearance of feet after metatarsophalangeal joint resections.

by Fowler[3] and the plantar incision of Hoffman[4] are both satisfactory. Multiple dorsal-interdigital incisions can also be used (Figs. 14-3 and 14-4).

In the foot with metatarsophalangeal subluxation without fixed severe deformities of the interphalangeal joints, metatarsal head resections alone are done (Fig. 14-5). The foot is better looking and the gait is usually better than after full joint resection (Fig. 14-6). The latter procedure is preferred, if there are fixed toe deformities, and recurrences of deformity will be less common (Fig. 14-7). Some surgeons feel it is important not to resect the fifth metatarsal head, though its removal will not impair foot function.

In a fore-foot affected severely enough to require these procedures, the great toe joint almost always requires reconstruction; the Keller procedure is most satisfactory.[5]

Hemostasis should be carefully maintained, and dressings which will harden on the skin should be avoided. The heavy pressure of elastic bandages may be troublesome. The patient is allowed to begin weight bearing on his heels with the support of walker or crutches as soon as he can do so comfortably. This is almost

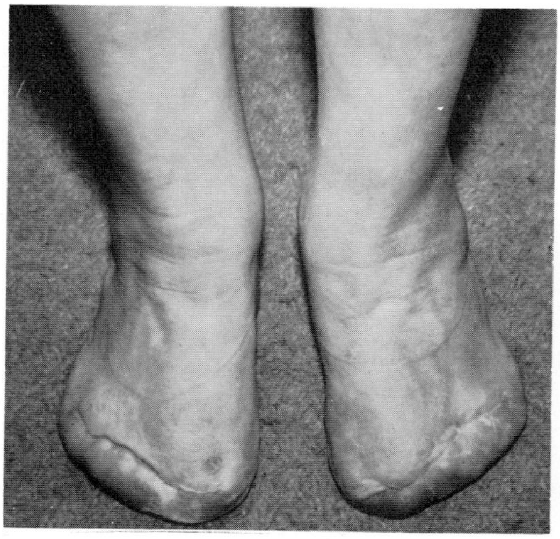

FIG. 14-8. Transmetatarsal amputation for recurrent failure of metatarsophalangeal joint resection. (Courtesy of Dr. Douglas Saville)

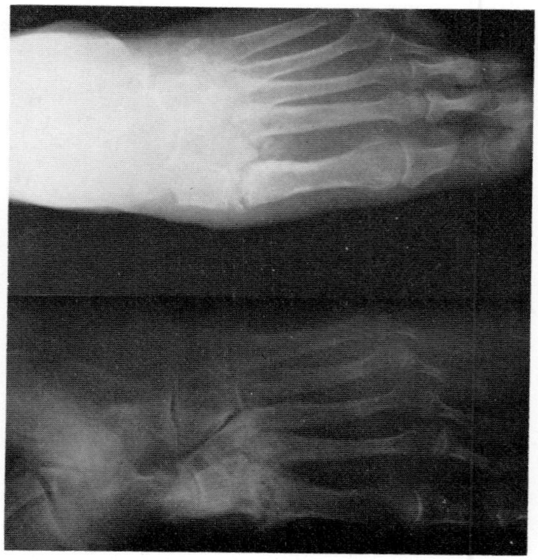

FIG. 14-9. X-rays of foot before (*top*) and after (*bottom*) excision of cuneiform-metatarsal with grafting. After the operation, the painful joint is fused without correction of the valgus deformity.

always by or before the fifth day. He should be encouraged to wear shoes early; cutting out the fore-foot portion of the upper shoe is necessary at first.

As noted earlier, the results of this procedure are very good. Symptoms requiring re-operation are said by Clayton to recur less than once in every ten operations. Recurrent severe deformity is seen occasionally, sometimes after a too-limited resection and usually in feet that had very severe deformities before operation. If after revision a fore-foot satisfactory for weight-bearing and wearing shoes is not obtained, transmetatarsal amputation can be done (Fig. 14-8). Saville in Edinburgh has found this a satisfactory treatment of the problem of recurrent, painful deformities and the patients indeed appeared pleased*. A toe-box is used in the shoes. Metatarsophalangeal disarticulations leave a very poor weight-bearing surface and are not done.

The Mid-Foot. Treatment of midtarsal arthritis ordinarily is conservative, the more so since symptoms can often be relieved by external supports. These must be shaped very carefully to allow room for prominences and sensitive local areas of inflammation or they will not be tolerated. Steroid joint injections occasionally will be a help but usually only temporarily; rest and systemic treatment, crutches, local heat, and other local palliatives are adjunctive.

Such treatment, of course, is not always effective, and joint destruction will progress with spontaneous fusion occurring infrequently except in juvenile patients. Fusion limited to the joints affected is recommended. In planning realignment of a lower extremity deformed at the knee level, it may appear that the foot position, rigid and adapted to a varus or valgus leg, will cause abnormal and painful weight bearing on one portion of the foot. While it is wise to make the patient aware of the possibility that foot realignment may also be necessary as a later procedure, in actuality this rarely needs to be done. With some even slightly mobile joints remaining, readaptation is surprisingly good. While fusions are very

* Saville, D. Personal communication.

useful in the rheumatoid foot, they should be limited to the least extent that will relieve local symptoms.

Often, the first resorption or destruction of bone contiguous with the joint surfaces is seen at the cuneiform-metatarsal joint (Fig. 14-9). Simple excision of the joint and plaster immobilization is not likely to result in fusion (fibrous ankylosis may occur), and graft bone should be added. A small tibial or iliac graft is superior to local bone. The foot is ordinarily flattened and rigid, and reconstruction of the arch is not possible. Twelve weeks of immobilization in a walking cast may be required. The treatment of the talonavicular joint is similar. With larger surfaces of cancellous bone opposed to one another, fusion usually occurs more rapidly; 6 weeks of cast support may be adequate.

When fusion of multiple midtarsal joints has occurred spontaneously, with the foot in fixed deformity (most often adduction-inversion in juvenile arthritis), painful pressure on the lateral border of the mid-foot can be disabling. Resection of a dome-shaped wedge of the midtarsal bone block from the lateral side in a closing fashion will realign the fore-foot (Fig. 14-10). Trimming of a medial protuberance through a medial incision may be necessary. Six weeks of plaster immobilization is probably adequate. Internal fixation is used if a wide wedge is resected. The cut is extended into the subastragalar joint area, if the heel is fixed and severely deformed.

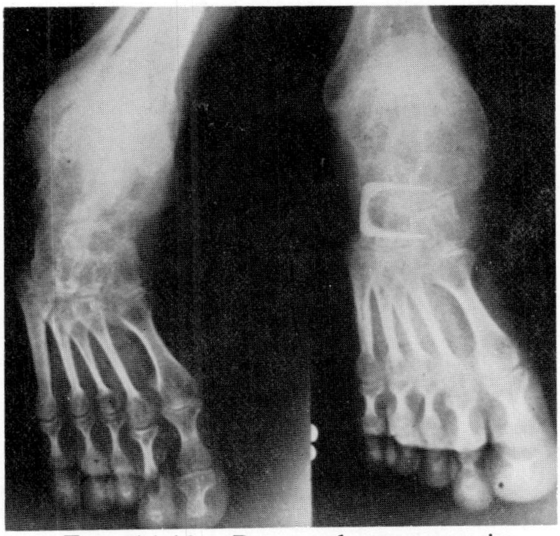

FIG. 14-10. Pre- and postoperative x-rays of a foot with severe adduction-inversion deformity which was corrected by midtarsal wedge osteotomy.

The Hind-Foot. As described earlier, the use of a Whitman plate with a flared heel and wedge is ordinarily effective in controlling heel position in a foot with active subastragalar disease. Spontaneous fusion, even in adult patients, is not uncommon, and when it occurs, pain is relieved.

Inversion or eversion of the heel will affect the foot distal to it, but unless midtarsal joints have also been involved, the deformity usually is tolerable and can be compensated by shoe corrections. Stress can affect the ankle if it too is involved by disease.

Subastragalar arthrodesis probably is rarely indicated. When it is, extra-articular fusion would be preferable unless the heel position is severely deformed and cannot be corrected or there has been extensive destruction of juxta-articular bone.

The Ankle. The ankle is commonly affected by rheumatoid disease; deformity in plantar flexion ordinarily occurs if joint destruction progresses. In adults it must be very rare for ankle fusion to occur spontaneously, whereas it is common in juvenile patients.

In the early phase of active synovitis without joint surface destruction, synovectomy should be considered. The author's limited experience has not been favorable. Possibly, this was influenced by selection of cases with more advanced joint disease than would be ideal. Cruess,* Gartland,† and Eyring and Bass (working with children)[8] have found ankle synovectomy of value.

* Cruess, R. L. Personal communication.
† Gartland, J. J. Personal communication.

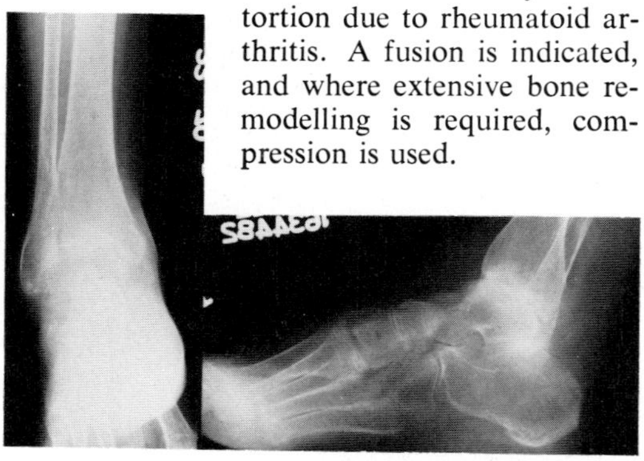

FIG. 14-11. Ankle joint distortion due to rheumatoid arthritis. A fusion is indicated, and where extensive bone remodelling is required, compression is used.

Ankle fusion is indicated after 12 to 18 months of continuing symptoms with x-ray evidence of joint deterioration. Though loss of ankle motion, if the foot joints remain mobile, is far less disabling than hip or knee fusion, in patients with rheumatoid arthritis, local improvement may occur. Early fusion is not recommended, because foot joints may be or may become involved.

Surgical arthrodesis is usually easy to achieve; almost any of the standard procedures are satisfactory. If the arthritis has destroyed considerable bone in the tibia or talus (Fig. 14-11), grafting and internal fixation, or compression by the Charnley apparatus should be used. Patients may be up in a walking plaster 5 to 7 days after operation. Plaster immobilization continues for about 8 weeks.

REFERENCES

1. Clayton, M. L.: Surgery of the fore-foot in rheumatoid arthritis. Clin. Orth., *16*:136-140, 1960.
2. Eyring, E. J.: The therapeutic potential of synovectomy in juvenile rheumatoid arthritis. Arthritis & Rheumatism, *11*:688-692, 1968.
3. Fowler, A. W.: A method of fore-foot reconstruction. J. Bone Joint Surg. [Brit.], *41*:507-513, 1959.
4. Hoffman, P.: An operation for severe grades contracted or clawed toes. Amer. J. Ortho. Surg., *9*:441-449, 1911/12.
5. Keller, W. L.: The surgical treatment of bunions and hallux valgus. New York Med. J., *80*:741-742, 1904.

CHAPTER 15

Surgery of the Spine in Rheumatoid Arthritis and Ankylosing Spondylitis

EDWARD H. SIMMONS, M.D.

ATLANTOAXIAL INSTABILITY

Gross fixed deformity is the main obvious clinical problem in ankylosing spondylitis of the spine. However, there is one area of instability which is sometimes overlooked in patients with rheumatoid arthritis and ankylosing spondylitis and which, when neglected, may give rise to grave consequences in its advanced stages. This is atlantoaxial subluxation and dislocation, which is particularly likely to occur when a solid column of the spine below places excessive stresses at the craniocervical junction; this stress is increased by the attritional effects of inflammation on the transverse ligament of the atlas or the associated effects of hyperemia on its bony attachments.

Atlantoaxial subluxation and dislocation may occasionally occur suddenly. Generally the onset is insidious and may go unrecognized, even in patients under routine observation and medical care by competent medical personnel. These patients invariably present symptomatology referable to the area, even in the early stages, but the symptoms may well be overshadowed by more severe complaints elsewhere.

The patient complains of soreness in the suboccipital area or upper portion of the cervical spine, with pain or discomfort radiating towards the occiput. The soreness tends to be aggravated by attempting full flexion or extension of the neck, and there is tenderness in the suboccipital area. In the more advanced phases of subluxation, vague paresthesias in the upper and lower extremities and a feeling of weakness and instability in an otherwise grossly disabled patient may also not give rise to any particular suspicion. Some observers feel that many deaths in the late or terminal phases may well have occurred for this reason.

The recognition of atlantoaxial instability or dislocation requires an awareness of its symptoms and the use of flexion and extension lateral radiographs of the upper cervical spine to indicate its presence. When gross instability is present, it almost invariably justifies stabilization.

Surgical Correction

Various methods have been described for achieving stability at the atlantoaxial level for dislocations of varying etiology. Mixter and Osgoode, in 1910, first described a procedure for stabilizing the first and second cervical vertebrae using a braided silk band.[8] In 1933, Bonet used an Albee graft to fix the occiput to the spine.[1] Willard and Nicholson, in 1941, reported a Mixter-Osgoode fascial stabilization in one patient; it later pulled free.[15] They then passed wire sutures around the posterior arches of the first and second cervical vertebrae with fusion by a modified Hibbs technique. Their patient was operated upon in 1937, and the result was presented to the American Orthopaedic Association in 1940.

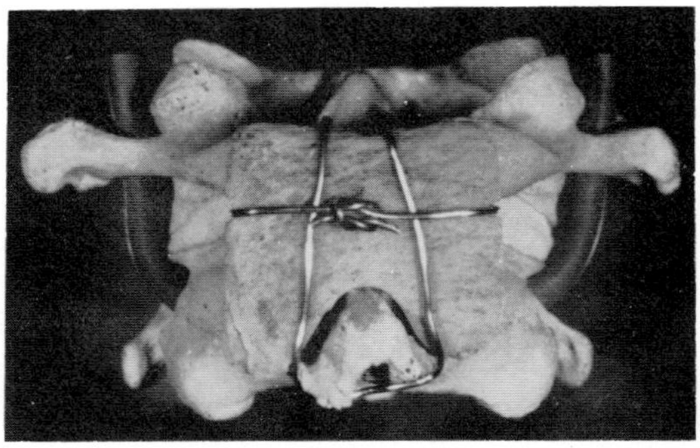

FIG. 15-1. The graft is in position with the cortical surface posteriorly. The Gallie wire is passed below the spinous process of C2 upwards over the graft on each side; it comes out below the arch of C1 and is tied firmly posteriorly.

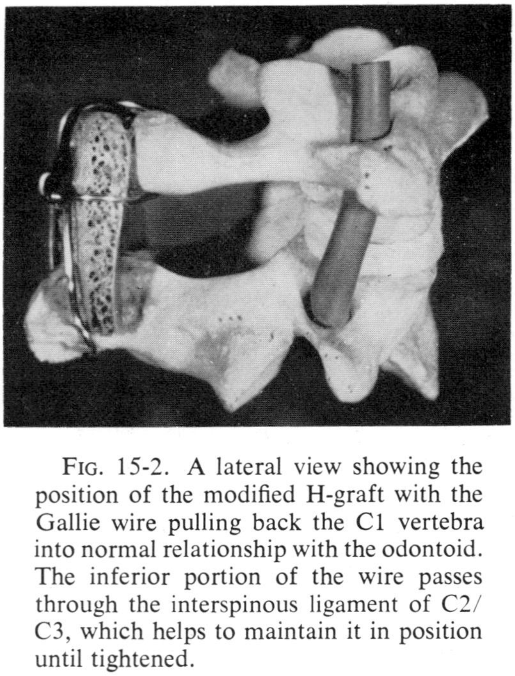

FIG. 15-2. A lateral view showing the position of the modified H-graft with the Gallie wire pulling back the C1 vertebra into normal relationship with the odontoid. The inferior portion of the wire passes through the interspinous ligament of C2/C3, which helps to maintain it in position until tightened.

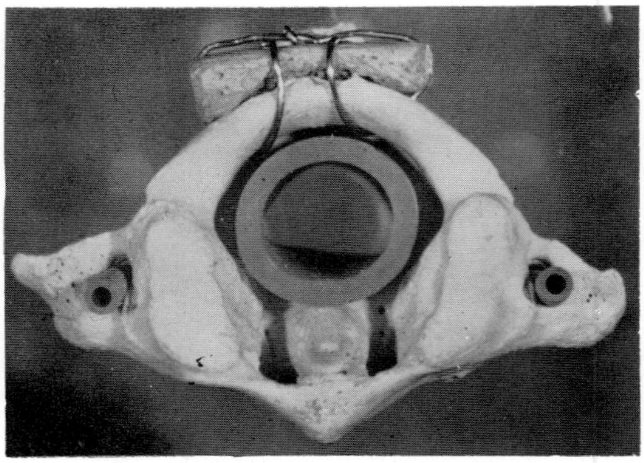

FIG. 15-3. The superior view shows the relationship of the contoured grafted bone and the wire to the vertebrae. Note the shape of the graft corresponding to the convex posterior surface of the arch of C1.

W. E. Gallie employed a technique of posterior atlantoaxial fusion which became known to his associates as a "Gallie fusion."* The exact circumstances under which he first carried out his procedure are not known. However, records are available of patients on whom this procedure was performed in 1939 and 1941. His procedure is a modification of a Willard-Nicholson fusion. Gallie employed a modified H-graft from the iliac crest contoured to fit over the posterior aspect of the arches of C1 and C2 sitting astride the spinous process of C2 (Fig. 15-1). A single piece of No. 22 stainless steel wire was then passed inferior to the spinous process of C2 through the interspinous ligament between C2 and C3. The two ends of the wire were carried upwards posterior to the graft, around a notch cut in its upper border, and then under the arch of C1 on each side of the graft. The two ends of the wire were tied over the posterior aspect of the graft locking it into position (Figs. 15-2 and 15-3) and pulling back the arch of C1 into normal relationship with the arch of C2. An essential instrument for the operation is a wire-tier like the one developed by the late R. I. Harris.[2] The wire-tier grasps the wire and allows one to put forceful tension on it, tying the knot quite firmly in the narrow confines of the wound with gentle pressure exerted by the hand (Fig. 15-4).

In addition to the main graft, cancellous bone chips are placed over the laminae on both sides as far laterally as possible. This procedure offers the advantages of rigidly immobilizing the involved segment. It avoids

* W. E. Gallie, Professor of Surgery, University of Toronto, 1929 to 1947. Personal communication.

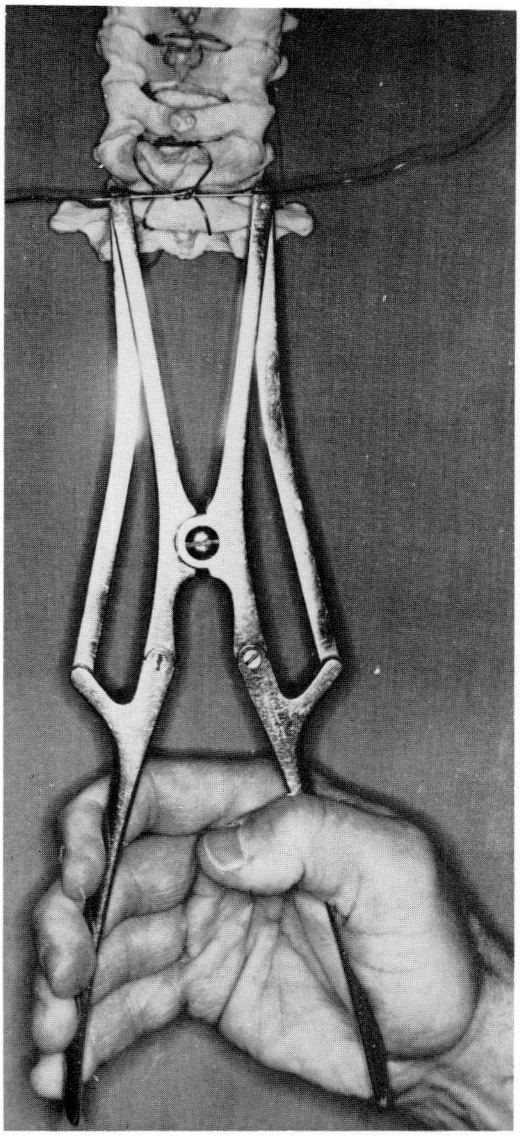

FIG. 15-4. The Harris wire tier tightening the second throw of a square knot. The first knot can be tightened quite firmly, pulling the graft and two vertebrae into firm apposition, the knot being held with a needle driver. The knot can then be completed.

the necessity of fusing to the occiput for lesions at the atlantoaxial junction, avoiding the higher pseudarthrosis rate of occipital-cervical fusions and at the same time preserving the very important motion at the atlantooccipital junction. The latter is all the more necessary in a patient who already has major stiffness and loss of function of the spine. The firm fixation of the graft to the atlas and the axis omits the necessity of a three-vertebrae fusion. The fusion also allows early mobilization and ambulation, which are important advantages for the patient with rheumatoid arthritis and ankylosing spondylitis.

A clear knowledge of the anatomy of the area is essential. The vulnerability of the vertebral arteries and the neural elements must be recognized. The vertebral arteries are carefully avoided and care is taken in dissecting the ligamentum flavum from the anterior surface of the posterior arch of C1 and in passing the wire around the posterior arch of C1. A flat curved guide may be inserted between the arch and underlying ligament as a safeguard when the wire is being passed. The end of the wire may be bent back on itself to prepare a blunt end, and then directed around the arch with a needle driver.

Figure 15-5 shows the type of lesion which justifies Gallie atlantoaxial fusion. The subluxation is reduced on extension, but on forward flexion there is obvious subluxation forward of C1 on C2 due to loosening or attrition of the transverse ligament of the atlas. Figure 15-6 shows the complete stability achieved by successful atlantoaxial fusion. The configuration of the wire is well demonstrated in Figure 15-7.

Table 15-1. Indications for Gallie Atlantoaxial Fusions

Origin	*No. cases*
Traumatic	33
Congenital & developmental	11
Inflammatory	
Retropharyngeal infection with subluxation	1
Rheumatoid & ankylosing spondylitis	6
Total	51

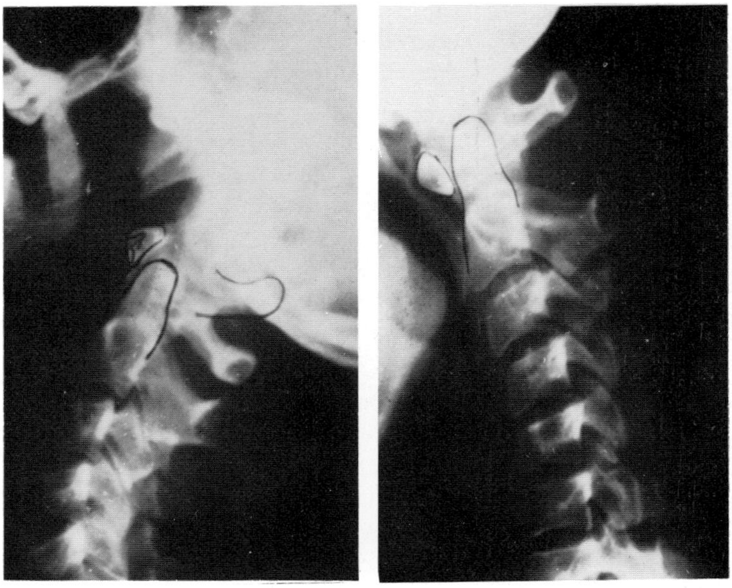

FIG. 15-5. Atlantoaxial instability due to attrition of the ligamentous components at the C1/C2 junction is evident on flexion (*right*) and extension (*left*). Forward subluxation is noted on flexion which corrects on extension. There is a slight upward or extension instability of C1 in relation to the odontoid.

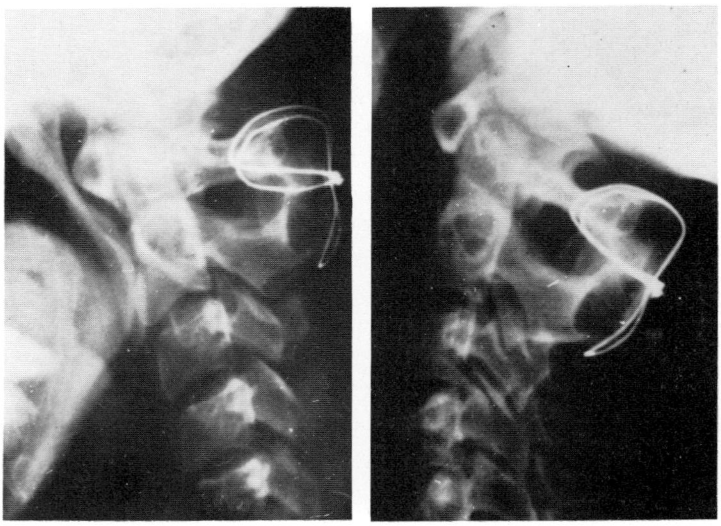

FIG. 15-6. Postoperative radiographs showing solid fusion with stability at the C1/C2 junction on full flexion and extension.

Results of Gallie Atlantoaxial Fusion

A total of 51 cases of atlantoaxial fusion of the Gallie type have been reviewed from 1939 to 1967 inclusive.[12] The indications are shown in Table 15-1. Although the bulk were traumatic or congenital, seven were inflammatory in origin. Of these seven, one was due to retropharyngeal infection with subluxation, and six were associated with rheumatoid arthritis and ankylosing spondylitis.

Table 15-2. Complications of Atlantoaxial Fusions in 51 Cases 1939-1967

Complication	*No. cases*
Operative mortality	0
Neurological complications	0
Infection	0
Nonunion	1
Fusion to occiput	2

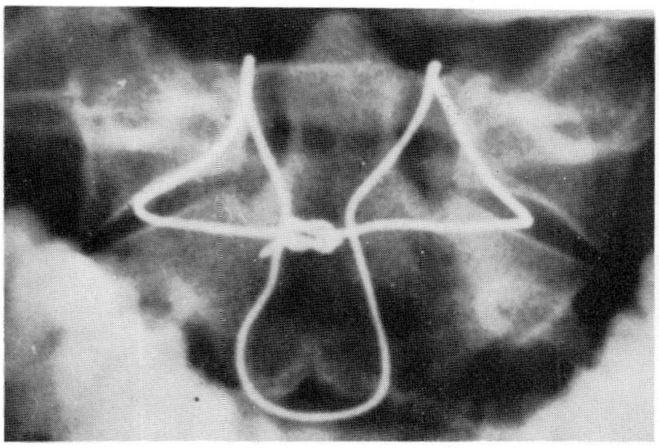

FIG. 15-7. Anteroposterior radiograph showing configuration of Gallie wire.

In the entire group of 51 cases no operative mortality occurred, nor has there been any neurological complication due to the operative procedure. No infections of the neck wound developed, probably because of the excellent vascularity of the area. A superficial infection of the iliac donor wound developed in one patient.

Only one recognizable pseudarthrosis has been found on clinical follow-up and routine flexion and extension lateral roentgenograms. This occurred in a patient in whom fusion was done for nonunion of a fractured odontoid. In retrospect, it was felt that C1 remained in some flexion, perhaps reducing the stability of the fixation. The patient did not splint his neck after discharge from the hospital, and he sustained a further neck injury when he was hit by a motor vehicle 1 week after leaving the hospital. He went on to nonunion. The wires were found to be broken at the time of reexploration when refusion was successfully carried out.

All of the inflammatory cases went on to solid union (Table 15-2). It is felt that the type of fusion, the excellent vascularity of the area, along with the firm fixation of the graft, are the major factors contributing to the very high rate of fusion.

Aside from the one pseudarthrosis, the only other complication was the extension of the fusion to the occiput in two cases.

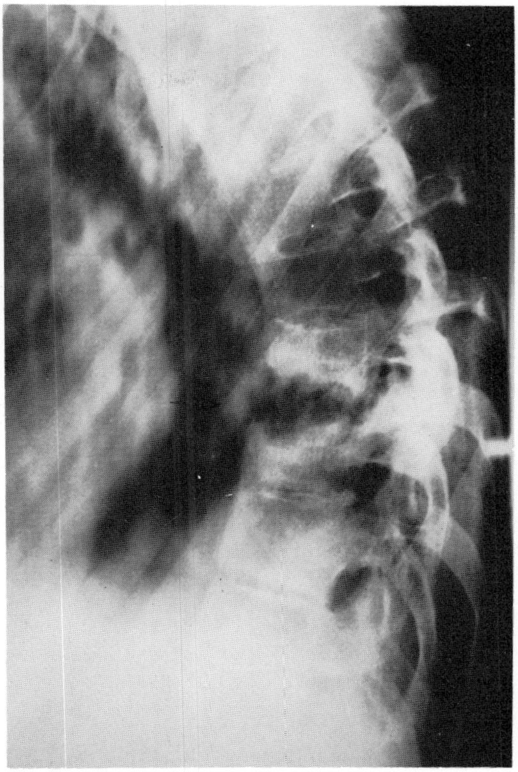

FIG. 15-8. Lateral radiograph of thoracic spine showing typical appearances of spondylodiscitis. Note erosive and sclerotic changes extending from disc space into adjacent vertebrae.

Fortunately, neither of these patients was in the inflammatory group. This complication can be avoided by not unduly exposing the occiput and by not extending the graft above the upper margin of the posterior arch of C1. Attention to these details is even more important in patients with inflammatory stiffness of the remainder of their spines.

SPONDYLODISCITIS

A radiological detectable characteristic of ankylosing spondylitis is the erosion and sclerosis of bone adjacent to the sacroiliac joint. The same erosion and sclerosis are commonly found on the anterior surface of the vertebral bodies. Occasionally the erosive sclerotic process will extend into the intervertebral disc and the adjacent bone. The condition is then called spondylodiscitis.

The radiograph of spondylodiscitis is fairly typical (Fig. 15-8). The erosive process widens the disc space, breaking down the subchondral bony plates. The surrounding bone becomes sclerotic and radiodense. Either erosion or sclerosis may appear more prominent. Both sides of the intervertebral disc are usually affected. The majority of the lesions develop in the lower thoracic area. Spondylodiscitis is unusual. Little, Urowitz and Rosen, in a prospective study of 128 cases, reported an incidence of five per cent.[7] This corresponds with the report of Shulitz of six per cent in his series.[10]

Of 11 patients studied by Little, Urowitz and Rosen, five presented because of unusually severe and persistent back pain. The remaining six were discovered on routine radiological review. The presence or absence of symptoms did not correlate with the severity of the radiological change.

Although one patient was treated with surgical stabilization early in the series because of disabling pain, all the others responded quite well to conservative management. It appears that the lesion generally follows a benign course and will usually respond to conservative management. Occasionally, surgical stabilization may be justified for intractable pain, particularly where there is an associated fracture posteriorly.

FLEXION DEFORMITIES OF THE SPINE IN ANKYLOSING SPONDYLITIS

It is well known that severe flexion deformities of the spine may occur in patients suffering from Marie-Strümpell spondylitis and ankylosing spondylitis associated with psoriasis. The prevention of these deformities by early recognition of the disease process, adequate medical treatment, and all the available preventive measures should still be the main aim of the medical profession in handling patients with specific spinal involvement.

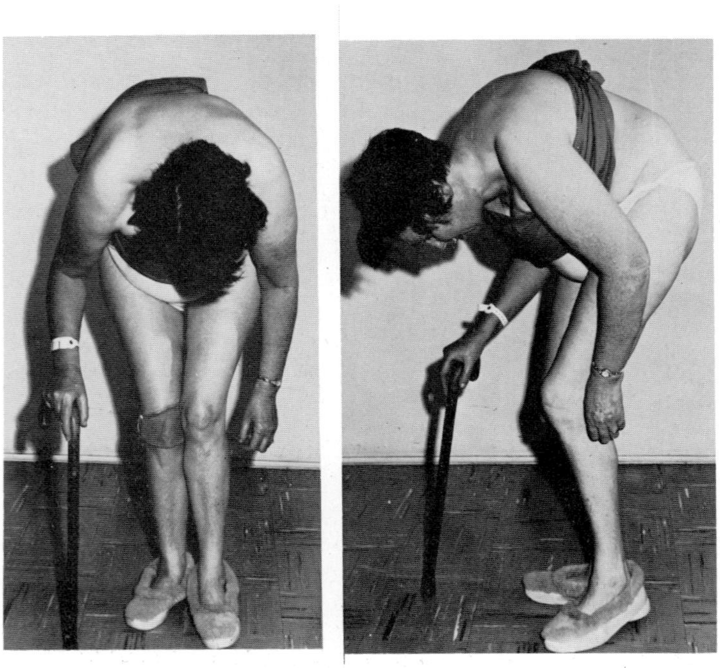

FIG. 15-9. (*Left*) Anterior "erect" standing view of 57-year-old woman referred for consideration of correction of spinal deformity. She had been held rigidly in this position for a period of 16 years. The distance between her nose and the floor was 32 inches. (*Right*) Lateral view of the patient giving outline of her deformity.

However, despite the recognition of this basic concept, all too often we still see patients with advanced fixed flexion deformities of the trunk who are very grossly disabled and who present a major problem for definitive surgical correction of their deformities.

Indications for Surgical Correction. The indications for surgical correction of deformity related to the trunk are variable and depend on the extent of the deformity, the degree of functional embarrassment, the age and general condition of the patient, the feasibility of correction, and (perhaps above all else) the morale and earnest desire of the patient to accept the risks and rehabilitative measures required for correction.

Assessment of the Deformity. In assessing these patients for possible surgical correction, it is most important that we recognize the primary site of their deformity. It is true that if the deformity is not severe we may occasionally compensate to a degree for deformity in one area by correction carried out a little removed from it. However, there is no doubt that if any major correction is to be carried out, then the correction must be made in the area of the main deformity. If this is not done, balance and the ability to walk and stand upright could be very materially affected. Patients who present because of apparent spinal deformity may in reality have the main deformity in the hip joints. The deformity may be in the lumbar spine, or to a degree in the thoracic spine, or it may be primarily cervical in situation.

Figure 15-9 shows a 57-year-old woman who was referred for correction of her spinal deformity. Once a woman of normal height, she was bent so that the distance from her nose to the floor was 32 inches. She had been held rigidly in this position for 16 years. Her knees were held rigidly together in adduction, and because of the impingement of one against the other, she wore a protective pad on her right knee.

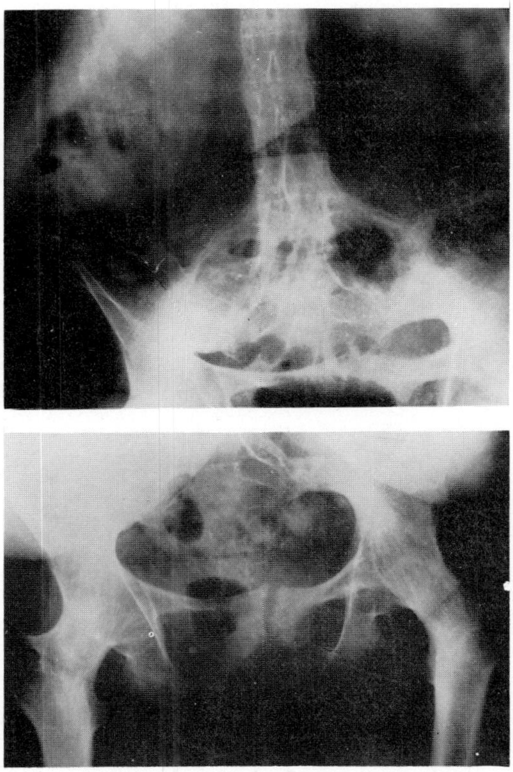

FIG. 15-10. Anteroposterior radiographs showing ankylosis of spine (*top*) and hip joints (*bottom*).

It is true that she had a forward curvature of her lumbar spine, her thoracic spine, and, to a degree, her neck. However, radiographs showed that her spine and hip joints were both solidly ankylosed (Fig. 15-10) so that she could be moved up and down in a teeter-totter fashion by either lifting up on her extremities or pushing down on her head. It is also evident that the main flexion deformity was at the hip joints, and if the lower limbs were placed below her, in line with her remaining trunk, then the main deformity would be corrected and she would undoubtedly be able to cope with the residual deformity of the spine. This woman was not treated by spinal osteotomy but by bilateral total hip replacement arthroplasties which mobilized the hips and corrected the hip flexion deformities by placing the limbs in more normal

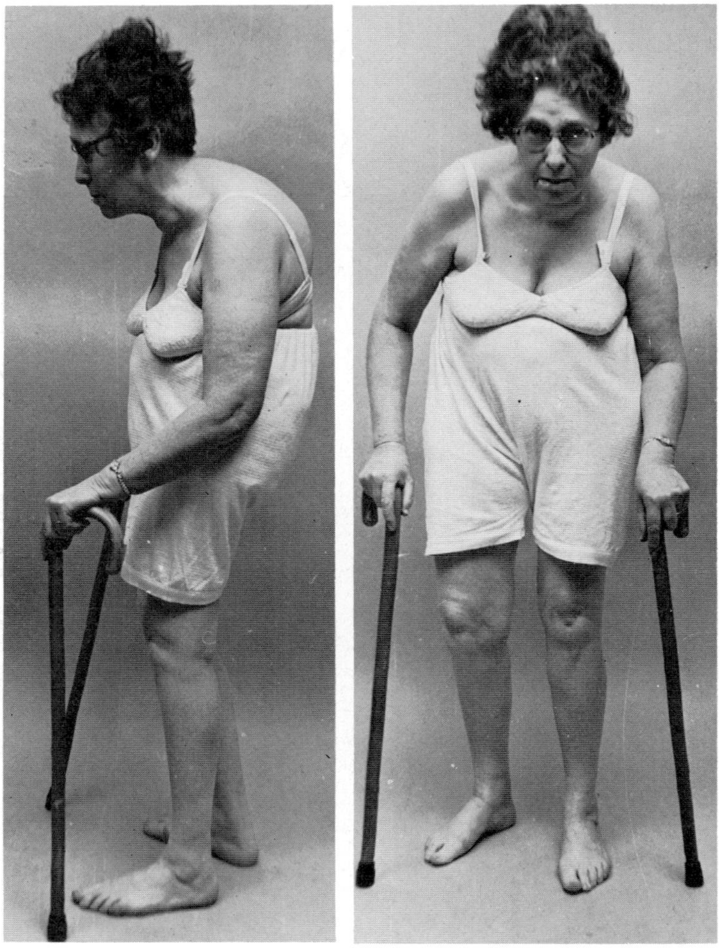

FIG. 15-11. (*Left*) postoperative lateral standing view of patient showing main skeletal deformity corrected. The patient is able to stand and look ahead with residual spinal deformity to which she is readily able to compensate. (*Right*) Postoperative standing anterior view.

alignment below the trunk. Following this she was able to stand and look ahead (Fig. 15-11), and she can now get in and out of a chair. As far as she is concerned, her major problem has been relieved.

Figure 15-12 shows a 41-year-old woman who first had intermittent symptoms of "rheumatism" in her early adult life. Over the years, gross stiffness of her spine developed which had an obvious diagnosis of ankylosing spondylitis. She had slight difficulty looking forward and tended to flex her hips and knees and hyperextend her neck to compensate for this. Her lower thoracic and lumbar spine ached. From the lateral view it is evident that the prime deformity was in the lumbar portion of her spine. Surgical correction of this patient's deformity was done in the lumbar portion of her spine with an extension osteotomy at the L2/3 level.

Surgical Correction of Flexion Deformity of the Lumbar Spine

In arthritic disease, the lumbar spine is one of the commonest areas of major deformity. Flexion deformity of the lumbar spine was the first deformity to be corrected surgically. The initial procedure by Smith-Petersen, Larson, and Aufranc was performed in 1945, with the patient under general anesthesia and lying prone.[13] This has been further reported by LaChapelle,[5] Herbert,[3] Nunziata,[9] Wilson,[16] Law,[6] and others. In all the

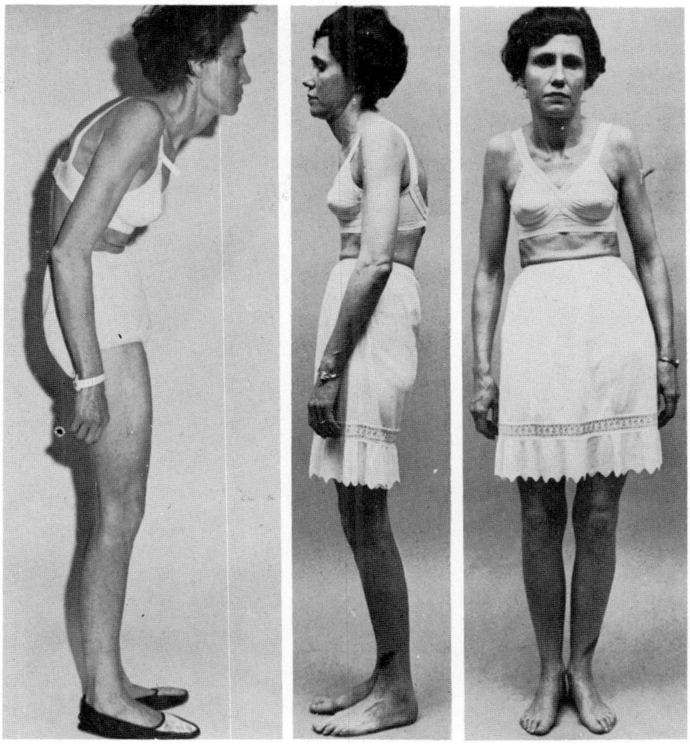

FIG. 15-12. (*Left*) Standing lateral view of 41-year-old woman with flexion deformity of thoracic and lumbar spine due to ankylosing spondylitis. It is evident that the prime deformity is in the lumbar portion of the spine. (*Center, right*) Postoperative standing anterior and lateral views of patient. Compensation has been achieved with restoration of lumbar lordosis. The patient has moderate rounding of dorsal spine but is functionally adequately aligned.

series reported, including Law's with a hundred cases, the operative mortality has been approximately ten per cent.

Some have recommended a two-stage procedure or double-exposure procedure with surgical division of the longitudinal ligament anteriorly. This is not usually required. In most instances correction can be done from the posterior approach alone. The double-exposure technique has the drawback of extending the operative procedure and anesthetic time.

A number of problems are encountered when trying to place a patient with acute flexion deformities of the spine in the face-down position. Adams has circumvented these problems by operating with the patient lying on his side and using a three-point rack to manipulate the spine and allow correction.

Major difficulties still exist, however, when a spinal operation on a patient with fixed deformity due to ankylosing spondylitis is done under general anesthesia. These patients usually have a rigid neck and intubation itself is a very difficult undertaking. Postoperatively the patients are not able to cough well, and accumulation of mucus with respiratory complications presents a real hazard.

Among the major complications or problems in straightening a spine by lumbar osteotomy are gastric dilatation and abdominal ileus. As the spine is extended the superior mesenteric artery is stretched over the third part of the duodenum, and this predisposes to gastric dilatation. If this hazard is not anticipated, the patients may vomit considerably, and with a stiff rigid neck, particularly when lying on the back, the danger of aspiration of vomitus is very real. As a result, it is wise to have a duodenal tube in position preoperatively, with suction drainage, until intestinal motility is established. The irritation of a duodenal tube and the accumulation of secretions caused by it, may also contribute to pul-

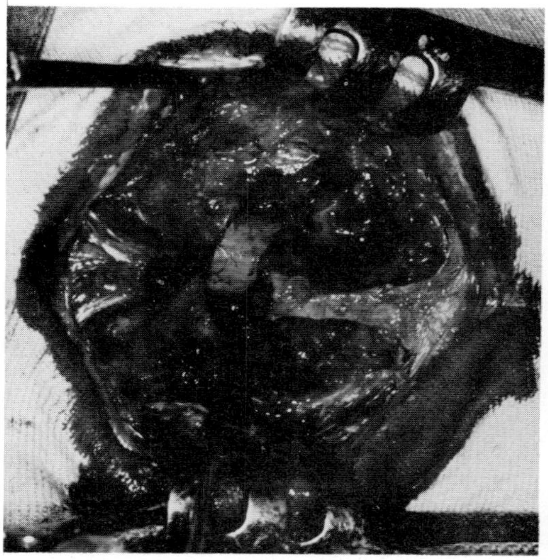

FIG. 15-13. Operative view showing V-shaped defect created with exposed dural sack. The superior portion of the V projects towards the head, the apex toward the pelvis. (Figures 15-13 through 15-16 pertain to the case of the patient pictured in Figure 15-12.)

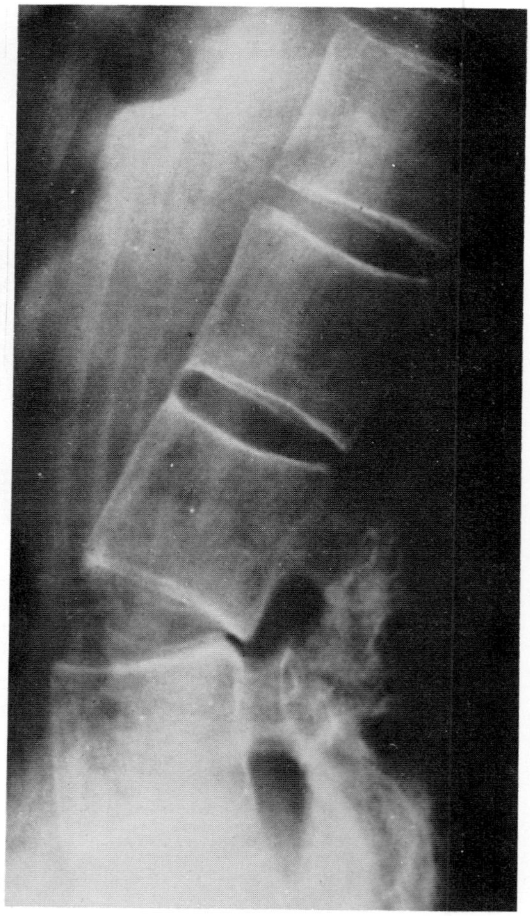

FIG. 15-14. Postoperative lateral radiograph of osteotomy site showing fracturing of the anterior longitudinal ligament and opening of the spine anteriorly at the L2/L3 level, with closing of the osteotomy defect posteriorly.

monary complications, particularly with general anesthesia.

The initial recommendation of Smith-Petersen et al. was to carry out a posterior resection osteotomy of the mid lumbar spine in a V fashion with manipulative fracturing of the anterior longitudinal ligament.[13] The spinous processes were resected and cut into small strips to be used for grafting. The level of osteotomy was identified and an elevator inserted beneath the lamina and the inferior articular facet, bringing it out through the superior articular facet of the vertebra below and the inferior facet of the vertebra above. The osteotomy was made in an oblique fashion, its angle being approximately 45° with the coronal plate. The obliquity of the osteotomy was to ensure locking of the vertebrae following correction—an effort to prevent serious displacement. The technique of the osteotomy as recommended by Smith-Petersen is sound and requires little alteration. However, it is undoubtedly an easier and safer procedure when done with the patient lying on his side, particularly when done under local anesthesia.

Operative Technique. As a result of experience with flexion deformity of the cervical spine, the possibility of carrying out correction in the lumbar spine under local anesthesia has been investigated and has been shown to be a safe, reliable, and practical procedure. After adequate discussion with one patient of the merits and the possible complications, it was done with the

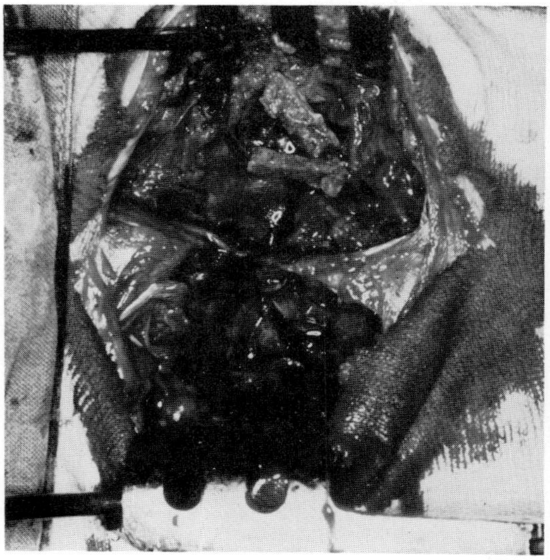

FIG. 15-15. Operative view showing defect closed posteriorly with removed portions of bone being inserted on each side as bone graft material.

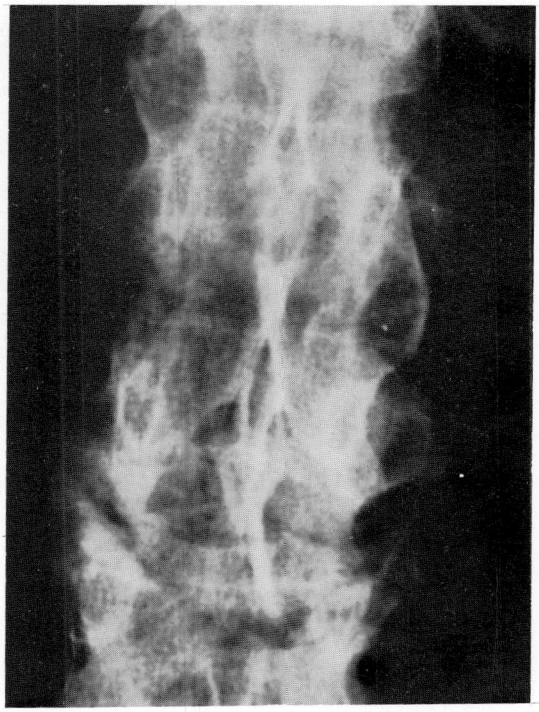

FIG. 15-16. Postoperative anteroposterior radiograph of osteotomy site showing closure and the V-shaped locking of the posterior elements.

patient on her side under local anesthesia. A duodenal tube was passed preoperatively with the patient awake, and it presented no problem. With the patient in the recumbent position on her side, Innovar could be used without fear of serious hypotension, since this could be readily controlled by tilting the table to offset any tendency in this direction.

Innovar is a very potent and effective drug and is ideally suited to supplement local anesthesia to allow the procedure to be carried out without the necessity of general anesthesia. Fentanyl is a synthetic opiate calculated to have one hundred times the analgesic potency of Demerol. Droperidol is a powerful tranquilizer and a strong antiemetic. Each milliliter of injectable Innovar contains 0.05 mg. of Fentanyl and 2.5 mg. of Droperidol. The two drugs may be obtained separately and used in different proportions if indicated. For local infiltration 0.8 per cent Xylocaine with Adrenalin 1 in 400,000 solution was used.

The type of correction described by Smith-Petersen was done at the L2/3 level with resection of a V-shaped wedge from the spine posteriorly at the L2/3 level. An electrical burr was used to cut through the inferior facet of L2 and the superior facet of L3 on each side and across the lamina of L2 in a V-shaped fashion (Fig. 15-13). The spine was straightened manually, the anterior longitudinal ligament fracturing at the L2/3 level (Fig. 15-14). The operative defect in the spine then closed posteriorly (Fig. 15-16). The patient tolerated this quite well and was able to cooperate by assuming a prone position while the wound was closed. A posterior plaster shell was applied in this position with the patient awake. She was turned over on her back in the shell, and an anterior plaster shell was made.

Postoperatively the patient was nursed in a Circo-Electric frame. She had no major

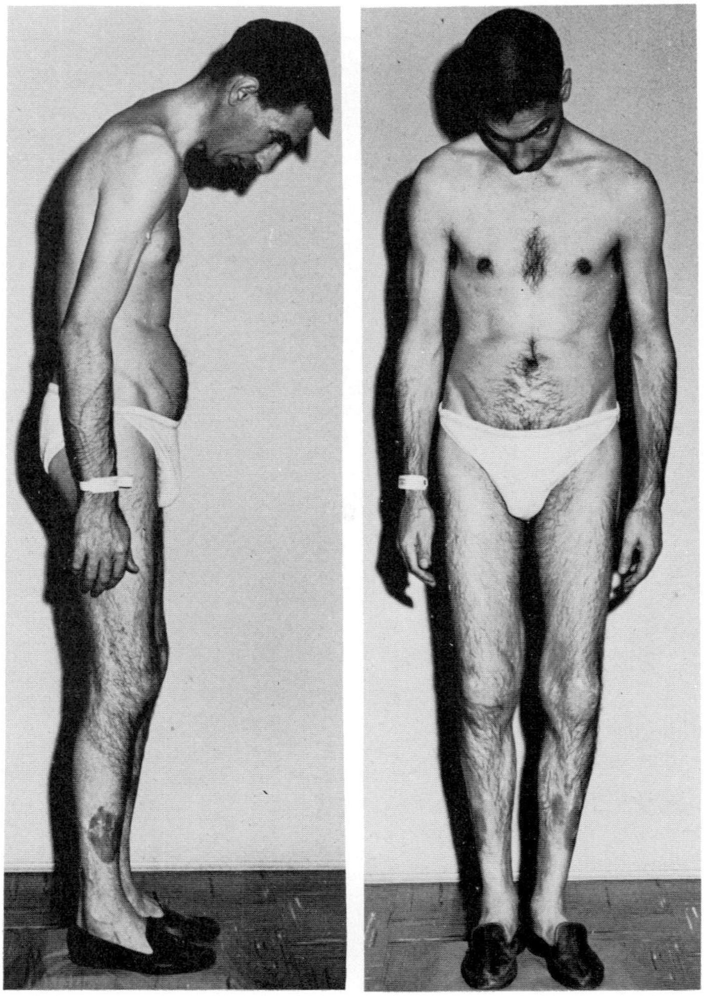

FIG. 15-17. Lateral and anterior views of 35-year-old man with 18-year history of ankylosing spondylitis, resulting in fixed flexion deformity of cervical spine. Patient had a grossly restricted field of vision.

discomfort. The duodenal tube was left in place for two to three days until bowel sounds were adequately established, and it was then removed.

The relative ease and freedom from complications with this modification of the usual technique for correction of flexion deformity in the lumbar spine has been most impressive. It is felt that this technique is the method of choice in most individuals.

The patient was immobilized in a plaster body jacket 6 weeks postoperatively and then allowed to walk. She was subsequently discharged to her home in plaster, which was removed 4 months postoperatively. Further splinting with a long spinal corset was done for an additional 3 months. Figure 15-12 shows the postoperative result. The patient had fairly normal functional alignment. Compensation has been achieved with the restoration of some lumbar lordosis. She still has moderate rounding of her dorsal spine, but it is not a functional handicap for her.

The Surgical Correction of Flexion Deformity of the Cervical Spine

There are a few patients with ankylosing spondylitis in whom flexion deformity occurs primarily in the cervical region. This deformity can be severely disabling and may progress to the point where it actually interferes with opening the mouth. The osteotomy of the lumbar spine is now a reasonably well understood and established procedure for correction of the most common deformity occurring in the spine in ankylosing spondylitis. The possibility and technique of correcting flexion deformity of the neck is less well understood. It has considerably greater hazard. For the few severely afflicted patients with this particular problem, it is important that the principles related to its possible correction and the indication should be clearly established.

Figure 15-17 shows a 35-year-old man who first experienced arthritic symptoms at the age of 17. They began in his knees and the sacroiliac areas and went on to involve his entire spine in an ascending progress. He also had some involvement of the hip joints. The entire spine became stiff, beginning in the sacroiliac area and ascending to the lumbar, dorsal, and cervical regions. A severe flexion deformity of the neck developed which made him unable to see more than 4 feet of the ground ahead of him. For over 4 years he had been unable to see the upper end of a door when entering a room or the upper portion of a person passing. He had been unable to work during this time. His general condition was relatively good, and the arthritic process appeared to be quiescent. He was considered a candidate for correction of his cervical deformity. The risks were explained to him, and he fully accepted them.

Operative Technique. Following the recommendation of Urist,[14] it was felt that the operation should be done under local anesthesia with the patient in the sitting position. The level between the seventh cervical and first thoracic vertebra was selected for correction of the deformity. As Urist indicated, this interspace is more receptive to surgical treatment than any other level in the cervical region. The spinal canal is relatively wide. The cervical cord and eighth cervical nerve roots have good flexibility in this area, and any weakness caused by injury to the eighth cervical nerve root is consistent with good function of the hand.

The passage of the vertebral arteries through the transverse foramina presents a unique anatomical situation, for fortunately the vertebral artery and veins usually pass in front of the transverse process of the seventh vertebra and enter the transverse foramen at the sixth vertebra (Fig. 15-18). The position of these blood vessels above the level of the first thoracic vertebra protects them from serious injury during osteotomy of the cervical spine. It was planned that an adequate excision would be carried out posteriorly at the cervical-dorsal junction with subsequent fracturing of the anterior longitudinal ligament and extension of the spine at the cervical-dorsal junction.

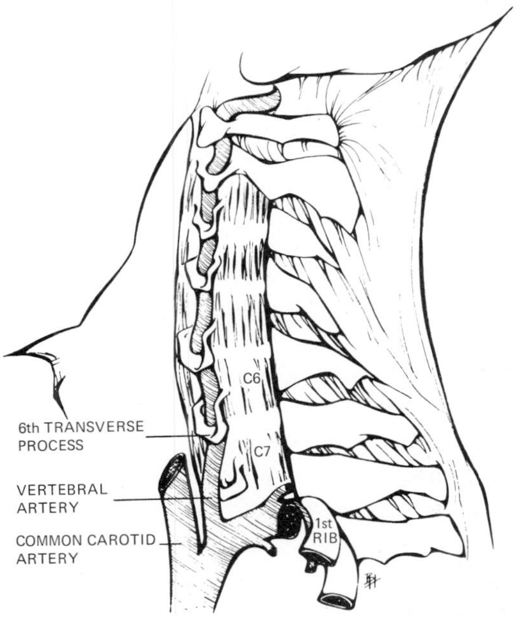

FIG. 15-18. Lateral anatomical view showing relationship of vertebral arteries to cervical spine. Vertebral artery and vein usually pass in front of transverse process of the seventh vertebra and enter the transverse forearm at the sixth vertebra. The position of these vessels above the level of the first thoracic vertebra protects them from serious injury during osteotomy of the spine at the C7/D1 level.

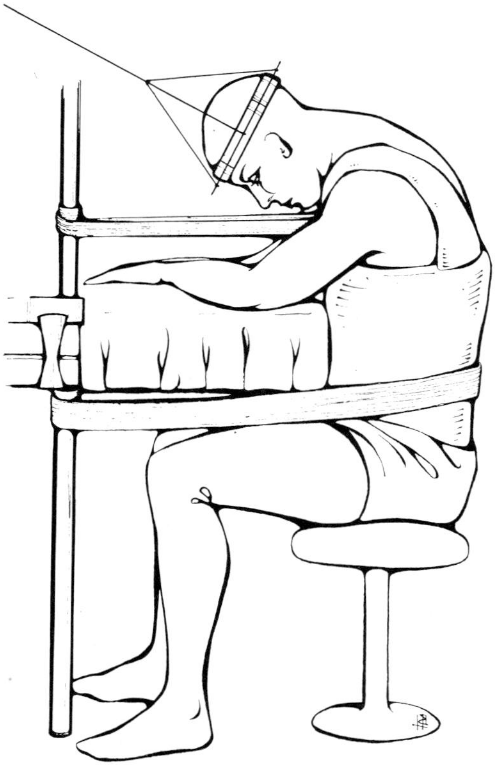

FIG. 15-19. Position of patient at operation, sitting on stool, resting arms on operating table with head suspended by halo unit.

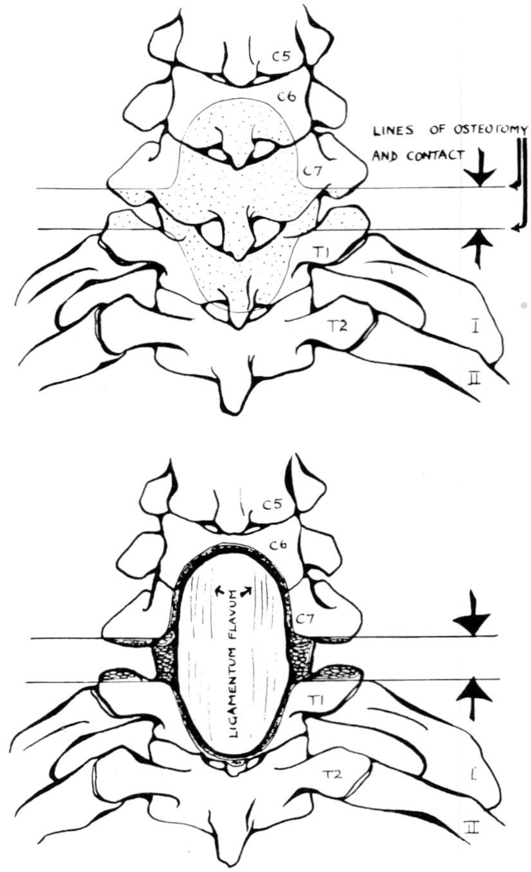

FIG. 15-20. Diagram showing posterior view of area of resection. Lateral resections are bevelled towards each other so that opposing surfaces will be parallel and in apposition following extension osteotomy.

Two to 3 days preoperatively the patient was fitted with a plaster body jacket incorporating the supports for a halo unit, in order to allow him to adjust to the plaster. The procedure was explained to him and he was brought to the operating room a day preoperatively so that he would understand what was going to occur and how he would be sitting at the time of operation. The operation was carried out with the patient in the sitting position; a stool was used to support the patient with his arms resting over the operating table. A halo unit was applied to his skull, the pins being inserted under local anesthesia. The halo unit was used to control the head during the procedure and to serve as a basis for stability immediately following the operative procedure. The halo was suspended by nine pounds balanced traction along the axis of his neck (Fig. 15-19).

Exposure was carried out posteriorly under local infiltration. The bifid spinous process of C6 was easily identified. The C7 spinous process and laminae were completely removed along with the inferior portion of the spine of C6 and the upper portion of D1 with their associated laminae. The spinal canal was opened, the dura and cord being protected with cottonoid patties. Removal of bone was carried out laterally through the fused area of the posterior joints, the eighth nerve root being thoroughly

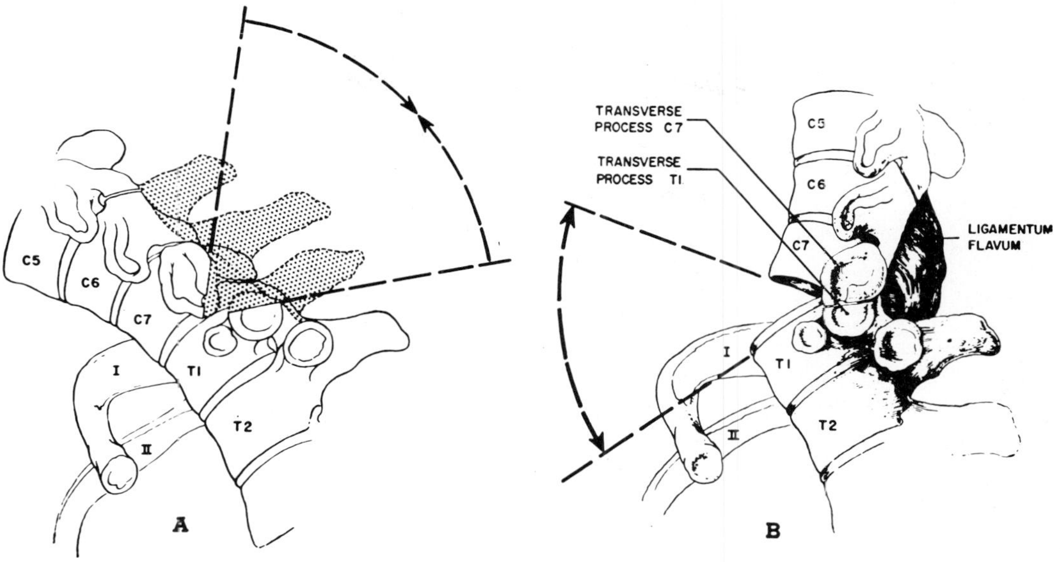

FIG. 15-21. Diagram of area of section before (*A*) and after (*B*) extension osteotomy.

decompressed. Approximately 1¼ cm. to 1½ cm. of bone was removed on both sides laterally, with slight beveling upwards and downwards so that following correction the two surfaces would be parallel and in apposition (Fig. 15-20). The patient was able to assist with operative localization, indicating at any time when the eighth nerve root was irritated. This was of real value during the course of the decompression. The cord was decompressed above and below posteriorly to avoid any impingement when the neck was straightened. The upper portion of the transverse process of D1 was ronguered away, as was the inferior portion of the transverse process of C7.

When the decompression had been completely carried out the patient was given a small amount of nitrous oxide and fluothane. He held the mask himself and when he was no longer able to hold it, his chin was then slowly elevated until the spine fractured in front (Fig. 15-21). The gap then closed up posteriorly on each side, the lateral masses coming together, the central portion being left open to allow buckling of the dura without any impinge-

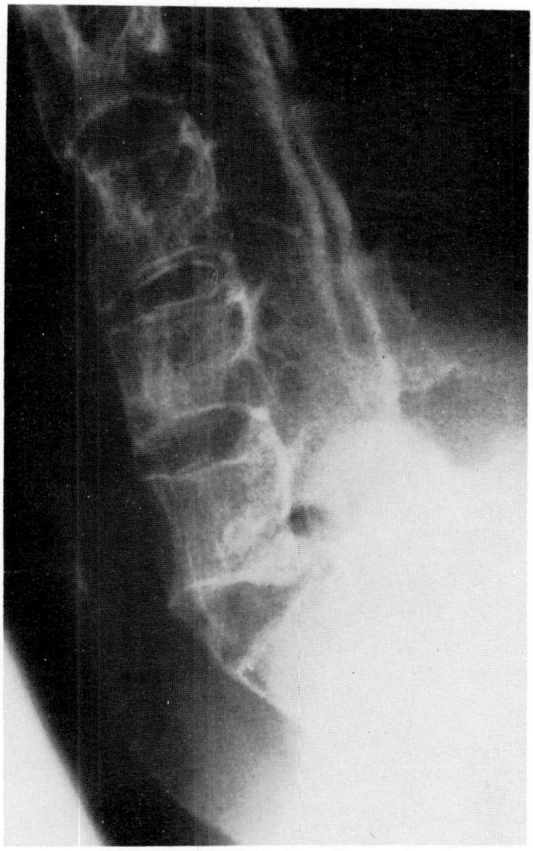

FIG. 15-22. Lateral radiograph of cervical spine showing postoperative correction and fusion at osteotomy site.

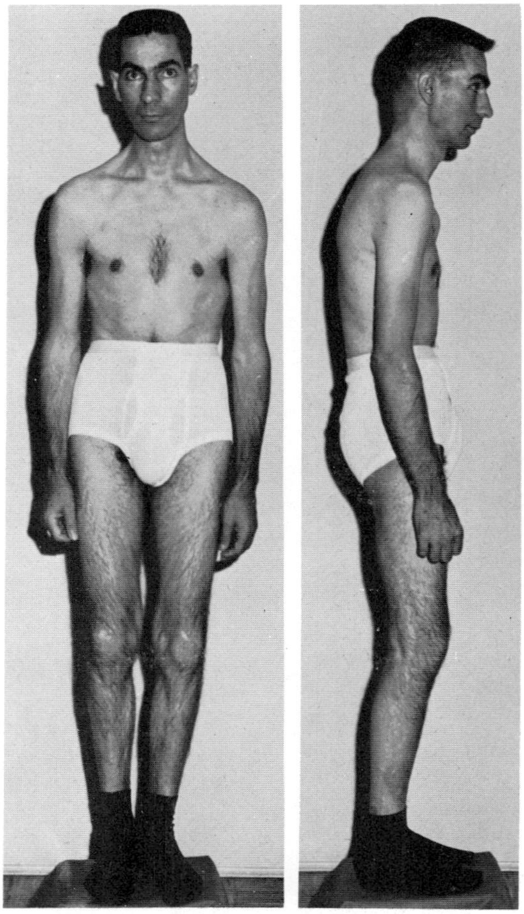

FIG. 15-23. Postoperative standing anterior and lateral views of patient. Compromise has been achieved between looking ahead for walking and being able to work at a desk. The patient selected the exact position in which he wished his head.

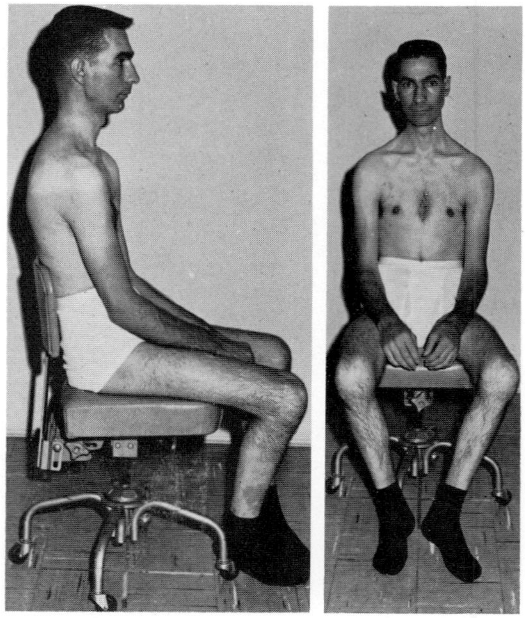

FIG. 15-24. Postoperative anterior and lateral sitting views of patient showing ability to sit effectively at his occupation as a clerk.

ment. The opposing bony surfaces came together posteriorly on each side quite well; this allowed adequate fusion later. Routine closure was carried out with suction drainage. The head was then stabilized with the plaster supporting unit incorporated into the halo apparatus. The patient was allowed to awaken. He was able to move all four limbs quite easily without any neurological complications. His neck was then further extended until adequate correction was obtained. With excessive correction he developed some numbness along the left fifth finger. This was eased by turning his head slightly to the right. The patient was then able to stand and walk over to his bed.

The postoperative course was quite uneventful. The patient was nursed on a Circo-Electric bed and was ambulant within a few days of his operation. He was discharged to a convalescent center 6 weeks postoperatively. His neck was splinted for 4 months postoperatively. He went on to solid bony union (Fig. 15-22). After discharge he was able to work as a clerk.

This patient illustrates the importance of not over-correcting the deformity. Such patients must have a compromise between looking ahead for walking and being able to work at a desk. The patient himself selected the position in which he wished to hold his head. He is now able to look straight ahead while walking and is able to work quite effectively at a desk (Figs. 15-23 and 15-24).

This technique has been applied to six consecutive patients without significant mod-

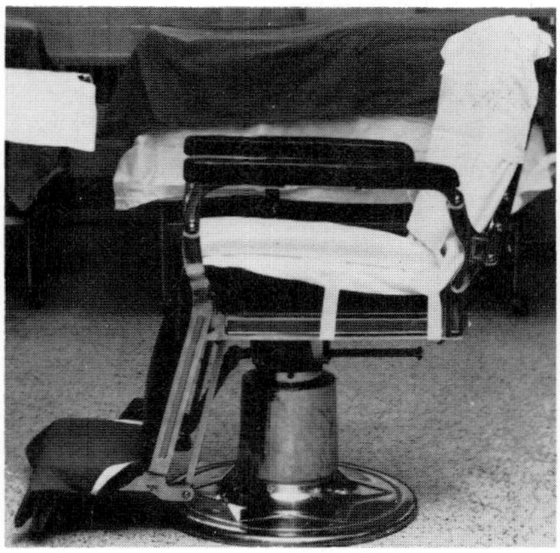

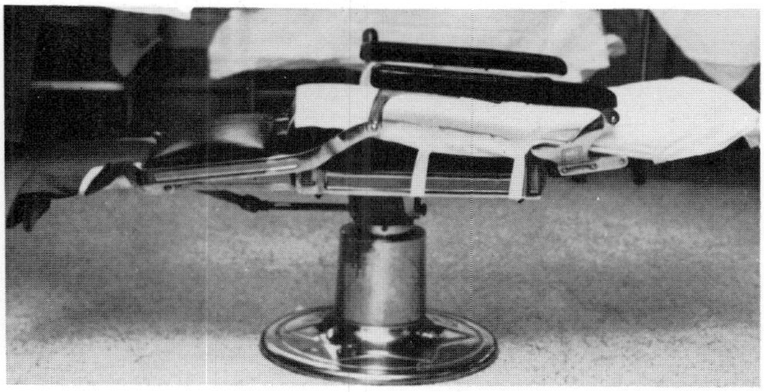

FIG. 15-25. Dental type chair allows patient to sit comfortably at operating table and can be readily put into recumbent position if needed.

ification and with equal success. Correction was carried out under local anesthesia. At the end of the procedure, each patient was able to walk from the operating table to his Circo-Electric bed. There has been no mortality and no major morbidity.

Special Technical Considerations. Further points concerning technique merit discussion. The bifid spine of C6 is a very valuable localizing anatomical sign, and in most instances it is sufficiently obvious so as to make anatomical localization very definitive. However, in one patient with a high dorsal forward curve as well as cervical deformity, difficulty was encountered with false localization of what appeared to be a bifid spine, this being at a lower level. When the neck did not straighten easily, the procedure was discontinued. The false localization was later indicated by radiographs; secondary correction was carried out. If there is any question about the localization of the level at operation, this should be confirmed radiographically. Before any correction of a flexion deformity of the cervical spine is carried out, it is important to check for radiographic evidence of instability at the atlantoaxial junction, since this could be aggravated by undue extension manipulation during operative correction.

Excessive force is not required to fracture the spine in front at the C7/D1 level providing adequate decompression has been carried out posteriorly. If the spine does not correct easily after what appears to be an adequate decompression posteriorly the operator must make sure that no bridge of bone has been left laterally which prevents the spine from closing behind and opening in front. He must also check that the correct level has been operated upon.

In an effort to avoid any undue force at the craniocervical junction, care is taken to direct the head and neck backward in a fairly straight fashion instead of forcefully angulating the head and neck upward into extension.

Because of concern on the part of the anesthetists over the fixed sitting position and the potential difficulties of placing the patient in the recumbent position in the event that resuscitation is required, we have adopted a dental-type chair which allows the patient to sit comfortably during the procedure and which can be readily straightened out to the horizontal position if required (Fig. 15-25).

Although an attempt is made to obtain full or nearly full correction at the time of the operative procedure, this may be limited by tightness of the anterior sternomastoid and strap musculature, by discomfort, or by fear on the part of the patient that he is going to be over-corrected. Further correction and adjustment can be carried out during the course of convalescence when the patient is over the initial discomforts and there has been some time for loosening of the anterior musculature. The latter may be facilitated by some gentle head and neck massage.

At this stage the patient can be rested in the recumbent position on his back and under Innovar sedation. The supports for the halo are detached while the operator carefully supports the head. The neck can then be fully extended to the desired position and the supports of the halo reattached.

REFERENCES

1. Bonnet, G.: Two cases of atlantoaxial dislocation without spinal or medullary symptoms; failure of orthopaedic treatment; bolting with Albee graft as a precaution. Internat. Abstr. Surg., *58*:358, 1934.
2. Harris, R. I.: New investigations: instrument for tightening knots in steel wire. Lancet, *1*:504, 1944.
3. Herbert, J. J.: Vertebral osteotomy, technique, indications, and results. J. Bone Joint Surg., *30*:680-689, 1948.
4. ———: Vertebral osteotomy for kyphosis, especially in Marie-Strümpell arthritis. A report on 50 cases. J. Bone Joint Surg., *41*:291-302, 1959.
5. La Chapelle, E. H.: Osteotomy of the lumbar spine for correction of kyphosis in a case of ankylosing spondylarthritis. J. Bone Joint Surg., *28*:851-858, 1946.
6. Law, W. A.: Lumbar spinal osteotomy. J. Bone Joint Surg. [Brit.], *41*:270-278, 1959.
7. Little, A. H., Urowitz, M. B., and Rosen, P. S.: Spondylodiscitis—an unusual feature of ankylosing spondylitis. Presented to the American Rheumatology Association, Detroit, Michigan, June 1970. (Submitted for publication)
8. Mixter, S. J., and Osgood, R. B.: Traumatic lesion of the atlas and axis. Ann. Surg., *51*:193-207, 1910.
9. Nunziata, A.: Osteotomia de la columna. Operacion de Smith-Petersen. Prensa med Argent, *35*:1536, 1948.
10. Schulitz, K. P.: Destruktive Veränderungen an Wirbelkörpern bei der Spondylarthritis ankylopoetica. Arch. Orthop. Unfallchir., *64*:116-134, 1968.
11. Simmons, E. H.: The surgical correction of flexion deformity of the cervical spine in ankylosing spondylitis. Presented to the Canadian Orthopaedic Association Meeting, Bermuda, June, 1968. (Submitted for publication.)
12. Simmons, E. H., and Fielding, J. W.: Atlantoaxial arthrodesis by the Gallie technique. J. Bone Joint Surg. (Abstr.), *49*:1022, 1967. (Submitted for publication)
13. Smith-Petersen, M. N., Larson, C. B., and Aufranc, O. E.: Osteotomy of the spine for correction of flexion deformity in rheumatoid arthritis. J. Bone Joint Surg., *27*:1-11, 1945.
14. Urist, M. R.: Osteotomy of the cervical spine, report of case of ankylosing rheumatoid spondylitis. J. Bone Joint Surg., *40*:833-843, 1958.
15. Willard, D., and Nicholson, J. T.: Dislocation of the first cervical vertebra. Ann. Surg., *113*:464-475, 1941.
16. Wilson, M. J., and Turkell, J. H.: Multiple spinal wedged osteotomy: its use in a case of Marie-Strümpell spondylitis. Am. J. Surg., *77*:777-782, 1949.

CHAPTER 16

Synovectomy in Children

ALICE L. GARRETT, M.D., AND CRAIG CAMPBELL, M.D.

Although medical literature throughout the world reflects the surge of interest in synovectomy in rheumatoid arthritis, most of the reported subjects are adults, although some children have been studied.[5-15] This may possibly be explained by the lower incidence of the disease and its different manifestations in children.[1-4]

INDICATIONS

The indications for the operation are easy to state but difficult to apply. Synovectomy is indicated before permanent damage has occurred but after the possibility of a remission has passed. The problem lies in determining the prognosis of a patient. Statistics from various studies show that approximately one-half of the patients will have no residual joint problems, whereas one-quarter to one-third will have a chronic, progressive course. However, in the early stages it is difficult to know just which course the disease will pursue in a particular child.

The ideal candidate for synovectomy is one who has persistent synovitis with excessive fluid in a few joints. The patient with the worst prognosis is one who has little excess synovial fluid and who has had no remissions. The conditions of the vast majority of patients are somewhere between these two stages.

In children, pain is not as reliable an index of disease activity as it is in adults; children may avoid pain by automatically decreasing their activity. When they or their parents are questioned about pain, they may deny it; yet, when asked to move the extremity through a full range of motion or to perform a forceful activity, they will experience pain. Therefore, loss of function or a contracture may be a better indicator than pain.

A STUDY OF SYNOVECTOMIES IN JUVENILE RHEUMATOID ARTHRITIS

During the past 8 years at Rancho Los Amigos Hospital, 41 synovectomies were done on 13 children wtih juvenile rheumatoid arthritis. One patient refused to return for evaluation, and one patient moved from the area after only 1 year of follow-up. This left 11 patients with 34 synovectomies for study. These patients were reviewed in an attempt to answer the following questions:

1. Does synovectomy halt the disease process locally?
2. Will joint stiffness follow synovectomy in children?
3. Does synovectomy affect growth?
4. Is this much surgery justified in children with juvenile rheumatoid arthritis?

There were eight girls and three boys in this group of 11 patients. The age of onset varied from 1½ years to 12 years, with eight of the children being younger than 6, and only one over 10. All had a severe form of the disease. All had multiple joint involvement; none had complete remissions. Only one had a hemoglobin that did not fall to ten or less at some time. Only four did not have at least one of the following manifestations: subcutaneous nodules, positive serology, or proteinuria.

The follow-up period varied from 2 to 7½ years. A clinical examination was made of each surgical area for pain, range of motion, and function, and this evaluation was compared with the preoperative status. Pre- and postoperative x-rays were also compared, and an attempt was made to correlate these with the findings at surgery.

The 34 synovectomies performed and evaluated reflect the pattern of joint involvement in children. Thirteen were performed on the upper extremities. Seven involved the dorsum of the wrist; four, the proximal interphalangeal joints of the hand, including the interphalangeal joint of the thumb; one, the metacarpophalangeal joints of the hand; and another, the flexor tendons of the hand. In the lower extremities, the 21 procedures included 13 knees, six hips, and two multiple ankle tendons.

Upper Extremity Joints

There were seven synovectomies of the tendons of the dorsum of the wrist in four patients. Through a curvilinear incision, the diseased synovium was removed from the involved tendons. The joint was not entered. In closing, the dorsal carpal ligament was placed deep to the extensor tendons. The follow-up period of these patients was from 2 to 6 years. Pain was abolished or markedly diminished in all. Strength of grasp and function increased in all but one wrist. One patient has had a recurrence of synovitis and has lost a few degrees of extreme flexion; however, pain and function remain markedly improved. The remaining five wrists maintained their preoperative range or gained slightly.

The one patient who had flexor tendon synovectomy is now 2 years postoperative with no recurrence of synovitis. Pain was abolished and function increased, but at the present time her index-finger MCP and IP joints have lost 15° to 20° of flexion.

Five synovectomies were performed in hands. This included bilateral PIP and thumb IP joints in two patients and the MCP joints in one patient. Follow-up was between 3 and 4 years. All five had continued partial relief of pain and slight improvement in function. Improvement was not as dramatic in this group as in those who had synovectomy of the dorsum of the wrist, but disability was also not as severe preoperatively. Four of the five hands either gained in range or maintained their good preoperative range. The flexion range of the PIP joints decreased in one hand with recurrence of synovitis 4 years later. The patient's range of motion with this hand is 60° of flexion, and she has mild pain on heavy activity.

Lower Extremity Joints

One patient had synovectomies of the tendons about both ankles. Two years later there was no recurrence or pain, and the preoperative deformities on the ankles had decreased.

The 13 cases of knee synovectomy in eight children formed the largest group. The follow-up was from 2 to 7½ years, with the majority followed for over 4 years. Prior to surgery, all patients had pain at rest or pain on motion, and all had swollen knees with active synovitis. The procedure was done through a medial parapatellar incision. All the children had diminution of pain. Six knees in four children are now pain-free. The remaining seven knees in four children have pain only intermittently or after walking a distance.

The knee joint was the most difficult of all to mobilize postoperatively. Over half of the patients had manipulation of the knee under general anesthesia 3 to 4 weeks postoperatively in addition to a concentrated exercise program both before and after surgery. The range of flexion was either increased slightly or the same as before in 11 knees. The other two lost flexion range, but only one did not obtain at least 90°. This

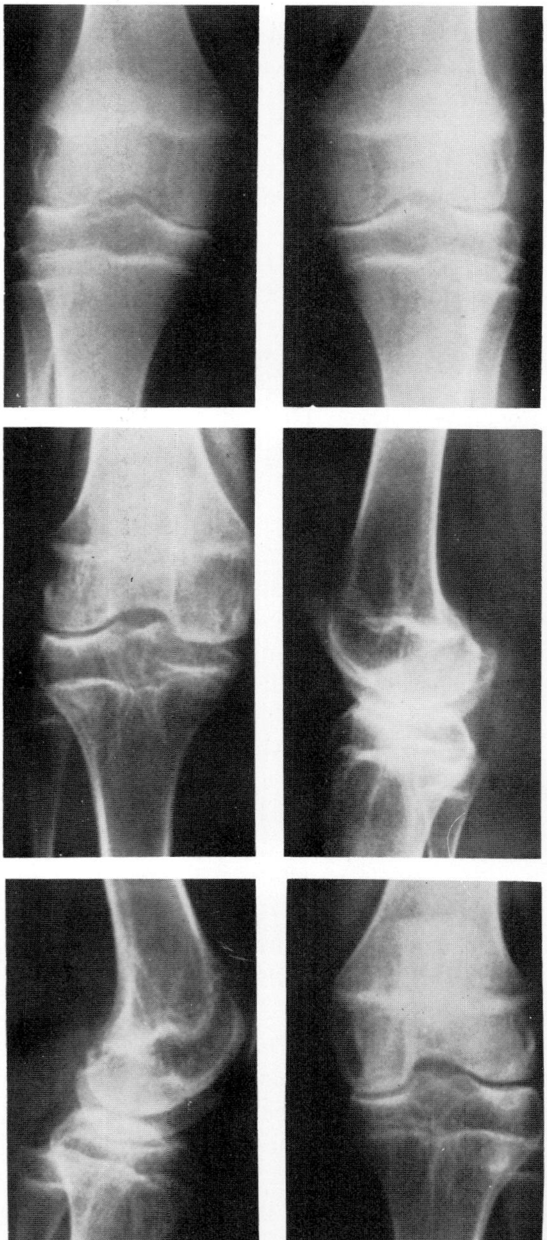

FIG. 16-1. (*Top*) Preoperative x-rays of knee of 14-year-old girl. Right knee moderately destroyed, left slightly. (*Center*) Right knee, 2½ years postop; marked diminution of pain, slight limitation in flexion to 90°, but not a normal knee. (*Bottom*) Left knee 2½ years postop; good range of motion, no pain, good preservation of knee joint.

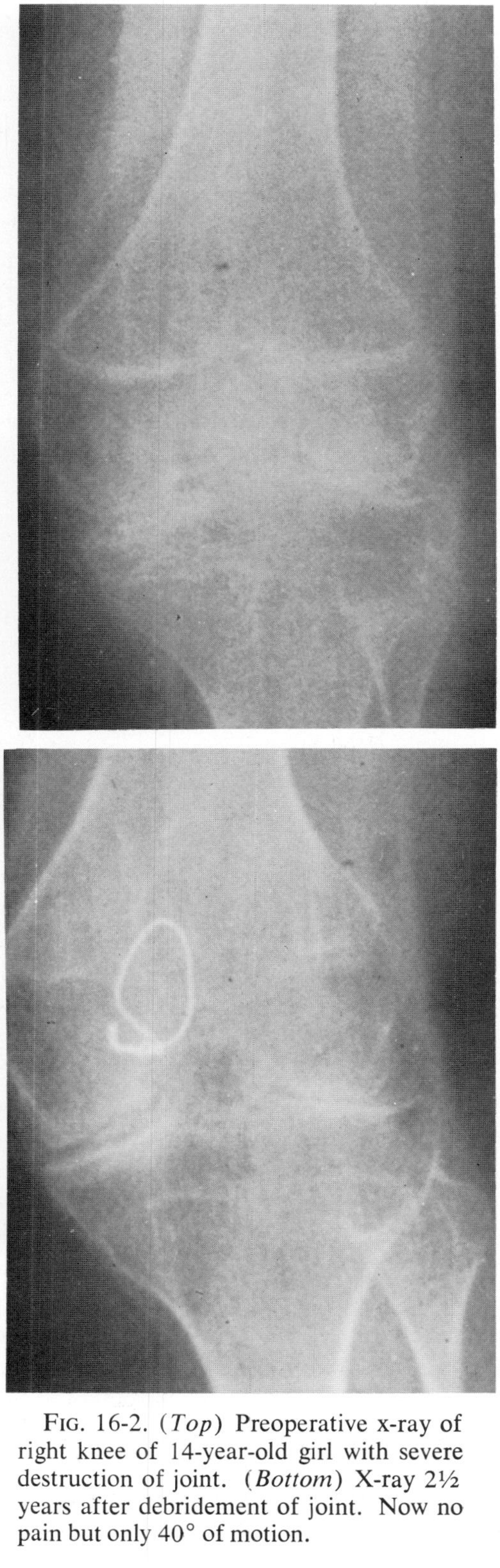

FIG. 16-2. (*Top*) Preoperative x-ray of right knee of 14-year-old girl with severe destruction of joint. (*Bottom*) X-ray 2½ years after debridement of joint. Now no pain but only 40° of motion.

knee had a range of only 40° and was pain-free. Full extension was obtained in three knees, and five knees lacked only 5° of extension. The remaining five had flexion contractures of 15° to 35°; one had the same contracture preoperatively, one gained 10° from a 30° contracture, but three lost range. There were, therefore, five knees which lost range of motion either in flexion or extension. These five knees had moderate to severe destruction of the joint apparent at surgery.

At the time of surgery no joint was normal, but in seven, erosions were present only around the cruciate and collateral ligaments and not on the weight-bearing surface (Fig. 16-1A). Of these seven, five were pain-free and all seven either maintained a good range of motion or increased their range (Figs. 16-1B, and C). Six knees showed moderate to severe changes (Fig. 16-2) including loss of cartilage on the weight-bearing surface and ligamentous and meniscus destruction. Of these, only one was completely pain-free and only one did not lose some range of motion.

Change in function was difficult to assess because of other joint involvement. However, it can be stated that those children in whom walking was limited only by knee pain all improved. The others who had limitation in walking were restricted by hip pain.

Hips

Six synovectomies were performed on the hips of four patients. Preoperatively, the patients all had pain that prevented ambulation or caused marked limitation of motion. An anterior Smith-Petersen approach was used in the first four. In the other two, lateral U-shaped incisions were made and the abductor muscles were taken down and reattached after the synovectomies were completed. These were all partial synovectomies with approximately 75 per cent of the synovium removed. None had the joint dislocated, and the posterior capsule was not disturbed in order to preserve the retinacular blood supply to the femoral head. All of the other joints had moderate to abundant amounts of pannus. In one case, abundant rice bodies were found.

The first patient had had pain in the right hip for several years, but in the left for only 3 to 4 months; as a result of the involvement of the second hip, she was nearly bedridden. At surgery, the synovium of the right hip was found to be fibrotic and adherent to the femoral neck. It was felt that the time for synovectomy had long since passed, so the procedure done was actually a flexion contracture release, including excision of the anterior capsule but without an iliopsoas release. The range of motion of this hip was restored quickly and easily, and pain was markedly relieved. Three weeks later the left hip was opened and 75 per cent of the abundant synovium was removed. Pain was relieved and range of motion readily improved. For about 3½ years, her hips continued to do well despite recurrent severe exacerbations of the disease. During the last 1½ years, range of motion has decreased, pain has recurred, and her x-rays are showing degenerative changes.

The second patient had a right hip synovectomy 5 years ago and has maintained a good range of motion without pain. His x-ray 5 years later showed some deterioration (Fig. 16-3).

The third patient had surgery at the age of 20 years. His joint was filled with rice bodies and the synovial fluid was under pressure. There was marked destruction of the articular cartilage but no pannus in the area of destruction. His pain was not relieved, and he had a cup arthroplasty 1 year later.

The last patient had bilateral synovectomies 2 years ago through a lateral U-shaped incision which permitted a complete excision of synovium. She has maintained range of motion and has no pain. One year later, x-rays showed a good joint space. Films taken 2 years after operation, however, showed a decrease in joint space and early cystic degeneration (Fig. 16-4).

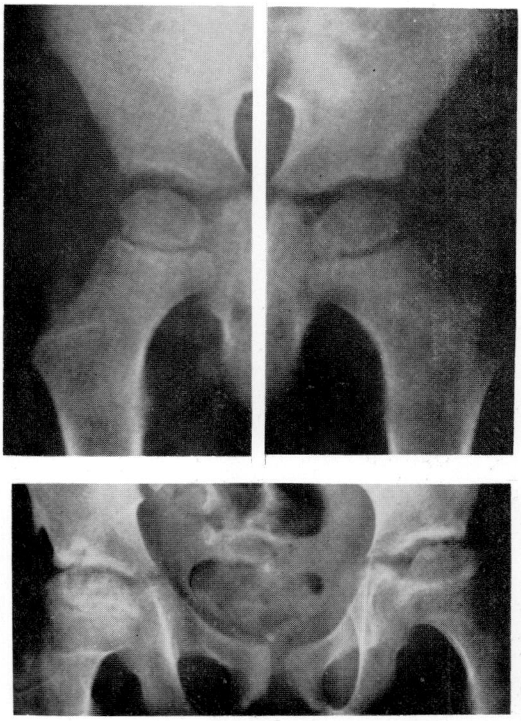

FIG. 16-3. (*A*) Radiographs of a right hip before synovectomy. (*B*) Five years after the operation there are degenerative changes, but the patient remains asymptomatic.

EVALUATION OF RESULTS

To return to the original four questions:

Does synovectomy halt the disease locally? With recurrence of swelling and fluid in two hands and ten knees, this claim cannot be made. However, it must be noted that despite this, function has been maintained and pain at least partially relieved. Even the hip and knee joints showing deterioration on x-ray are still improved over the preoperative status. The progressive deterioration of the hips seen on x-ray is discouraging. The use of the lateral incision, enabling removal of more synovium and release of the iliopsoas may improve the results. Ambulation was prolonged in the first patient for 4 years and the second has no difficulty at 5 years. If this procedure only enables a patient to be active until the age when an arthroplasty can be performed, it will still be useful.

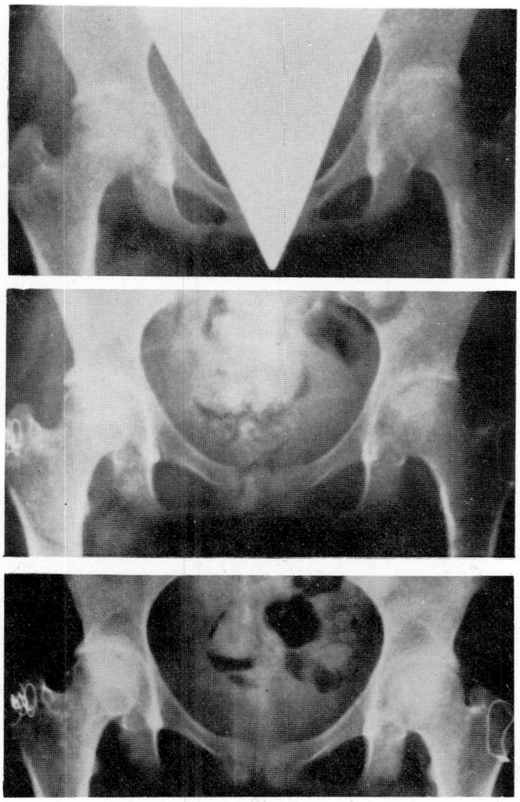

FIG. 16-4. (*Top*) Preoperative hip x-rays; patient was non-ambulatory because of hip pain. Bilateral hip synovectomy was indicated. (*Center*) One year after surgery; patient asymptomatic. (*Bottom*) Two years after surgery the patient remains asymptomatic.

Will joint stiffness follow synovectomy in children? This small series does establish that an adequate range of motion can be obtained in children following synovectomy. The knee joint appears to be the most difficult to mobilize, but even in this joint a good range of motion is possible if the surgery is not delayed too long and if an intensive pre- and postoperative exercise program is employed.

Does synovectomy affect growth? Firm conclusions cannot be drawn from so few patients. The only leg-length discrepancy found is in a child who had a synovectomy 7 years ago on the right knee and bilateral hip synovectomies 5 years ago. The hip joint changes also present account for most of the discrepancy. One hip and three knee synovectomies, all unilateral, produced no leg-length discrepancy.

Is this much surgery justified? Every patient has a limit to the number of surgical procedures that he can tolerate. In polio patients the limit is high. The consistent pain relief and increase in function would indicate the level is equally high for rheumatoid children.

REFERENCES

1. Ansell, B. M., and Bywaters, E. G.: Rheumatoid arthritis (Still's Disease). Pediat. Clin. N. Amer., *10*:921-939, 1963.
2. Brewer, E. J., Blattner, R. J., and Wing, H.: Treatment of rheumatoid arthritis in children. Pediat. Clin. N. Amer., *10*:207-224, 1963.
3. Calabro, J., and Morchesano, J. M.: The early natural history of juvenile rheumatoid arthritis. Med. Clin. N. Amer., *52*:567-591, 1968.
4. Juvenile Rheumatoid Arthritis. *In* Christian, Charles L. (ed): 18th Rheumatism Review, Review of American and English Literature for Years 1965-1966. Arthritis Rheum. (Suppl. 3), *2*:568-570.
5. Eyring, E. J.: The therapeutic potential of synovectomy in juvenile arthritis. Arthritis Rheum., *11*:688-692, 1968.
6. Fink, C. W., Beum, J., Paradies, L. H., and Carroll, B. C.: Synovectomy in juvenile rheumatoid arthritis. Ann. Rheum. Dis., *28*:612-616, 1969.
7. Gulish, E.: Synovectomies performed on children with Still's Disease. Resident's paper at Rancho Los Amigos Hospital.
8. Hanson, V., and Kornreich, H.: The rheumatic diseases of childhood. Postgrad. Med., *45*:192-197, 1969.
9. Jakubowski, S., and Ruszczynska, J.: The possibility of surgical treatment in cases of juvenile rheumatoid arthritis. Acta Rheum. Scand., *13*:113-118, 1967.
10. Laine, V.: Early synovectomy in rheumatoid arthritis. Ann. Rev. Med., *18*:173-183, 1967.
11. Laurin, C. A., and Favreau, J. C.: Rheumatoid disease in children. Canad. Med. Ass. J., *89*:288-301, 1963.
12. London, P. S.: Synovectomy of the knee in rheumatoid arthritis. J. Bone Joint Surg. [Brit.], *37*:392-399, 1955.
13. Martel, S., Holt, J. F., and Cassidy, J. T.: Roentgenologic manifestations of juvenile rheumatoid arthritis. Amer. J. Roentgen., *88*:400-423.
14. Polakowa, I., Ruszczynska, J., and Duchowska, H.: The dynamics of the disease process in cases of juvenile rheumatoid arthritis when surgical treatment is applied. Acta Rheum. Scand., *12*:287-290, 1966.
15. Sbarbaro, J. L., and Vance, P.: Early synovectomy in juvenile rheumatoid arthritis. J. Med. Soc. N.J., *65*:504-506, 1968.

CHAPTER 17

The Rheumatoid Shoulder

CHARLES S. NEER II, M.D.

The shoulder is one of the more frequent sites of rheumatoid arthritis. Yet, while much attention has been given to the hand, wrist, hip and foot, there has been a conspicuous silence regarding the surgical management of the rheumatoid shoulder. There are several reasons for this: (1) the onset of the disease in the shoulder is often insidious; (2) the glenohumeral joint is deeply seated and escapes notice unless specifically examined; (3) the importance of the influence of the protective posture of the shoulder upon the upper extremity unit (neck, elbow, wrist and hand) has not been adequately appreciated; (4) patients who suffer disabling arthritis of their weight-bearing joints are, in general, rather complacent about their shoulders; and (5) since the shoulder is comprised of four joints with great mobility, complex muscle couplings, and a number of gliding surfaces and bursae, all of which may be involved in the disuse, its postoperative rehabilitation can be especially discouraging.

Insidious nature of onset. The shoulder occupies a considerable segment of the anatomy between the neck and the hand, and any one of a number of structures may be affected. The onset of the disease is variable but initially tends to be subacute and transitory rather than constant and destructive. With each attack the painful joint is splinted against the chest. This leads to disuse and stiffness with loss of external rotation and abduction. The reduction in range is the basis of a second source of pain, that felt at the extremes of movement when the shortened ligaments and muscles are brought under tension. The patient learns to avoid these positions and to function within a limited range, which subsequently leads to more stiffness and more pain. The vicious cycle of a "frozen shoulder" continues until eventually the arm is fixed to the chest. This process is usually reversible by conservative treatment based on functional exercises and whatever analgesic and anti-inflammatory modalities are needed. Characteristically, many months are required before granulation tissue offers a significant impediment to recovery or roentgen evidence of bony changes becomes apparent.

Detection of shoulder arthritis. Shoulder arthritis early in the reversible state—prior to bone atrophy and fixed postural deformities—has too often gone unrecognized. The patient should be examined sitting on a low stool in a well-lighted room, stripped to the waist. The neck, both shoulders, elbows and hands should be evaluated. Swelling and tenderness over the superficially located sternoclavicular and acromioclavicular joints should be noted. Referred pain on tilting or rotating the cervical spine is an important indication for further investigation at that level. The most sensitive index of glenohumeral arthritis is limitation of external rotation along with joint-line tenderness posteriorly as well as anteriorly.

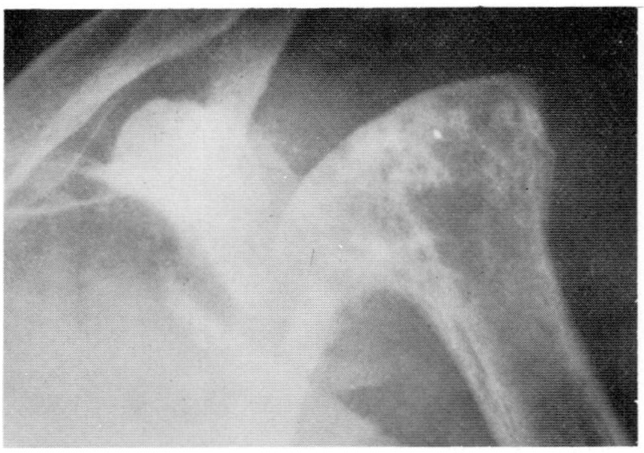

FIG. 17-1. Steroid arthropathy following repeated intra-articular injections of hydrocortisone. Note the Charcot-like changes. Pain and disability were relieved by replacement arthroplasty, which differed from the usual procedure in that the distended capsule was plicated and the arm was immobilized for 5 weeks following surgery.

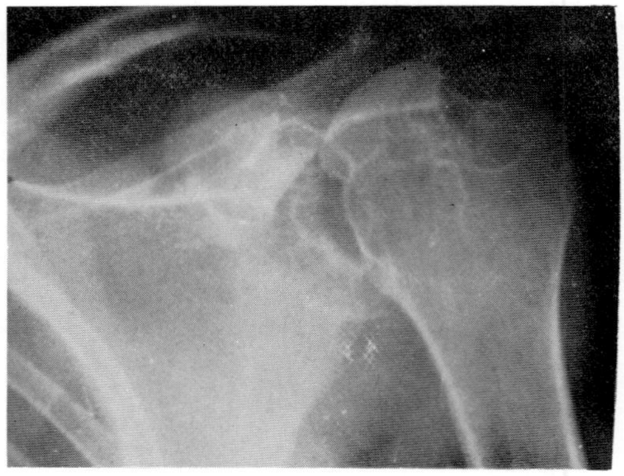

FIG. 17-2. The typical roentgen appearance of marginal erosion of the head in a 29-year-old woman with severe generalized disease, shoulder pain of 5 years duration, and ankylosis of the opposite shoulder. At surgery, the joint was filled with proliferating synovial and granulation tissue, and the articular surface had been completely destroyed.

Influence on the upper extremity unit. The protective position of the shoulder, with the arm at the side in internal rotation, is accompanied by flexion of the elbow, flexion and ulnar deviation at the wrist, and ulnar drift and extension of the fingers. Thus, the painful shoulder enhances the development of deformities throughout the length of the extremity.

Attitude of the patient. It is always much more difficult to rehabilitate patients with bilateral shoulder disease, as is often present in rheumatoid arthritis, than those with one good upper extremity. If in addition the patient is distracted by disabling lower extremity arthritis and more conspicuous hand deformities, it becomes even more difficult to obtain the cooperation that is so essential to the proper management of shoulder problems. Any program of stretching or strengthening exercises must be realistic and workable, and the patient should be encouraged by the surgeon when he sees even minor progress.

Role of surgical treatment. Since the onset of shoulder arthritis is usually low grade, the reversible state extends over a long period of time. If recognized early, fixed contractures can usually be eliminated by medical and physiotherapeutic measures. The surgeon must appreciate the value of judicious steroid injections (Fig. 17-1) and the importance of stretching and strengthening exercises during this period. In a few patients, accumulation of granulation tissue acts as a mechanical barrier to the recovery of range of motion and threatens the articular surfaces (Fig. 17-2); this is the irreversible state. In these patients, when conservative treatment has failed and boggy synovial thickenings are palpable, synovectomy and, in the case of the glenohumeral joint, capsular releases are indicated. In the advanced stages, when the articular surfaces have been destroyed, arthroplasty should be considered and can be of great benefit (Figs. 17-2, 3).

INDICATIONS AND CONTRAINDICATIONS

Glenohumeral Joint. Except for loss of motion following surgery, we see no place for manipulation under anesthesia in the treatment of the rheumatoid shoulder. The osteoporotic bone may fracture. If adequate conservative measures fail, capsular release and synovectomy are preferred.

We no longer believe that bicipital tenosynovitis alone constitutes a barrier to recovery by conservative means. The tendon sheath of the long head of the biceps is a part of the glenohumeral joint space, as can be readily demonstrated in an arthrogram. Inflammatory changes and granulation tissue here are only a small portion of the disease process within the remainder of the joint. It is only the visible peak of the iceberg. Surgery limited to this site has been inadequate and disappointing. A capsular release and synovectomy is thought to be more thorough and rational.

The subacromial bursa is rarely involved as an isolated problem. Chronic thickening of this bursa is usually associated with attrition and disruption of the supraspinatus tendon which may communicate with an arthritic joint. In rare cases enlargement of this bursa may act as a deterrent to recovery and require excision, but more often this procedure is done in conjunction with synovectomy and cuff repair.

If fixed contractures and chronic synovial thickening are preventing recovery after adequate conservative treatment, synovectomy and capsular release is indicated. During this procedure the sheath for the tendon of the long head of the biceps, the subacromial bursa, and the outer clavicle may or may not require excision. Attrition defects in the rotator cuff can usually be repaired by direct suture. The subscapularis tendon may require lengthening for adequate external rotation.

If the humeral articular surface has been destroyed by granulation tissue or its contour altered to prevent movement, in addition to synovectomy and capsular release and what other local procedures are indicated, a replacement prosthesis is inserted.[1] When the head has been destroyed by granulation tissue (see Fig. 17-2), it is obvious that a prosthesis is needed. In low-grade or burned-out disease with secondary osteoarthritic changes, it is at times tempting to remove the ridges and excrescences and simply reshape the head. However, the results of this procedure have been disappointing, and we now prefer a prosthesis in this situation as well. In bilateral shoulder disease, we perform the arthroplasty on the most disabled side and give that shoulder time for advanced recovery before considering surgery on the other shoulder.

Arthrodesis is no longer performed in rheumatoid patients, because it entails an undesirable period of immobilization of the elbow and ablates the rotary movements of the shoulder that are so important for personal hygiene, especially since movement of both shoulders is usually restricted. Radical acromionectomy weakens the deltoid and is contraindicated.

Acromioclavicular Joint. Swelling, tenderness, and pain on adduction of the arm across the chest indicate arthritis at this site. This may be controlled by steroid injection and medical therapy. If symptoms persist, synovectomy and excision of that portion of the clavicle distal to the coracoclavicular ligaments is indicated.

Sternoclavicular Joint. The indication for resection of the inner end of the clavicle (proximal to the costoclavicular ligament) and synovectomy is persistent pain on movement of this joint that cannot be relieved by steroid injection and conservative treatment.

Shoulder Syndromes. Disabling tenderness and pain along the medial border of the scapula, *scapulocostal syndrome,* may be relieved by local steroid injection. Referred pain from the cervical region can be differentiated by the relation of pain to cervical motion and the relative lack of local tenderness.

Vasomotor changes and stiffness of the hand, *shoulder-hand syndrome,* may be augmented by shoulder disease. We have observed improvement in the rheumatoid hand

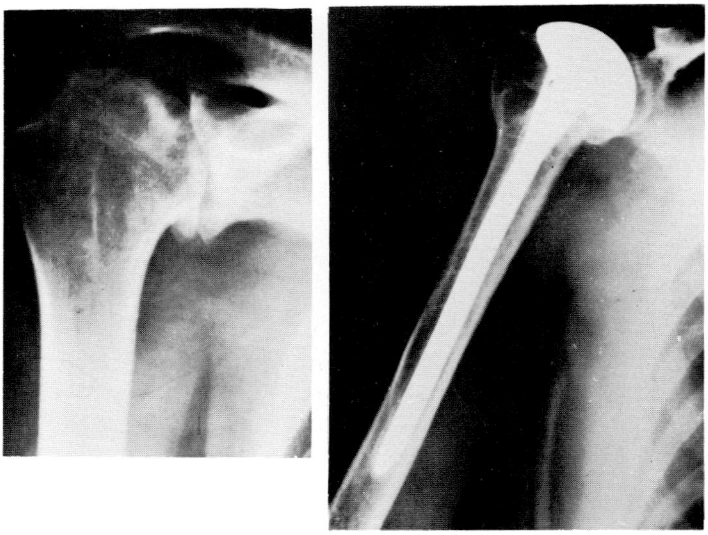

FIG. 17-3. Anteroposterior films to show secondary osteoarthritic changes in the glenohumeral joint, acromioclavicular arthritis, and the successful arthroplasty in a 47-year-old woman with "burned-out" rheumatoid arthritis. (*Left*) The humeral and scapular joint surfaces were eroded, and motion was blocked by osteophytes, which were largest along the inferior and posterior margins of the head. (*Right*) Postoperative film after excision of the outer end of the clavicle and glenohumeral arthroplasty.

in some patients following arthroplasty or correction of shoulder contractures. Sympathectomy has not been employed for this purpose.

It must be emphasized that we do not consider *bicipital tendinitis* as an isolated entity, especially in the treatment of rheumatoid arthritis.

OPERATIVE TECHNIQUES

Glenohumeral Arthroplasty

It is expedient to discuss the complete procedure, because this can be adapted to the individual case, depending upon the pathology and structures involved. The steps in the procedure of capsular release and synovectomy are the same as those when a prosthesis is used.

Because preoperative preparation of the skin is usually handicapped by pain and contractures, a scrupulous cleansing and adherent plastic drapes are important steps. A 5-inch curved incision is made, starting at the anterior acromion, passing just lateral to the coracoid, swinging lateral to avoid the axillary skin creases, and stopping just below the level of the circumflex vessels. The deltopectoral interval, just medial to this incision, is spread. The cephalic vein is ligated, and the anterior three inches of the deltoid is detached from the clavicle and anterior acromion.

If the acromioclavicular joint is diseased, the lateral end of the clavicle is excised (Fig. 17-3). The underneath edge of the anterior process of the acromion is usually prominent and an "anterior acromioplasty" is performed. In this procedure, the anterior edge of the acromion with the attachment of the coraco-acromial ligament is removed by beveling horizontally with a thin three-quarter inch osteotome. The subacromial space is increased as much as possible. The coraco-acromial ligament is excised with this wedge shaped fragment. This type of acromioplasty removes the anterior impingement and does not interfere with reattachment of the deltoid. Radical acromionectomy is now thought to be harmful. If the acromioclavicular joint was symptomatic or is enlarged, the lateral end of the clavicle is excised at the time of the acromioplasty. The thickened subacromial bursa is next removed along with any bony irregularities of the greater tuberosity.

The clavipectoral is divided just lateral to the coracoid muscles. With the arm externally rotated, the subscapularis tendon is identified with a stay-suture and detached about 1 inch medial to the lesser tuberosity, leaving sufficient tendon attached to the

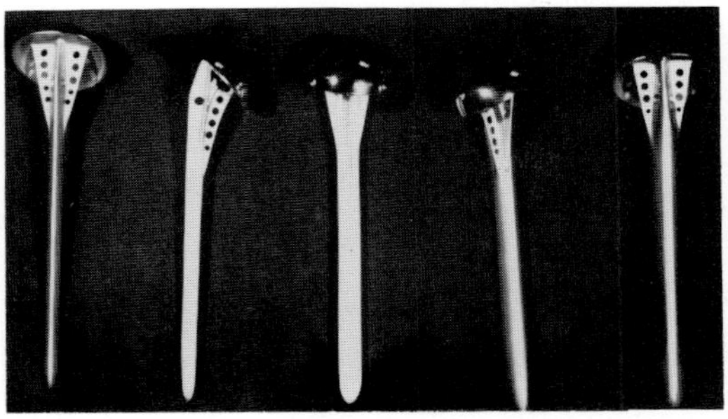

FIG. 17-4. The Vitallium prosthesis used to replace only that portion of bone normally covered by articular cartilage. It is made with five graduated stem sizes, each with drill specifications. A snug fit of the stem in the medullary canal and 30° to 40° retroversion are important.

lesser tuberosity to facilitate lengthening it at the time of closure, if necessary. The capsule is then dissected free anteriorly, inferiorly, and superiorly, with care to avoid injury to the axillary nerve. Three-quarters of the capsule is thus exposed and divided transversely (Fig. 17-5). With further external rotation the articular surface is delivered into the wound.

At this point, a complete synovectomy is performed with a curette or scissors. It may or may not be necessary to excise the intra-articular part of the long head of the biceps and to withdraw its stump from the bicipital groove. This tendon is often adherent, and prolongations of proliferative synovial tissue along its sheath are removed.

When the humeral articular surface has been destroyed by granulations or its contour altered by osteophytes, a prosthesis is used. That small portion of bone normally covered by articular cartilage is removed with a broad osteotome. The normal intra-articular calcar is meticulously saved to ensure preservation of the length of the neck (Figs. 17-3 and 17-5). Since the rotator cuff is often loose and attenuated, it is important to save a long lever arm. The Vitallium prosthesis is currently supplied with five stem sizes, each with drill specifications, if needed, for reaming the medullary canal (Fig. 17-4). Reaming

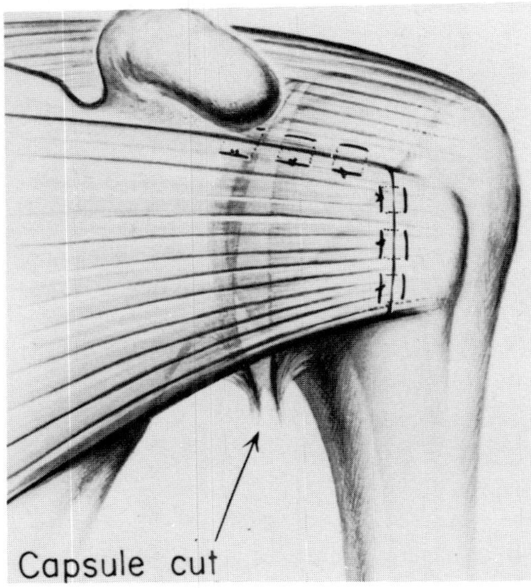

FIG. 17-5. Drawing of shoulder following glenohumeral arthroplasty. The anterior three-quarters of the capsule has been released, a synovectomy performed, and the capsule left open. If the subscapularis muscle is contracted, its tendon is lengthened prior to reattachment to allow full external rotation. When the articular surface has been altered, it is replaced with a prosthesis, with care to preserve the length of the neck. The coraco-acromial ligament and anteroinferior edge of the acromion have been excised. Concomitant procedures may include excision of the outer clavicle, subacromial bursa, tendon sheath for the biceps, or osteophytes on the greater tuberosity, as well as suture of the rotator cuff, depending upon the pathology of the individual case.

is rarely necessary. That stem is selected which allows seating to within 2 inches by hand. It is imperative that a tight fit of the stem within the medullary canal be obtained. The prosthesis is seated in 30° to 40° retroversion. The bicipital groove faces anteriorly. It and the humeral epicondyles can be used as reference points to ensure proper retroversion. This angle is important in providing stability against dislocation.

It should now be possible to move the joint through a full range. After thorough irrigation the subscapularis is repaired, but the capsule is left open (Fig. 17-5). If the subscapularis is contracted, its tendon on the lesser tuberosity is lengthened by splitting it in the coronal plane, detaching the superficial part laterally (leaving the deep portion attached to the lesser tuberosity), and rotating the superficial portion medially. Ample length for full external rotation can be obtained this way. Complete attrition in the supraspinatus is surprisingly rare and, if present, can be repaired with the arm at the side by direct suture and shifting the subscapularis tendon superiorly. If the intra-articular part of the biceps tendon was excised, the remaining stump is sutured in its groove on the humerus. The anterior deltoid is carefully reattached to the outer clavicle through drill holes using interrupted zero chromic catgut sutures for the tendons.

Following surgery, the arm is placed in a sling and swath. This is removed within 48 hours so that the arm may be brought to 80° abduction and neutral rotation in removable lateral suspension. During the first week the patient sleeps and is allowed out of bed with the arm in a sling from the first day, but is replaced in suspension when in bed during the daytime. It is, of course, important that the medical regimen be reinstituted immediately postoperatively. Assisted exercises are begun on the fourth day with the object of regaining lateral rotation and forward elevation. Elbow and hand exercises are encouraged. After 1 week the arm is placed in the sleeve, allowed complete freedom, and the sling is discarded. At 10 days, when the deltoid and subscapularis have reattached, progressive active exercises are added to the limbering exercises. It seems important to concentrate early on recovering motion and much later on regaining strength. Patients are discharged from the hospital between the second and third week. By this time they have been instructed in stretching exercises, isometric exercises, and the value of light, purposeful use.

Acromioclavicular Resection

As mentioned, this may be done at the time of glenohumeral arthroplasty or as a separate procedure. It is important to preserve the coracoclavicular ligaments. For this procedure alone, a 1½-inch incision is made obliquely in Langer's lines over the outer clavicle. The outer clavicle is stripped of soft tissue until a flat instrument can be placed beneath it against the coracoclavicular ligaments. The clavicle is divided with an osteotome obliquely in such a way as to remove more bone posteriorly than anteriorly; otherwise, there is a tendency for impingement posteriorly. The distal one inch of the clavicle is removed retrograde by dividing the capsule. A synovectomy is then performed. Before closure, the trapezius muscle is sutured to the deltoid to obliterate the dead space. The skin is closed loosely, and exercises are deferred for a few days to minimize hematoma formation.

Sternoclavicular Resection

A 2-inch horizontal incision is made below the bony prominence. With care to avoid injury to the great veins posteriorly, the clavicle is stripped of soft tissue until two flat instruments can be positioned, one behind it and one beneath it and against the costoclavicular ligament. Again with caution to avoid the great veins, the clavicle is then cut across and the medial end removed retrograde. Proliferative synovial tissue is removed. The clavicular head of the sternocleidomastoid is sutured to the sternum to obliterate dead space. The skin is closed loosely to minimize hematoma formation. It is important to preserve the costoclavicular ligament.

RESULTS TO BE EXPECTED

It is possible to standardize the procedures for rheumatoid arthritis but not possible to standardize the disease. Neverthe-

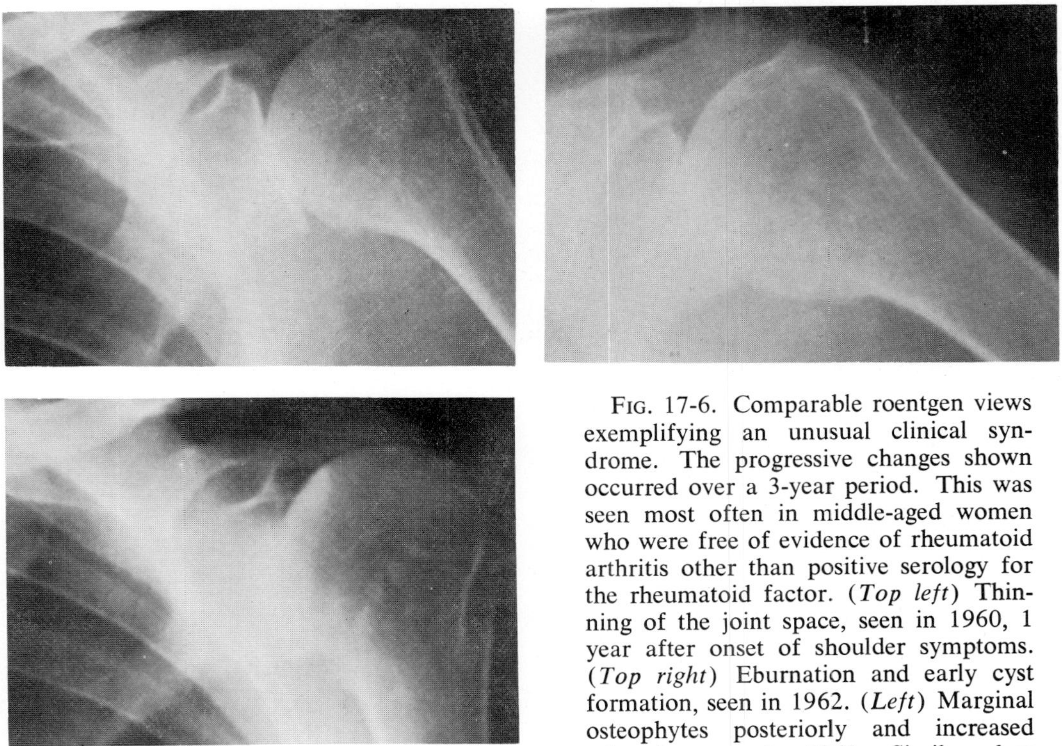

FIG. 17-6. Comparable roentgen views exemplifying an unusual clinical syndrome. The progressive changes shown occurred over a 3-year period. This was seen most often in middle-aged women who were free of evidence of rheumatoid arthritis other than positive serology for the rheumatoid factor. (*Top left*) Thinning of the joint space, seen in 1960, 1 year after onset of shoulder symptoms. (*Top right*) Eburnation and early cyst formation, seen in 1962. (*Left*) Marginal osteophytes posteriorly and increased sclerosis, seen in 1963. Similar slow changes have been noted in a number of middle-aged women in whom only the glenohumeral joints were involved, a clinical syndrome of atypical rheumatoid arthritis.

less, in properly selected patients with a single joint involved, such as the acromioclavicular or sternoclavicular, we can expect that resection and synovectomy will relieve pain, arrest the local disease, and restore the reversibility of any residual contractures elsewhere in the shoulder. However, the results of 36 glenohumeral arthroplasties have varied with the activity of the systemic disease during the postoperative period.

We have encountered a special group, all women between 40 and 60 years of age, who have low grade rheumatoid arthritis that predominately affects the glenohumeral joint (Fig. 17-6). It has been possible to observe their progressive roentgen changes from normal, to thinning of the joint space, to spotty irregularities in the head, and finally loss of contour and secondary osteoarthritic changes. Since patients in this group have little other evidence of rheumatoid arthritis (apart from uniformly positive serology), they have been ideal candidates for arthroplasty, and their results all approach normal. At the other end of the spectrum are patients with severe defects in their elbows, hands, and opposite shoulders, who are distracted during the period of rehabilitation by an unfortunate flare of activity in their lower extremities. These patients can be expected to be relieved of their shoulder pain, but they fail to recover the desired range of motion. Prior to surgery some of these patients were unable to do their hair, eat, or care for their personal hygiene. Even though their functional rating was insufficiently improved to be graded satisfactory, they were most appreciative of the comfort and minor improvements in range.

Patients with longstanding and advanced glenohumeral arthritis have weakened musculature. Improvement in strength is slow, but can be expected to increase over many months with a few stretching exercises to preserve range and useful strength.

These conclusions have been reached on the basis of 36 procedures on 34 glenohumeral joints. A numerical rating based on points was utilized. The rating scale is reproduced below.

The average initial rating was 27 points and the average rating at the last follow-up was 77 points. Patients with mild disease achieved excellent or satisfactory results. Most patients with severe polyarthritis were rated below 70. They were usually satisfied, however, because pain relief was good,

Table 17-1. Criteria for Evaluation of Results*

1. *Pain (35 units)*	
a. None/ignores	35
b. Slight, occasional, no compromise in activity	30
c. Mild, no effect on ordinary activity	25
d. Moderate, tolerable, makes concessions, uses aspirin	15
e. Marked, serious limitations	5
f. Totally disabled	0
2. *Function (30 units)*	
a. Strength	
Normal	10
Good	8
Fair	6
Poor	4
Trace	2
Zero	0
b. Reaching	
Top of head	2
Mouth	2
Belt buckle	2
Opposite axilla	2
Brassiere hook	2
c. Stability	
Lifting	2
Throwing	2
Pounding	2
Pushing	2
Hold overhead	2
3. *Range in Motion (25 units)*	
Flexion (sagittal plane)	
180	6
170	5
130	4
100	2
80	1
less	0
Extension	
45	3
30	2
15	1
less	0
Abduction (coronal plane)	
180	6
170	5
140	4
100	2
80	1
less	0
External rotation (from anatomical position with elbow bent)	
60	5
30	3
10	1
less	0
Internal rotation (from anatomical position with elbow bent)	
90 (T-6)	5
70 (T-12)	4
50 (L-5)	3
30 (gluteal)	2
less	0
4. *Anatomy (10 units)* (rotation, angulation, joint incongruity, retracted tuberosities, failure metal, myositis, non-union, avascular necrosis)	
None	10
Mild	8
Moderate	4
Marked	zero to 2
Total points	100 units

* Excellent, above 89 units; satisfactory, 80 units; unsatisfactory, 70 units; failure, below 70 units. (Neer, C. S. II: Displaced proximal humeral fractures. J. Bone Joint Surg., *52A*:1087, 1970)

although range of motion was very restricted.

Of ten shoulders treated by capsular release and synovectomy, two were later treated by prosthetic replacement, and only four had good results.

Of 26 shoulders treated with prostheses the functional results were characteristically good in patients with low grade disease, but the range of motion was usually poor in those with severe systemic disease. There were no postoperative wound infections, and no prostheses dislocated.

COMMENTARY

In the past, radical acromionectomy has received much attention. Since this procedure weakens the leverage of the deltoid, the prime motor of the glenohumeral joint, and since subacromial impingement is rarely the seat of the problem, we now believe that this procedure is contraindicated, especially in rheumatoid arthritis. An adequate space between the coracoacromial arch can be provided, without weakening the deltoid, by removal of the coracoacromial ligament and anterior, horizontal acromioplasty. However, when the glenohumeral joint is the seat of the disease, this procedure alone is inadequate.

In the future, total joint replacement will be given much attention. In this chapter, we have not mentioned the glenoid. Unlike the acetabulum, the glenoid articular surface is only one-quarter that of the humeral head. Its arc does not match that of the humeral articular surface, and a tight fit has been found undesirable. Normally the stability of this loosely connected joint is dependent upon ligaments, muscles, and the inclination of the humeral head. We have had no problem with dislocation after division of the ligaments but would welcome a method of preventing periarticular adhesions and eliminating the need of the short rotators. Rheumatoid patients often have attenuated, weak rotator muscles which allow upward displacement of the humerus as the arm is elevated. It is challenging to consider a total joint replacement that would stabilize the head against the deltoid, thereby eliminating the necessity for rotator cuff muscles. A prototype has been drawn, and much thought has been given to a means of anchoring this prosthesis, which is of non-anatomical design, to the scapula. This non-weight-bearing joint enjoys a unique mechanical advantage so far as the humeral element is concerned, but anchorage to the scapula will entail greater mechanical problems. Unfortunately, the scapula is a frail bone and not easily adapted to total joint replacement.

The importance of the team approach in rheumatoid surgery, especially in such a complex joint as the shoulder, has not been adequately emphasized. Medical supervision should continue before, during, and after the procedure, and the value of an understanding and knowledgeable physiotherapist cannot be overstated. The surest deterrent to improvement following these procedures is a gloomy surgeon who provides inadequate aftercare.

REFERENCES

1. Neer, C. S. II: Articular replacement for humeral head. J. Bone Joint Surg., *37*:215-228, 1955.

CHAPTER 18

Synovectomy of the Elbow and Excision of the Radial Head in Rheumatoid Arthritis

LEWIS D. ANDERSON, M.D., AND MALCOLM HEPPENSTALL, M.D.

Until recently published results of synovectomy of the rheumatoid elbow have occupied scant space in the medical literature. Apparently, those interested in rheumatoid arthritis have directed their attention toward surgery of the more obviously affected joints, such as the wrist, hand, knee, and hip. However, 13 patients who initially presented themselves to see if something could be done about their stiff and painful elbows have been followed at the Campbell Clinic in Memphis, Tennessee. Radial head excision and subtotal synovectomy were performed on 15 elbows and were followed by substantial improvement. The technique and the results of these operations are reported in this chapter.

J. S. Speed[11] stated that recognition for the first synovectomy probably should go to Volkmann, who performed the procedure as early as 1877 for tuberculous arthritis. Geens[4] credits Schuller with performing the first synovectomies for rheumatoid arthritis; he reported four such cases in 1887. The operation did not become popular until 1923, when Swett presented a series of patients who had undergone synovectomy with favorable results.[13] He emphasized that the operation should not be limited to the knee and reported what is probably the first case of synovectomy of a rheumatoid elbow. In 1943, Smith-Petersen and his associates noted that radial head excision combined with subtotal synovectomy gave excellent relief of pain and significantly increased pronation when performed on elbows affected with rheumatoid arthritis.[10] The elbows in their series showed moderate to severe degenerative changes at the time of surgery, and they thought the benefits of the operation would have been increased if the procedure had been performed before the joint destruction was so severe. Good results after synovectomy of the elbow have been confirmed by other authors, including Mori,[9] Wilkinson and Lowry,[15] and Torgerson and Leach.[14] Laine and Vainio[8] recently reported a large series of patients with synovectomy of the elbow. Overall results were very good in 92 elbows. Motion was increased in 39 per cent after the operation, remained the same in 48 per cent, and was decreased in only 13 per cent. Pain was completely relieved in 48 per cent. Twenty-nine per cent reported occasional pain after strenuous use, and 23 per cent had some degree of constant pain. Prior to 1966, Laine and Vainio performed the operation through a single lateral approach. After reviewing their results, they found that most patients who had residual pain localized it to the medial aspect of the elbow. Because of this, they now advocate an additional medial incision in order to carry out a more complete synovectomy and to transplant the ulnar nerve anteriorly. These authors concluded that 80 per cent of their patients benefited from the procedure and advised early synovectomy with excision of the radial head when crepitation is first felt in the radiohumeral joint.

The only article in which generally disappointing results were reported was that of D'Aubigne and Delbarre.[2] They reported a small series in which synovectomy was performed on four elbows. Function was decreased in two and unchanged in two. Pain was initially decreased in three but recurred in two after a few months. It is not clear from their article whether the radial head was resected or not. Apropos this discussion, it is interesting that Mori[9] in his early cases performed synovectomy alone, without excision of the radial head. A number of these patients experienced loss of motion. Subsequently, he combined excision of the radial head with the synovectomy, and the results improved significantly. It appears that there are two reasons for radial head removal. First, the radiohumeral joint almost always shows destructive changes if there is significant synovitis, even though roentgenograms may appear normal. Second, excision of the radial head makes it technically possible to do a more complete synovectomy.

RATIONALE OF SYNOVECTOMY

The rationale of prophylactic early synovectomy as it applies to joints generally has been discussed by others in this volume and need not be repeated here (see Chaps. 2, 3, 8). The prophylactic benefit of synovectomy is lost on joints with significant destruction of cartilage and bone.[3] However, most investigators agree that after synovectomy of the elbow relief of pain is the most prominent postoperative finding. This is so even in joints that are severely affected. This is in contrast to the knee, a weight-bearing joint, where the results of late synovectomy are usually poor. Perhaps this lessening of discomfort is secondary to partial denervation of the joint, since the synovial nerve endings are obviously removed at the time of surgery. It is unlikely that this is the complete explanation, because a significant number of pain receptors remain in the capsule, ligaments, and adjacent bony structures. Individually Key,[6] in 1925, and Wolcott,[16] in 1927, showed that the synovium regenerates almost completely within 60 days of synovectomy in experimental animals. Branemark[1] confirmed these findings and also found that regeneration of the nerve endings accompanies the regeneration of the new synovial lining. Perhaps there is some change in the quality of the regenerated pain receptors, for it is obvious that relief of pain persists long after the joint lining has been re-formed. Another possible explanation for the pain relief obtained is that the pressure within the joint is reduced. Although the synovium is regenerated, it is unusual to see hypertrophy to the degree present before synovectomy.

Improved motion following elbow synovectomy may be partially due to decreased muscle spasm secondary to relief of pain. Probably of more importance is the mechanical effect of joint debridement and excision of the radial head. Several authors have noted that severe degenerative changes may be present in the radiohumeral articulation, while the articulation of the humerus and olecranon may be relatively well preserved. Goodfellow and Bullough[5] have confirmed these observations by examining a large number of elbows in subjects without rheumatoid arthritis in the older age group. These authors noted that the pattern of cartilage aging and destruction in the elbow shows primary involvement of the capitellum and radial head; they suggest that this pattern of degeneration is secondary to the mechanical effect of simultaneous rotating and gliding movements present in this portion of the elbow.

METHODS AND MATERIALS

From 1962 through 1969, 13 patients with rheumatoid arthritis were treated by the Campbell Clinic staff with synovectomy of the elbow and excision of the radial head. In two patients the operation was performed bilaterally, making a total of 15 operations. All of the patients had classic rheumatoid arthritis with multiple joint involvement. Eleven of the patients were women and 2 were men. Ages ranged from 35 to 68 years; the average age at the time of surgery was 46 years. Duration of disease involving the elbow ranged from 6 to 20 years, with the average being 12 years. The average length of follow-up was 17 months.

Each elbow showed moderate or severe involvement according to the American Rheumatism Association's classification of anatomical stages. None of the elbows showed early or terminal involvement. Six of the 15 joints had marked synovial activity and the remainder demonstrated moderate activity. One patient had symptoms of ulnar nerve compression at the elbow because of herniation of the synovium behind the medial epicondyle. None had symptoms of median nerve involvement at the elbow. Instability of the joint was demonstrated in one elbow, which showed clinical and radiographic evidence of subluxation of the radial head prior to surgery. The primary complaint in all patients was pain that increased with movement of the joint. A second complaint, also present in all patients, was loss of motion. Each patient had received steroids at one time or another, but only three were taking some form of steroid at the time of surgery.

At the time of follow-up, the range of motion of the elbow, including pronation and supination, was carefully recorded by the standard techniques. The degree of inflammatory activity was estimated by the extent of effusion, synovitis, redness, heat, tenderness, and pain. Numerical values on a scale of four grades from 0 to 3 were recorded for each of these findings, and they are shown in Table 18-1. Pre- and postoperative roentgenograms were compared to determine the extent of joint narrowing and bony destruction.

Each patient was asked to evaluate the elbow in terms of pain, function, and general overall result. The degree of pain was classified as none, mild, moderate, or severe. Through enquiries into activities of daily living, including the use of crutches if they were required, we were able to elicit details of any changes in function. The patients were asked to categorize their results as: worse, no improvement, some improvement, or marked improvement.

Since pain was the primary indication for surgery in all 15 elbows it is necessary to include the patient's own estimate of improvement in any classification. Therefore, we have classified the results in two ways. First, the patient's own evaluation of pain

Table 18-1. Eighteen-Point Scoring of Local Inflammatory Activity in Rheumatoid Arthritis of the Elbow*

Points	*0*	*1*	*2*	*3*
Effusion	Little or none	Minimal	Moderate	Marked
Synovitis	None	None to mild	Moderate	Marked
Heat	None	Mild	Moderate	Marked
Redness	None	Mild	Moderate	Marked
Tenderness	None	Mild	Moderate	Marked
Pain	Little or none	Mild	Moderate	Marked

* Modified from a table proposed by the ARA Committee on Diagnostic and Therapeutic Criteria, 1962, Dr. Evan Calkins.

Table 18-2. Patient Evaluation of Results of Synovectomy and Radial Head Excision

Pain	*Number of cases*
None	4
Mild	11
Moderate	0
Severe	0
Overall result	
Marked improvement	9
Some improvement	6
No improvement	0
Worse	0

relief and overall result (Table 18-2) and second, a classification combining the patient's subjective evaluation with the more objective measurements of range of motion and decrease in the inflammatory activity score (Table 18-3).

RESULTS

Patient Evaluation. From the subjective viewpoint, none of the patients thought that their elbows showed no improvement or were worse (see Table 18-2). Six patients thought there was some improvement and nine reported marked improvement. Relief of pain was the most frequent comment by patients during the subjective evaluation. All patients noted relief of pain after the operation: four had no pain, 11 had mild pain, and none complained of moderate or severe pain. Those having mild pain noted it mainly after strenuous activity. Subjective evaluation of function was difficult to separate from relief of pain. Patients frequently commented that they were now able to perform such activities as ironing clothes or washing dishes, which they had been unable to do before, because the pain had been too severe. One patient had taught typing and had been forced to stop because of her elbow. She returned to this occupation 6 weeks after surgery; 46 months later, she was continuing her work without difficulty.

Before gaining experience with elbow synovectomy and radial head excision we were concerned that patients might have difficulty using crutches or a walking cane after the operation. This has not proved to be the case. The greater ease in using these devices appears due principally to decreased pain. In some patients, increased motion is also a factor.

Joint Motion. The average range of motion for all 15 elbows and the average gain in motion after surgery is shown in Table 18-4. Without exception, all ten elbows rated excellent (Table 18-5) showed greater range of motion after surgery. The average increase in motion for these ten patients was 19° flexion, 11° extension, 23° pronation, and 30° supination. The maximum gains in extension and flexion were 20° and 45°, respectively. The maximum gain in pronation was 55° and, in supination, 60°. One

Table 18-3. Classification of Results of Synovectomy of the Elbow and Radial Head Excision

	Excellent	*Good*	*Fair*	*Poor*
Patient evaluation of improvement	Marked	Marked or some	Some	None or worse
Range of motion	Increase or no change in all 4 planes	Increase, no change, or loss in only one plane	Increase, no change, or loss in two planes	Loss in more than two planes
Decrease in Activity Score	At least 10 points	5 to 10 points	5 to 10 points	Less than 5 points

Table 18-4. Range of Motion in 15 Elbows Before and After Surgery

	Before	*After*	*Gain*
Average Flexion	110°	126°	16°
Average Extension	40°	32°	8°
Average Pronation	40°	64°	24°
Average Supination	40°	61°	21°

Table 18-5. Results of Elbow Synovectomy and Radial Head Excision*

Rating	*Number of cases*
Excellent	10
Good	4
Fair	1
Poor	0

* Classified according to Table 18-3.

patient with a subluxation of the radial head before the operation demonstrated a dramatic increase of 55° of pronation and 45° of supination. Before surgery, motion in each of these planes was only 5°.

Two patients had an increase in their flexion contracture following surgery. Of these, one lost 10° extension from 35° to 45° but gained 30° of pronation and supination. The other patient lost 20° of extension but gained 20° pronation and 15° supination. The results in these two patients were classified as good.

Only one elbow demonstrated loss of motion in more than one plane. This patient lost 35° of flexion and 45° supination; he gained 20° extension, and pronation remained unchanged. This was the only patient classified as fair. Only 6 months has elapsed between surgery and his most recent evaluation. It is hoped that he will regain additional motion with more time.

Inflammatory Activity Score. All elbows demonstrated a decrease in the inflammatory activity score (Table 18-6). Twelve elbows showed an improvement of more than 10 points. Three elbows showed decreases of 8, 7, and 6 points, respectively. As seen in Table 18-3, a decrease of 10 or more points is compatible with an excellent result, a decrease of 5 to 10 points with a good or fair result, and a decrease of less than 5 points with a poor result.

Over-all Results. When the 15 elbows were rated according to the criteria outlined in Table 18-3, ten were classified as excellent, four as good, and one as fair. None were considered poor.

Table 18-6. Eighteen-Point Score of Local Inflammatory Activity: Averages in 15 Elbows

	Before	*After*	*Decrease*
Effusion	2.27	.33	1.94
Synovitis	2.53	.40	2.13
Heat	2.00	.33	1.67
Redness	1.47	.13	1.34
Tenderness	1.93	1.00	.93
Pain	2.67	.73	1.94
Total (Mean)	12.87	2.92	9.95

OPERATIVE TECHNIQUE

Several different surgical approaches and techniques have been reported. As noted previously, Laine and Vainio[8] initially used only a lateral approach and excised the radial head. They now use both the original lateral approach and a medial approach and routinely transplant the ulnar nerve anteriorly. Mori[9] originally did not excise the radial head but later found motion was improved if it was resected. Straub[12] uses a posterior approach with osteotomy of the olecranon to provide wide exposure. He resects the radial head and replaces the olecranon with a wire loop or a long screw after the synovectomy is completed.

In all 15 elbows in this series a lateral approach was used. We believe an additional medial approach is indicated if there are symptoms of ulnar nerve entrapment or if significant synovitis is noted about the medial epicondyle. There was one such patient in our series.

Make a lateral incision 2 inches proximal to the capitellum along the epicondylar ridge to a point 2 inches distal to the radial head. Then curve it distally and medially to end at the subcutaneous border of the ulna. Separate the plane between the triceps muscle posteriorly and the brachioradialis and extensor carpi radialis muscles anteriorly and identify the capsule of the joint. Distal to the radial head, separate the plane between the extensor carpi ulnaris and the anconeus. Using a knife, divide the capsule of the joint in line with the incision, but attempt to stay outside the synovium. Flex the elbow to relax the anterior capsule and separate the plane between the capsule and synovium proximally, distally, and as far medially as possible, before entering the synovium. (When the synovium is adherent, this may not be possible.) Now incise the synovium and expose the radial head and neck. Excise the radial head in the usual manner. Remove as much as possible of the synovium of the anterior compartment in one block of tissue. Then complete the anterior part of the synovectomy by sharp dissection and by using a sponge to strip away the final remnants. Dissect the posterior capsule from the epicondylar ridge with a knife. Cut the lateral collateral ligament leaving a small tag attached to the humerus for subsequent repair. Now, extend the elbow and retract the capsule posteriorly to expose the olecranon fossa. Complete the posterior synovectomy with sharp dissection and by using a sponge as described previously.

If there are symptoms of ulnar nerve compression, make a second incision medially, beginning 2 inches proximal to the epicondyle and curving posteriorly and distally to a point 2 inches below the epicondyle. Reflect the anterior flap and expose the common origin of the flexor muscles. Identify the ulnar nerve and free it from the surrounding soft tissue; take care to protect the branches to the flexor carpi ulnaris and flexor profundus muscles. Retract the nerve and excise any synovium from the groove. Incise the capsule and inspect the joint for any remnants of synovium. Free the nerve proximally and transplant it anteriorly. Place a few interrupted catgut sutures between the subcutaneous tissue of the skin flap and the deep fascia of the anterior forearm to maintain the nerve in the desired position. Now, suture the capsular incisions with medium chromic catgut, repair the lateral collateral ligament, and close the subcutaneous tissue and skin routinely.

Apply a posterior plaster splint to hold the elbow at 90° and the forearm in neutral pronation-supination. Encourage active finger and shoulder exercises during the time the elbow is immobilized. Remove the plaster splint at 2 weeks and begin active elbow exercises.

SUMMARY

As stated previously, none of the synovectomies in this series was done in a patient with early disease. All elbows demonstrated moderate or severe destruction of the joint at the time of surgery. In spite of this, the result of the operation was excellent in ten, good in four, and fair in only one; none were considered poor. All patients thought they were improved, and there were no serious complications.

Relief of pain was the most rewarding result. Four of the 15 patients stated they had no pain, and 11 had only mild pain. None complained of moderate or severe discomfort.

Joint motion was increased in all but three patients. Of the three who showed a loss of motion, two lost a few degrees of extension but gained motion in two other planes. Only one elbow had loss of motion in two planes.

We were concerned that loss of stability in the elbow might be a problem after the operation, particularly in patients who used crutches or canes. Happily, this has proved unfounded, and significant instability has not been seen following the procedure.

The activity of the disease decreased in all 15 elbows following the operation. Details about the inflammatory activity index are shown in Tables 18-1 and 18-6.

How long will the good and excellent results last? We do not claim to know the answer. Since we have been doing this procedure for only a few years, the follow-up period is relatively short, ranging from only 6 months to 46 months. Thus far, we are encouraged that none of the patients has demonstrated a deterioration in the overall result with the passage of time.

What are the contraindications to synovectomy of the elbow with resection of the radial head? We think they are few. We would expect the results to be best in early cases, though none in this series was truly an early synovectomy. The favorable results reported above were all in patients with moderate or severe joint destruction according to the A.R.A. classification. These stages of involvement or long duration of active disease in the elbow are still compatible with a good result. Probably the operation should not be done when there is total destruction of the elbow and terminal involvement by the A.R.A. standards.

This procedure is primarily indicated in classical rheumatoid arthritis. With end-stage disease and fibrous or bony ankylosis following Still's disease or in Marie-Strümpell arthritis, synovectomy and radial head resection would not be expected to benefit the patient; a classical fascial arthroplasty as described by Knight and Van-Zandt[7] would be much better. Of course, excision of the radial head is contraindicated in a growing child. We have had no experience with synovectomy of the elbow alone in children but believe it might be beneficial if done early.

REFERENCES

1. Branemark, P. I., and Goldie, I.: Physiological aspects of the timing of synovectomy in rheumatoid arthritis. *In* Hijmans, W., Paul, W. D., and Herschel, H. (eds.): Early Synovectomy in Rheumatoid Arthritis. Amsterdam, Amsterdam Exerpta Medica Foundation, 1969.
2. D'Aubigne, R. Merle, and Delbarre, F.: Synovectomy of elbow in rheumatoid arthritis.
3. Gariépy, R., Demers, R., and Lanvin, C. A.: Prophylactic effect of synovectomy of the knee. Canad. Med. Ass. J., *94*:1349-1352, 1966.
4. Geens, Staf: Synovectomy and debridement of the knee in rheumatoid arthritis. Part 1, Historic review. J. Bone Joint Surg., *51*: 617-623, 1969.
5. Goodfellow, J. W., and Bullough, P. G.: The patterns of aging of the articular cartilage of the elbow joint. J. Bone Joint Surg. [Brit.], *49*:175-181, 1967.
6. Key, T. A.: The reformation of synovial membrane in the knee of rabbits after synovectomy. J. Bone Joint Surg., *7*:793-813, 1925.
7. Knight, R. A., and Van Zant, I. L.: Arthroplasty of the elbow. An end result study. J. Bone Joint Surg., *34*:610-618, 1952.
8. Laine, V., and Vainio, K.: Synovectomy of the elbow. *In* Hijmans, W., Paul, W. D.,

and Herschel, H. (eds.): Early Synovectomy in Rheumatoid Arthritis. Amsterdam, Amsterdam Exerpta Medica Foundation, 1969.

9. Mori, M.: Surgical Experience of Synovectomy in the Rheumatoid Elbow. Read at the Eleventh Congress of the International Society for Orthopaedic Surgery and Traumatology, Mexico City, Mexico, October 6-10, 1969 (in press).
10. Smith-Petersen, M. N., Aufranc, O. E., and Larson, C. B.: Use of surgical procedures for rheumatoid arthritis involving joints of the upper extremity. Arch. Surg., *46*:764-770, 1943.
11. Speed, J. S.: Synovectomy of knee joint. J.A.M.A., *83*:1814-1820, 1924.
12. Straub, L. R.: A discussion of Laine-Vainio. *In* Hijmans, W., Paul, W. D., and Herschel, H. (eds.): Early Synovectomy in Rheumatoid Arthritis. Amsterdam, Amsterdam Exerpta Medica Foundation, 1969.
13. Swett, P. P.: Synovectomy in chronic infectious arthritis. J. Bone Joint Surg., *3*:110-121, 1923.
14. Torgerson, W. R., and Leach, R. E.: Synovectomy of the elbow in rheumatoid arthritis. J. Bone Joint Surg., *52*:371-375, 1970.
15. Wilkinson, M. C., and Lowry, T. H.: Synovectomy for rheumatoid arthritis. J. Bone Joint Surg. [Brit.], *47*:482-488, 1965.
16. Wolcott, W. E.: Regeneration of the synovial membrane following typical synovectomy. J. Bone Joint Surg., *9*:67-68, 1927.

CHAPTER 19

Surgery in Rheumatoid Arthritis of the Wrist

D. KAY CLAWSON, M.D., AND F. RICHARD CONVERY, M.D.

The wrist is one of the most frequently affected regions in rheumatoid arthritis. The wrist joint is at least three joints (the radiocarpal, the radioulnar, and the intercarpal joints) and is surrounded by some 21 tendons encased in synovial sheaths. The wrist is readily inspected and palpated, making it possible to follow minor changes in disease activity, and it is easily approached surgically. Surgery will certainly not arrest the arthritic process, yet few will deny that synovectomy, arthroplasty, and arthrodesis are all excellent procedures if properly applied in selected individuals. Early synovectomy may prevent local destruction and hence preserve function. Early disease has yet to be clearly defined. Certainly the disease process may be advanced before there is any evidence of x-ray changes. Cineradiography reported by Arkless[1] has demonstrated abnormal motion of the carpal bones in the arthritic wrist when no other roentgen changes are visible. Ranewat et al have shown through arthrography that synovial disease may be very advanced, with destruction of the articular disk and ligaments about the joint, before x-ray changes can be appreciated.[5]

Surgical intervention must be planned according to the pathology present. The pathologic stages of disease can be divided as follows:

Stage 1—Synovitis. The disease is an inflammatory response in synovial tissue. An effusion is present in joints, and there is excess fluid in synovial sheaths. Destruction occurs from pressure which stretches the capsule and ligaments or possibly from interference with normal cartilage and tendon nutrition. The changes are largely reversible, and, therefore, there would seem to be no indication for surgical interference.

Stage 2—Proliferative response. At some time during the inflammatory stage, the synovium takes on a proliferative character and invades tendon, ligaments, cartilage and bone. When this type of response is persistent, it seems justified to remove the proliferative synovium before it can seriously destroy the joints or tendons. As the anatomy of each area differs so does the ease and completeness of synovial removal. Hence, each joint must be treated individually when considering the appropriateness of prophylactic synovectomy. Satisfactory statistics are not available on the recurrence rate after prophylactic synovectomy. We have yet to take into account the natural history of the disease, the stage of the disease at the time of operation, and the completeness of synovectomy in assessing and following a significant number of individuals. Brown reports a 6.5 per cent recurrence rate in 1 year after synovectomy of the joints of the wrist and hand.[2] We have observed recurrences later than 1 year, and hence the recurrence rate is perhaps somewhat higher than this figure.

Stage 3—Destruction. By this time the cartilage and ligaments have been destroyed

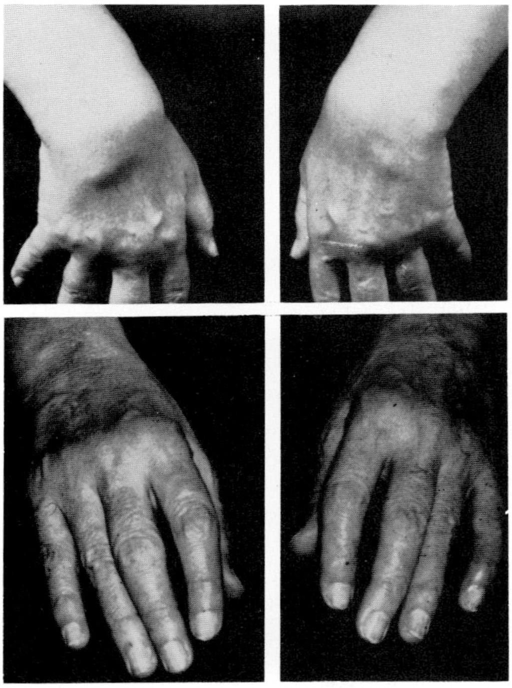

FIG. 19-1. (*Top*) Preoperative wrists of patient with proliferative rheumatoid tenosynovitis on the dorsum of the wrist. (*Bottom*) Postoperative photographs. Note the lack of swelling. The scars are difficult to see at 6 (*right*) and 18 (*left*) months.

and only reconstructive procedures or arthrodesis can be of significant value. Tendon ruptures are not infrequent and occur at sites of friction.

INDICATIONS FOR SURGERY

The literature does not provide clear guidelines as to when operative intervention is indicated. We have never regretted having operated early. Yet many times we have felt negligent for not advocating operative intervention forcefully enough before destructive changes occurred that finally mitigated an excellent result. Good medical management, including high levels of salicylates, other anti-inflammatory drugs, and splinting, should have proved unsuccessful in a trial of at least 3 months before prophylactic surgery is recommended.

The frequent use of corticosteroids injected into tendon sheaths and joints must be condemned, because these drugs have been shown to interfere with cartilage metabolism.*[4] The use of the steroids in tendon sheaths is probably a contributing factor in many tendon ruptures.

Studies conducted at the University of Washington have shown that in a three-year follow-up of 84 hands not treated surgically, 40 per cent improved and 16 per cent showed no change.[3] A significant number of individuals diagnosed as rheumatoid arthritics will have a lasting remission. These persons must be excluded before one assesses the effectiveness of prophylactic surgery.

OPERATIVE PROCEDURES

Dorsal Wrist Surgery

Proliferative tenosynovitis of the extensor tendons is readily appreciated on physical examination. The reaction extends from the myotendinous junction to the insertions of the wrist tendons and the metacarpal region on the common extensor tendons where the synovial sheath is lost. Proximal and distal bulging around an intact extensor retinaculum are usually evident. Physical examination should also document the extent of the disease around the distal radioulnar joint. This joint should be examined for abnormal motion, pain, and limitation on supination. Subluxation of the radiocarpal joint is also common. It can be diagnosed by carrying out a push-pull examination of the wrist in the long axis of the forearm. In the authors' experience there has been considerable disease of the distal radioulnar joint, with destruction of the articular disk and the distal radioulnar capsular ligaments, by the time operative intervention was contemplated. The extent of involvement of the radiocarpal and intercarpal joints in early disease is only now being fully appreciated.

---

* Salter, Robert. Personal communication.

We have occasionally attempted limited synovectomies on the dorsum, or ulnar aspect, of the wrist. The subsequent appearance of proliferative disease in adjacent areas of the wrist has led us to conclude that the minimal recommended procedure for dorsal wrist surgery is a tenosynovectomy of all extensor tendons, transfer of the tendons superficial to the extensor retinaculum and excision of the synovium and 1.5 cm. to 2.0 cm. of the distal ulna (Fig. 19-1). We have not felt that a complete enough synovectomy of the carpal joints could be carried out to warrant this as a routine prophylactic procedure (as is advocated by Straub[7]). However, it is certainly indicated where there is gross evidence of proliferative synovium, some instability of the radiocarpal joint, and good articular cartilage and joint motion remaining.

Surgical Technique. Standard techniques for carrying out this procedure have been extensively recorded in the literature. Certain points seem worth stressing. The lazy-S incision, starting on the ulnar side of the forearm extending to the radial side of the hand, will give complete exposure on the dorsum of the wrist. The extensor retinaculum should be divided at its ulnar border and carefully preserved. Tenosynovectomy should be carried out on *all* involved tendons (Fig. 19-2). The paratenon should be carefully preserved, even if it is invaded by rheumatoid granulation tissue. Handling of the tendon with sponges or forceps or attempts to remove this material will only cause increased scarring and delayed postoperative recovery. The extensor pollicis longus should be rerouted away from the dorsal tubercle of the radius. The remnants of the radioulnar articular disk should be preserved and reconstructed so far as possible. Failure to do so will increase the chance of ulnar displacement of the carpus. The distal 1.5 cm. to 2.0 cm. of ulna should be excised subperiosteally. Care should be taken to preserve any ligament still present.

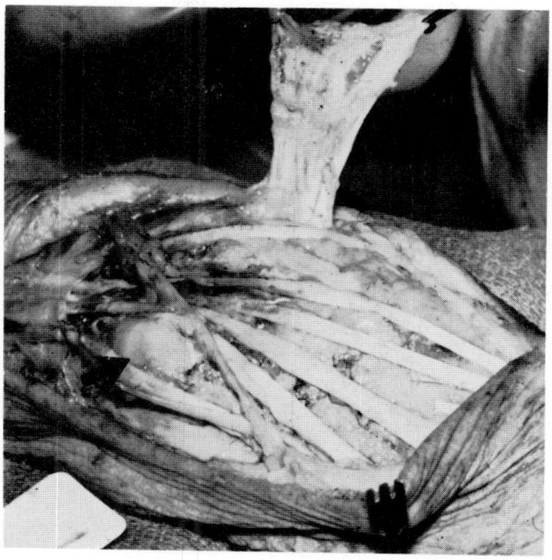

FIG. 19-2. Complete tenosynovectomy has been carried out with preservation of the dorsal retinacular ligament. Note the position of the dorsally subluxated distal ulna (arrow) in relation to extensor tendons prior to its excision.

The periosteum and ligaments should be reconstructed to stabilize the distal ulna. Hypermobility of the ulna is not uncommon and will result in symptoms on pronation and supination. In an effort to improve the stability, we have used a Kirschner wire across the distal radius and ulna in the early postoperative period. Complications from the wire and occasional failures to achieve stability have led us to conclude that if good stability is not present from ligament reconstruction, stabilization of the distal ulna should be carried out by a figure-8 tendon graft around the ulna and into the radius (Fig. 19-3). Before closure, the extensor retinaculum is routinely transferred beneath the extensor tendons (Fig. 19-4). This reinforces the dorsal joint capsule and places the tendons in a new bed adjacent to healthy fat.

A tendon rupture of extensor pollicis longus can occasionally be repaired by direct suture or the insertion of a very small segment of tendon graft after rerouting. Usually more extensive procedures are nec-

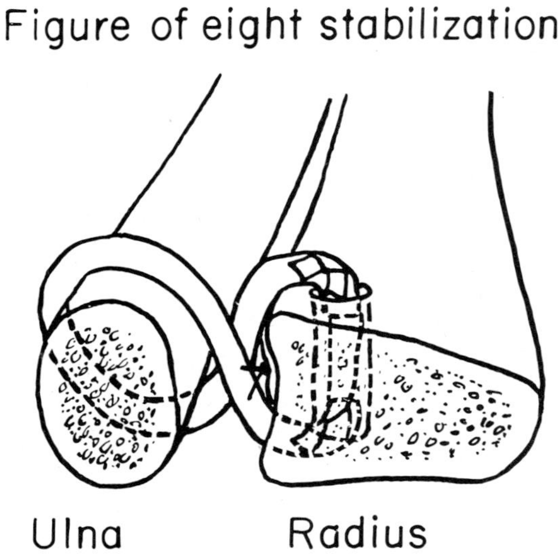

FIG. 19-3. The distal ulna can be quickly stabilized with the use of a palmaris longus tendon or a portion of the extensor carpi ulnaris passed extraperiosteally around the distal ulna. The tendon ends are passed through a previously drilled anteroposterior hole in the radius and fixed using a criss-crossing Bunell-type suture.

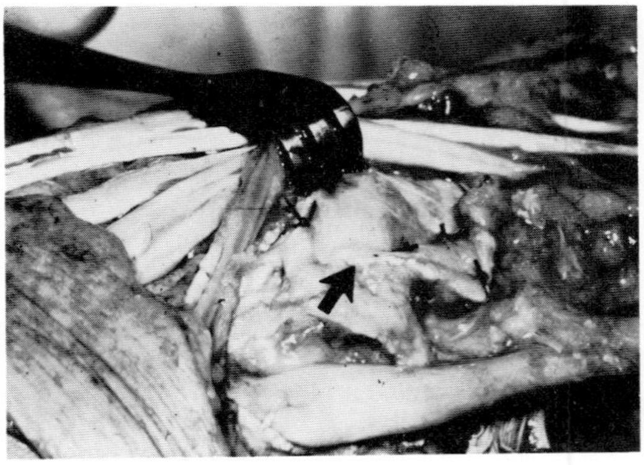

FIG. 19-4. The extensor net retinaculum has been transferred beneath the extensor tendon and sutured to reinforce the radiocarpal joint and stabilize the distal ulna (arrow).

essary for repair of extensor pollicis longus or extensor communis ruptures. Our experience confirms the literature; transfer of the extensor indicis proprius is usually the procedure of choice. Attempts at suturing the distal stump of the tendon into the next adjacent functioning tendon have resulted in a limitation of flexion. Hand function is improved due to a tenodesis effect rather, not because normal tendon function has been restored.

Results. Dorsal wrist surgery has been carried out on 38 wrists in 30 patients with rheumatoid arthritis who have been followed from 1 to 8 years. Four patients had limited procedures; all have experienced extension of the disease. Of the 34 complete procedures, 18 have shown significant improvement in function with relief of pain when it was present. Ten are relatively unchanged insofar as function is concerned, but they show no recurrence of the proliferative tenosynovitis. Six individuals have shown steady deterioration. A more complete evaluation is not possible, since the exact stage of the disease was not satisfactorily documented preoperatively in all cases. Nine patients experienced instability and pain at the site of resection of the distal ulna. Three have subsequently had the figure-8 repair, which provided good stability and complete relief of symptoms. No case of postoperative tendon rupture has been noted. Three individuals have had ruptures of extensor tendons on the opposite wrist while awaiting dorsal synovectomy or after having refused surgical treatment.

Volar Wrist Surgery

Because of the very heavy flexor retinaculum (volar carpal ligament), rheumatoid disease has not been as successfully detected in the flexor compartment as in the extensor compartment. Tenosynovitis of the flexor tendons can be suspected when there is a fullness in the distal forearm or in the palm just distal to the carpal tunnel. Weakness of grip from flexor tenosynovitis frequently goes unrecognized. The usual indication for surgical intervention has been median nerve compression. In addition to weakness of grip, pain on the volar aspect of the wrist (occasionally extending into the thumb, index, or long finger) is not uncommon. Numbness and tingling in the median nerve distribution is a relatively late complaint. These symptoms frequently occur an hour or two after going to bed. In many patients, the complaints are minor compared with the over-all disease and may be overlooked. Forced palmar flexion of the wrist (Phalen's test) will accentuate the symptoms, provided the wrist disease is not too advanced to allow full flexion. Delay in nerve conduction is a relatively late finding, and many patients will be denied considerable symptomatic relief from minimal surgery if this is the criteria for operative treatment. Wrist splints are usually beneficial in relieving symptoms but rarely provide lasting relief. The injection of hydrocortisone into the carpal tunnel should be limited to one or two treatments. Surgical treatment varies from a simple division of the flexor retinaculum and a limited tenosynovectomy to a more complete procedure that opens the proximal palm, the wrist, and forearm with a careful tenosynovectomy from the myotendinous junction to the palm. Straub also recommends inspection and synovectomy of the carpal joints from this approach.[6] Simple release of the flexor retinaculum and limited tenosynovectomy has many advantages over more extensive surgery. The wrist disease is only one aspect of the multiple problems confronting the patient. The simpler the surgical procedure, the more readily it can be accepted and the more useful it becomes in managing the patient. Carpal tunnel release and limited synovectomy have resulted in functional improvement as good as that obtained with the more extensive operations. The functional improvement is recognized immediately and hospitalization is brief. To date, the improvement has been lasting.

Carpal Tunnel Release. A palmar incision is made parallel to the ulnar side of the thenar crease extending from the distal wrist crease to a line extended across the palm with the thumb in 90° of abduction (Fig. 19-5). The incision allows for visualization and excision of the flexor retinaculum. The proliferative synovium can be removed from the midpalm to 1½ inches proximal to the distal wrist crease. The paratenon is left intact, and the wound closed. The procedure can be done bilaterally. The patient leaves the hospital the following day. Immediate use of the hand provides the best form of rehabilitation, and this is encouraged. The only dressing is a small volar splint for a week to 10 days. One of our patients, a physician's wife, had one wrist done with the standard approach and the other through the limited approach. The postoperative discomfort and the time required for rehabilitation was significant on the side with the more extensive surgery. The patient has now been followed 6 years, and there is no difference on the two sides except for the prominent scar from the more extensive procedure.

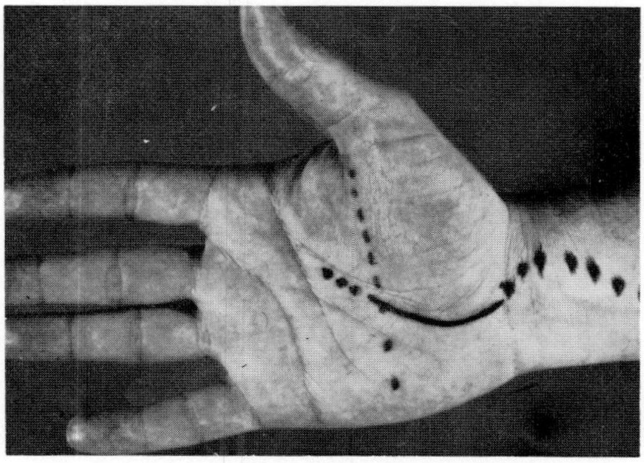

FIG. 19-5. Solid black line indicates the extent of the incision for carpal tunnel release and limited tenosynovectomy. The dashed line extending from the base of the thumb indicates the distal margin of the carpal tunnel. The dotted line extending from the solid line indicates the extension of the incision for complete visualization of the flexor tendons.

Standard Volar Synovectomy. An incision extending from the proximal palmar crease

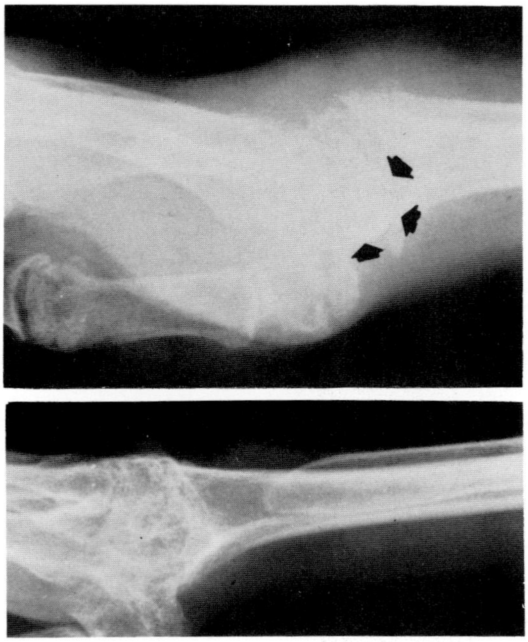

FIG. 19-6. Pre- and postoperative wrist fusion. Note the severe volar subluxation and shortening of the carpals on the radius (black arrows). The soft tissue swelling can be compared between the preoperative (*top*) and the one year postoperative (*bottom*) x-rays. Note in the postoperative film the correct position of wrist fusion of 0° to 10° of extension.

crossing the wrist in a lazy-S fashion (Fig. 19-5), curving up the forearm to the myotendinous junction is advocated by most authorities. The flexor retinaculum is excised and a careful synovectomy is carried out from the myotendinous junction to the midpalm. Full early finger flexion and extension are essential to prevent adhesions of the flexor superficialis and flexor profundus tendons from limiting full flexion of the distal interphalangeal joints.

Results. Sixteen operations in 13 patients have been reviewed. All patients have been relieved of their preoperative median nerve symptoms. In none of the patients was there a deterioration in grip strength, and 50 per cent of those with satisfactory pre- and postoperative testing showed slight, but not statistically significant, improvement.

Arthrodesis

Many orthopedists look upon arthrodesis of a joint as an admission of defeat and refuse to recognize the tremendous functional benefits that can be achieved by a painless stable joint. Patients are extremely gratified by the relief of pain and the improved function resulting from this stabilizing procedure. On a number of occasions, we have reluctantly done a dorsal synovectomy and debridement and later regretted that we had not done a wrist arthrodesis. Therefore, we believe that radiocarpal arthrodesis is indicated for all patients who are seen at the stage where there is gross bone and cartilage destruction or where the carpal bones have marked volar subluxation (Fig. 19-6).

Arthrodesis in rheumatoid arthritis is a simple procedure and will result in considerable improvement in hand function. In addition to the relief of pain, the subluxed carpals can be placed in a more appropriate position on the radius, thus providing a better mechanical advantage for the finger tendons. Unlike patients with cerebral palsy and poliomyelitis, where the joint is normal and the patient can use the flexion and extension of the wrist to provide a tenodesis effect thus improving muscle function, the patient with rheumatoid arthritis does not have this advantage. Hence, considerations that weigh against wrist arthrodesis in other conditions are not applicable here.

Surgical Technique. The technique of arthrodesis is extremely important. The procedure is carried out through the same or a modification of the incision for dorsal tenosynovectomy. The operation is identical to that described for dorsal synovectomy until the joint is opened. Any cartilage or subchondral bone remaining is removed along with the proliferative synovium. A small V is made in the distal radius just volar to the dorsal cortex. The volarly subluxated carpal bones are then placed in this groove (Fig. 19-7). A

$\frac{9}{64}$-inch K wire is inserted between the index and long finger metacarpals, through the carpals, and into the medullary canal of the radius (Fig. 19-8). The wire is divided subcutaneously. Chips of the distal ulna are placed about the fusion site. The transverse carpal ligament is sutured over the fusion site and the extensor tendons transplaced superficially as for the dorsal synovectomy. The patient is placed in a "boxing glove" compression dressing and plaster splints are applied to the forearm and are extended to form a long-arm cast. The bulky dressings are removed in about 5 days, and usually a long-arm cast is applied. At 6 weeks this is changed to a short-arm cast for an additional 6 weeks, after which all immobilization is removed. The patient is encouraged to use the hand and arm during the entire postoperative period. The K wire is removed when it becomes symptomatic or at 4 months.

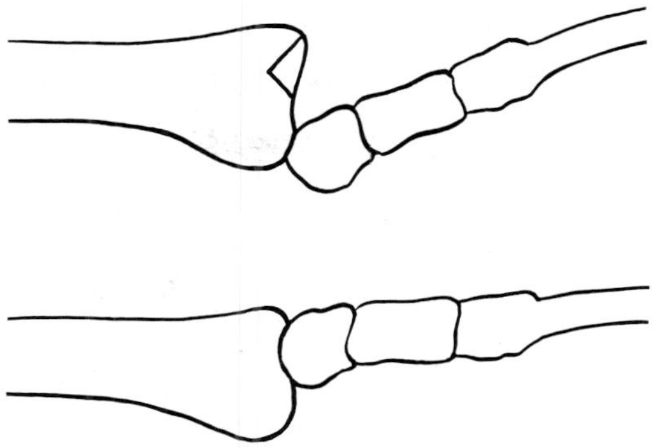

FIG. 19-7. This line drawing emphasizes the correct positioning of the subluxated carpus on the radius for wrist function.

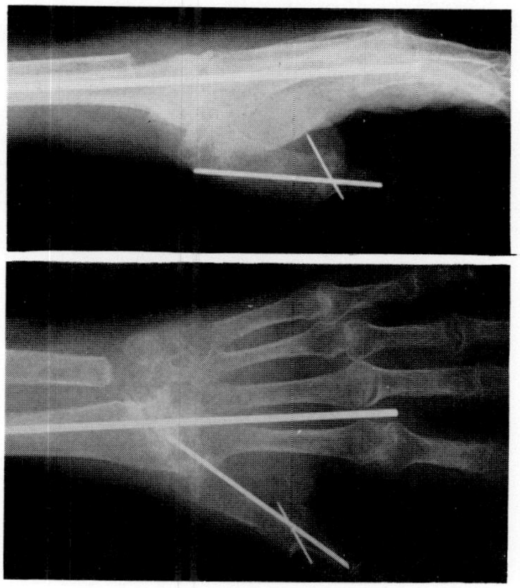

FIG. 19-8. The 9/64-inch Kirschner wire is shown in the correct position for wrist function. A subluxated metacarpal phalangeal joint of the thumb was fused at the same procedure accounting for the extra pins.

Position of Function. Classically it is stated that the position of function of the wrist is 25° to 30° of extension. This position may be ideal for heavy labor but is of no value for a person trying to care for his personal needs with limited adaptive capacity from adjacent joints. For this reason the dominant wrist is fused in the neutral position or at most with 10° of extension. When there is bilateral disease, the nondominant hand *must* be fused in 15° to 20° of flexion. This allows the patient to reach all portions of his body and still provides a very satisfactory grip.

Results. Despite our enthusiasm for this procedure, its general condemnation in the literature has made it difficult to obtain patients from rheumatologists and orthopedists for wrist fusion. We can report only eight procedures in six patients. All wrists united and were out of plaster within 3 months. Seven of the eight patients showed an immediate functional improvement. Four patients more than doubled their grip strength, despite extensive disease elsewhere in the hand. One patient was functionally unchanged but relieved of pain. No patients were worse by objective or subjective assessment.

SUMMARY

The wrist is commonly affected with rheumatoid arthritis. Because of its superficial nature, the wrist joint lends itself to careful follow-up; however, the multiplicity of problems affecting the wrist and hand make objective assessment of improvement difficult.

Tenosynovectomy of the extensor tendons with transfer superficial to the transverse carpal ligament and limited excision of the distal ulna can be expected to provide lasting relief of symptoms and prevent extensor tendon rupture. The role of synovectomy in prevention of destruction of the radiocarpal joint is still being evaluated. Either limited or complete synovectomy and release of the carpal tunnel will provide considerable relief for patients with volar wrist disease and median nerve compression. Wrist arthrodesis will eliminate pain and provide a significant increase in grip. We consider it the procedure of choice when the radiocarpal joint has been severely disrupted.

REFERENCES

1. Arkless, R.: Rheumatoid wrist. Cineradiography. Radiology, *88*:543-549, 1967.
2. Brown, P. W.: Early recurrence of rheumatoid synovium after early synovectomy in the hand and wrist. *In* Hijmans, W., Paul, W. D., and Herschel, H. (eds.): Early Synovectomy in Rheumatoid Arthritis. pp. 201-206. Amsterdam, Exerpta Medica Foundation, 1969.
3. Clawson, D. K., Souter, W. A., Carthum, C. J., and Hymen, M. L.: Functional assessment of the rheumatoid hand. Clin. Orthop. Related Res. (to be published).
4. Mankin, A. J., and Conger, K. A.: Effect of intra-articular hydrocortisone on articular cartilage in rabbits. J. Bone Joint Surg., *48*:1383-1388, 1966.
5. Ranewat, C. S., Freiberger, F. H., Jordan, L. R., and Straub, L. R.: Arthrography in the rheumatoid wrist joint. J. Bone Joint Surg., *51*:1269-1281, 1969.
6. Straub, L. R., and Ranewat, C. S.: The wrist in rheumatoid arthritis. J. Bone Joint Surg., *51*:1-20, 1969.

CHAPTER 20

Pathogenesis of Rheumatoid Deformities in the Hand*

A. B. Swanson, M.D., G. A. de Groot, M.D., R. W. Hehl, M.D., T. J. Waller, M.D., and N. R. Boeve, M.D.

Rheumatoid arthritis is one of the enigmas of medicine. It is a systemic disease whose most characteristic lesion is inflammation of the synovial membranes of joints and tendon sheaths. The most widely held theory of the pathogenesis of rheumatoid arthritis involves an immunological response taking place in the synovial tissues. This inflammatory reaction is the basis of the swelling, redness, heat, and pain of arthritis. It is the cause of the resultant damage to joints, supporting soft tissue structures, and tendons.[8,18] The inflammatory reaction is chronic and persistent in two-thirds of the cases.[15]

Recent hypotheses suggest that rheumatoid arthritis may be the result of a confusion of the body's normal defenses.[1] There are probably two mechanisms involved in the chronicity of the arthritic inflammation.[12] The first is attributable to the initiating antigen, which is presumably exogenous. The second relates to development of an autoimmune response to a new antigen from the host tissues. Normally, when a foreign antigen enters the body, it comes in contact with a defender cell, the lymphocyte. The lymphocyte is transformed into a larger plasma cell. The plasma cell manufactures antibodies[21] that have surfaces precisely keyed to fit the surfaces of the antigen so that the two can lock together. As antibodies lock in with and immobilize antigens, a blood substance called complement is attracted and combines with them. The three-part combinations formed in this way are called complexes. The scavenger phagocytic cells then engulf the complexes. The phagocytic cells have small sacs called lysosomes which contain enzymes. The enzymes destroy the complexes, thus disposing of the intruder. In arthritis, the phagocytic cells become confused or are incapable of handling the antigen-antibody-complement complex. Some of the lysosomes escape from the cells and attack the synovium and cartilage of the joints. Destruction of cartilage adds to the requirement for more phagocytic activity to dispose of the resulting debris. The phagocytic cells pour out more of their enzymes and trigger further inflammation. Thus, once triggered, arthritic inflammation becomes self-perpetuating.[27]

The inflamed synovium forms a pannus, a granulomatous mass which grows over the surface of the cartilage, into and around the tendons, and into ligament attachments.[22] If unchecked, this invasion results in the loosening of ligaments, destruction of joint surfaces, and the inability of tendons to function, all of which are typical of the advanced rheumatoid process.[4,7,11] Every derangement or deformity of the musculo-skeletal system seen in rheumatoid arthritis is the result, either primarily or secondarily, of this synovial invasion.[30] The pathogenesis of deformities in the hand, therefore, is the result

* A survey of the incidence of deformity in 1,000 digits.

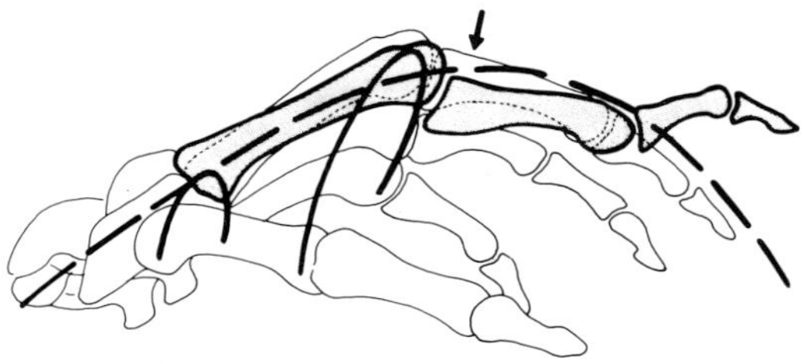

FIG. 20-1. The normal arch system of the hand is frequently disturbed in rheumatoid arthritis. This drawing illustrates how palmar subluxation of the MP joint causes collapse of the longitudinal arch. (Redrawn after Tubiana, R.: The Rheumatoid Hand, G.E.M. Monograph No. 3. p. 25. Paris, l'Expansion, 1969)

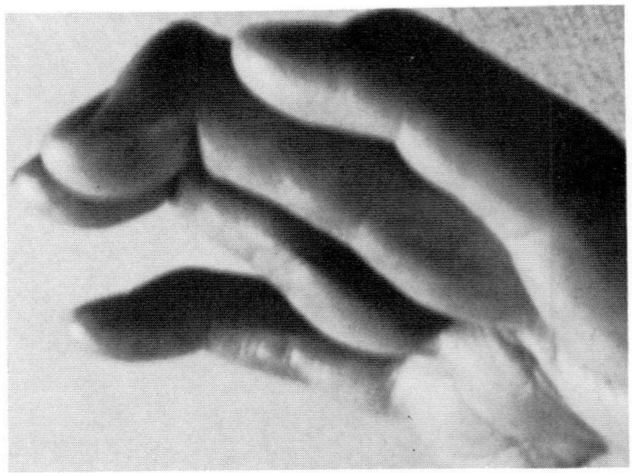

FIG. 20-2. Isolated mallet finger is an uncommon deformity in rheumatoid arthritis. Distal joint deformities are usually secondary to either boutonniere or swan-neck deformities.

of the disturbed anatomy caused by this destructive process. Specific deformities are related to the location and intensity of the involvement.[8,17]

In the normal hand, there is a fine balance between the muscle system and the bones and joints through which they act.[10,19] If the restraining ligamentous structures of the joints are lengthened by rheumatoid disease, this vulnerable balance is compromised. The normal arch system of the hand is disturbed, and the stability and equilibrium necessary for prehension is lost (Fig. 20-1). In the presence of these deranged mechanical factors the use of the hand in functional adaptations contributes to the progress of deformity.

PATHOMECHANICS OF FINGER AND THUMB DEFORMITIES

Deformities at the Distal Interphalangeal Joint

Synovial invasion of the distal joint resulting in specific deformities in rheumatoid arthritis is uncommon. Loosening of the distal attachment of the extensor may cause a typical mallet or drop finger (Fig. 20-2). Loosening of the collateral ligament system and erosive changes in the subchondral bone, cartilage destruction, and external forces may result in instability of the joint. The severe absorptive changes noted in arthritis mutilans may totally destroy the joint. Most of the deformities seen at the distal interphalangeal joint are secondary to the collapsing deformities of the boutonniere or swan-neck deformity (Fig. 20-3).

Deformities at the Proximal Interphalangeal Joint

The interphalangeal collateral ligament system consists of two parts: an oblique and a vertical component. The oblique component connects the middle and proximal phalanges by a ligament from the head of the proximal phalanx to the side of the middle phalanx. The vertical component, frequently called the accessory collateral ligament, is mainly a system for suspension of the palmar plate and the flexor tendon sheath. The flexor tendons are contained within this fibrous sheath. The extensor apparatus consists of the central tendon which inserts into the dorsal capsule and the base of the middle phalanx. It is flanked by lateral tendons of the intrinsic muscles. A synovial pouch from the joint extends proximally beneath the extensor tendons. A synovial pouch also extends proximally between the palmar plate and the overlying bone.

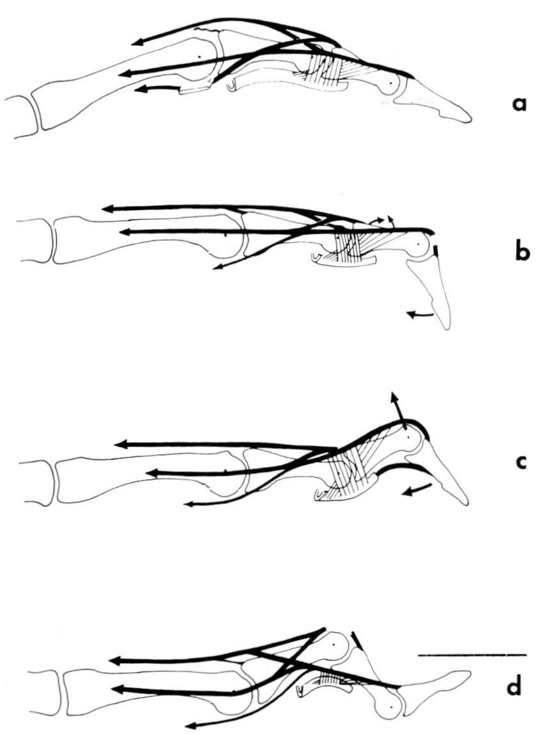

FIG. 20-3. Mechanisms of finger deformities after damage to the extensor apparatus, showing the altered relationship of the extensor tendons and bone and joint systems. (a) Normal finger, (b) mallet finger, (c) swan-neck deformity, (d) boutonniere deformity.

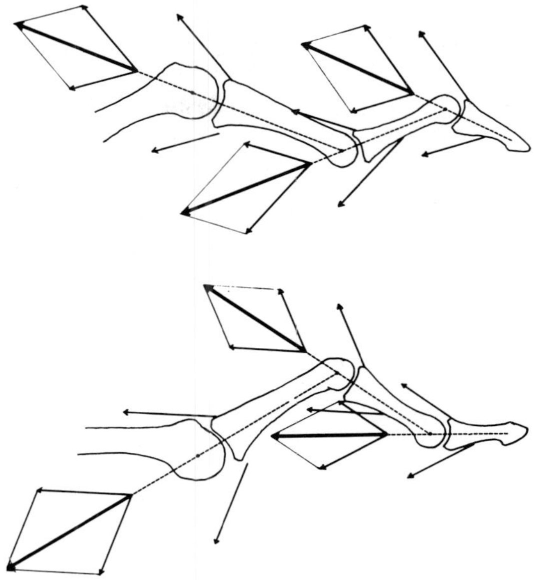

FIG. 20-4. Diagrams showing how axially applied deforming forces further aggravate the established collapse deformities. (*Top*) Swan-neck deformity, (*bottom*) boutonniere deformity.

Limited movement of the proximal interphalangeal joint may result from: (1) articular causes due to disorganization of the joint and fibrinous adhesions, (2) periarticular causes due to adhesions affecting the attachments of the collateral ligaments, and (3) tendinous causes, arising from involvement of the flexor tendons by hyperplastic synovial tissue which limits the gliding of the tendon and later forms adhesions.[14]

Collapse Deformities

Collapse deformity or the buckling phenomenon of the three-joint system of the digit is seen frequently in rheumatoid arthritis. This disturbance is characterized by hyperextension of one of the joints and reciprocal flexion of the contiguous joints. This zig-zag break in the normal flexion-extension pattern of the bony chain is ordinarily prevented by balanced tendon mechanisms and ligament restrictions to hyperextension. Claw finger, swan-neck, and boutonniere deformities are examples of this dysfunction. The latter two are seen frequently in rheumatoid arthritis. A vicious circle of deforming forces is established, and axially applied forces further aggravate the established deformity (Fig. 20-4).

The Boutonniere Deformity. The boutonniere, or buttonhole deformity usually occurs in rheumatoid arthritis through bulging of hyperplastic synovium between the central and lateral extensor tendons. The capsular and bony attachments of the central tendon are weakened, and a relative lengthening of the tendon occurs. The tendon is thus unable to effect normal extension of the middle phalanx. The transverse fibers, which connect the lateral tendons to the central tendon, are further lengthened by this synovial invasion. This allows the lat-

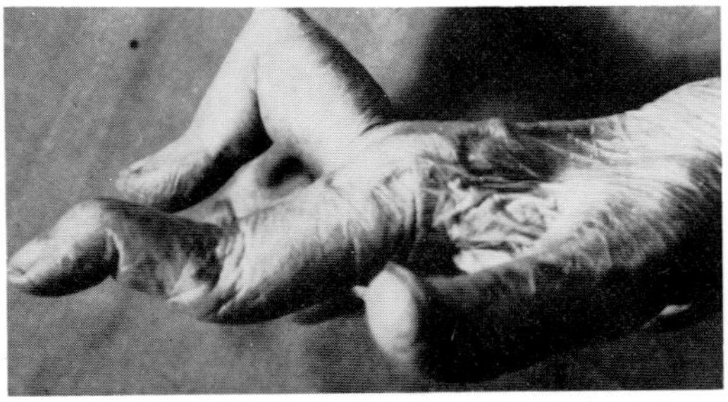

FIG. 20-5. Swan-neck deformities are more common than boutonniere deformities, though they may both be seen in the same hand.

eral tendons of the extensor apparatus to dislocate in a palmar direction. The lateral tendons cross the central axis of the proximal interphalangeal joint and become flexors of the proximal interphalangeal joint. Because they are relatively shortened by their displacement, increased pull is exerted on their distal insertion to the distal phalanx.[36] This results in hyperextension deformity of this joint. Once this collapse deformity is established, it becomes self-perpetuating. The joints may become stiff due to contracture of associated soft tissue structures, and the PIP joint may become further disorganized and subluxated if the disease process continues.

Swan-Neck Deformity. The swan-neck deformity is characterized by hyperextension of the PIP joint and flexion of the distal joint (Fig. 20-5). It probably has as its primary basis a synovitis of the flexor tendon sheath with restriction of interphalangeal joint flexion.[14,16] The main function of the long flexors is interphalangeal joint flexion, especially during the first part of finger flexion.[6] Patients who have flexor synovitis have difficulty in initiating or completing interphalangeal joint flexion either due to pain or the mechanical restriction of the flexor tendons. The flexor tendons then concentrate most of their power on the metacarpophalangeal joints. This posture of the digit facilitates the intrinsic muscle pull to the central tendon across the dorsal aspect of the PIP joint.[31] The failure of proximal interphalangeal flexion, therefore, gives more opportunity for the intrinsics to provide imbalancing forces to the extensor aspect of the joint. Hyperplastic synovium in the PIP joint and the volar pouch also prevent flexion and cause loosening of the attachments of the palmar plate and the accessory collateral ligaments, thus allowing hyperextension of the joint. Treatment programs for this severely disabling deformity must first be directed at the flexor tendon synovitis.[32] Correction of the hyperextension deformity of the PIP joint becomes the main problem once the imbalance of the joint system occurs.[34]

Once the collapse deformity is established, the tendency for perpetuation of the deformity is promoted by axially directed forces and a further disturbance of the linked motor system for the chain of joints.[33] As the hyperextension deformity is increased, the transverse fibers of the retinacular ligament are stretched out, allowing the lateral tendons to dislocate dorsally, which further magnifies the deforming power above the center of axis of rotation of the joint. The oblique retinacular ligaments are stretched and a relative lengthening of the lateral tendons occurs so that the distal joint is flexed from the pull of the flexor profundus tendon. Other deforming forces which can increase the mechanical advantage of the extensors (such as palmar subluxation of the MP joint or wrist joint, or a contracture of the wing-inserted intrinsics due to chronic flexion deformity of the MP joint) add to the swan-neck deformity.[28] The failure of the long flexor tendons to flex the PIP joint will result in permanent joint stiffness. Further destructive changes will result in complete joint disorganization and subluxation.

Deformities at the Metacarpophalangeal Joint

Deformities of the metacarpophalangeal joint in rheumatoid arthritis are usually manifested by increased ulnar drift or pal-

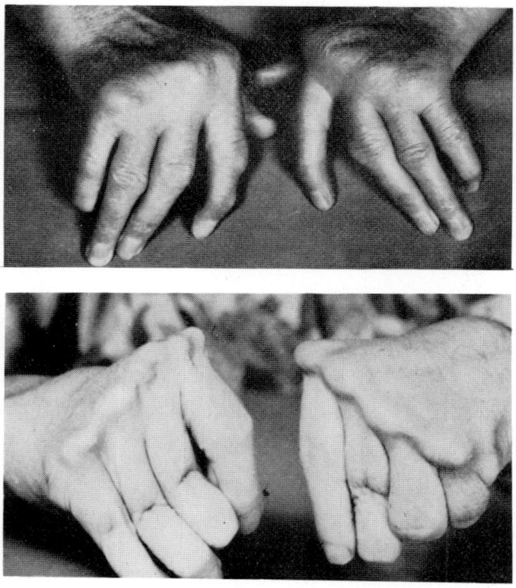

FIG. 20-6. The most common deformities present in rheumatoid hands requiring surgery are (*top*) ulnar drift and (*bottom*) palmar subluxation.

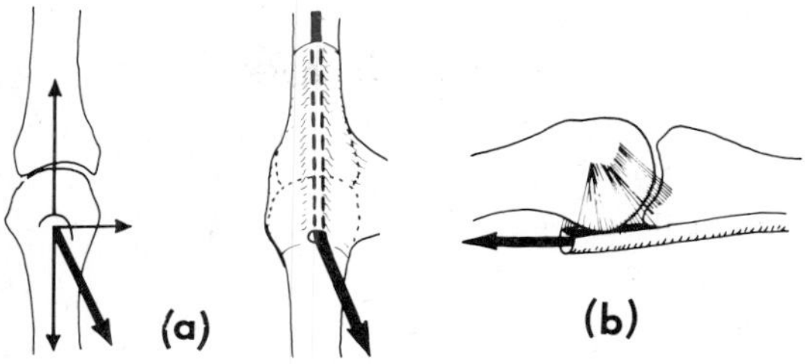

FIG. 20-7. Forces produced by the action of the common flexor in a normal digit cause little or no displacement effect. (a) Anterior view, (b) lateral view. (Redrawn after Tubiana, R.: The Rheumatoid Hand, G.E.M. Monograph No. 3. p. 37. Paris, l'Expansion, 1969)

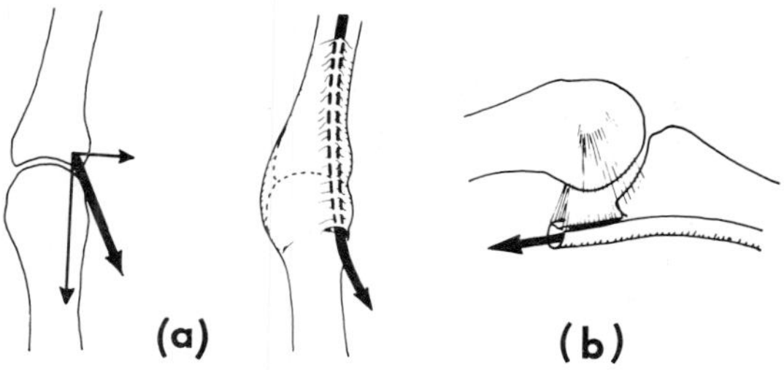

FIG. 20-8. Anterior (*a*) and lateral (*b*) views of MP joint. In rheumatoid arthritis, when the MP joints and ligaments become loosened by the synovial pannus, the fibrous sheath is displaced ulnarward and palmarward. Significant deforming forces result on contraction of the long flexor muscles. (Redrawn after Tubiana, R.: The Rheumatoid Hand, G.E.M. Monograph No. 3. p. 37. Paris, l'Expansion, 1969)

mar subluxation (Fig. 20-6). The MP joint is potentially unstable if normal muscle balance is lost or if the restraining structures of the ligamentous system are destroyed by rheumatoid disease. The MP joint differs from the interphalangeal joint in that its movements are not simply flexion and extension. Movements at this joint are associated with some degree of rotation, abduction, and adduction. The MP joint, because its complex movements are almost constantly in use during functional adaptations of the hand, is subjected to greater stresses.[13]

The extensor tendon expansion across the joint is loosely fixed and is vulnerable to disruption.[38] The flexor tendon mechanism and its supporting structures are more complex. Forces generated across the sheath during pinch and grasp may act adversely to produce elongation of the supporting accessory collateral ligaments.[25] The palmarly and ulnarly displaced flexor tendons are further deforming (Figs. 20-7, 20-8). The intrinsic muscles, which form a bridge between the extensor and flexor systems and at the same time offer direct flexor power across the MP joint, can become deforming once the restraining structures of the MP joint have been lengthened by the rheumatoid disease.

Increased mobility of the fourth and fifth metacarpals is seen frequently in rheumatoid arthritis (Fig. 20-9). It is due to ligamentous loosening at the carpometacarpal joints[40] and the dysfunction of the extensor carpi ulnaris action as seen in the caput ulnae syndrome.[3] The increased breadth of the hand in MP joint flexion causes ulnar displacement forces to be ap-

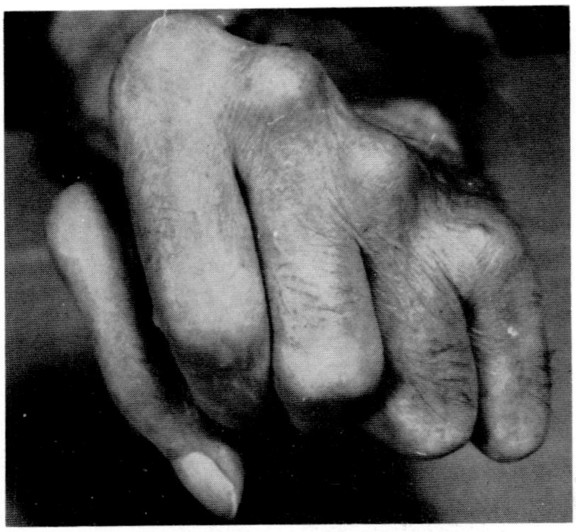

FIG. 20-9. Increased mobility of the fourth and fifth metacarpals is seen frequently in rheumatoid arthritis. The resulting increased breadth of the transverse arch can be a cause of ulnar displacement of the extensor tendons due to pull through their junctura tendonae.

plied on the extensor tendons through their juncture tendons. When the extrinsic extensor across the MP joint has become ulnarly displaced, the intrinsic extensor balance is lost. The intrinsics will then further increase the tendency for volar subluxation and ulnar drift. The ulnar-sided intrinsics seem normally to have a mechanical advantage.[5] This is markedly increased once deformity is established. The metacarpal heads are asymmetrical and show an ulnar-directed slope, especially in the index and middle fingers.[25,37] The collateral ligaments also show an asymmetry that allows ulnar drift to occur. Wrist deformities and ruptured extensor tendons play a secondary role in aggravation of MP joint disturbances.[24,39,40] After ulnar deviation and palmar subluxation occur, the effects of muscle action and the functional forces of digit activity and gravity accentuate the deformity.

Thumb Deformities

Boutonniere Deformity. The most common thumb deformity is a boutonniere deformity,[9] which starts out initially as a synovitis of the MP joint (Fig. 20-10). The joint capsule and extensor apparatus are stretched. The extensor pollicis longus tendon and adductor expansion are displaced ulnarward, and the lateral thenar expansions are displaced radially in relation to the MP joint.[20,23] The attachment of the extensor pollicis brevis to the base of the proximal phalanx is lengthened and becomes ineffective. The ability to extend the MP joint is diminished, and flexion deformity ensues. The combined displaced distal extensors produce hyperextension deformity

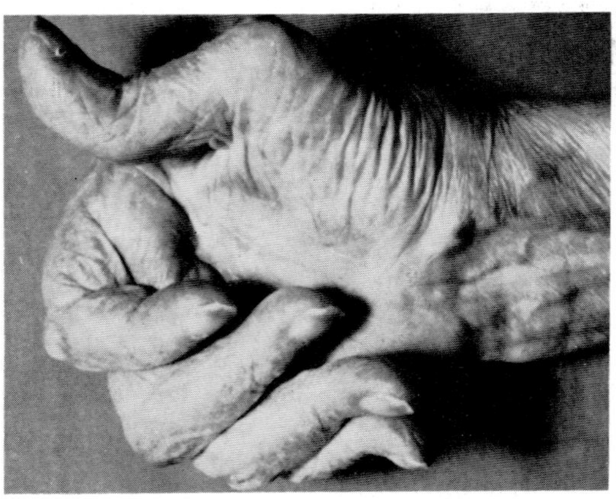

FIG. 20-10. The boutonniere deformity is the most common thumb disturbance in rheumatoid arthritis.

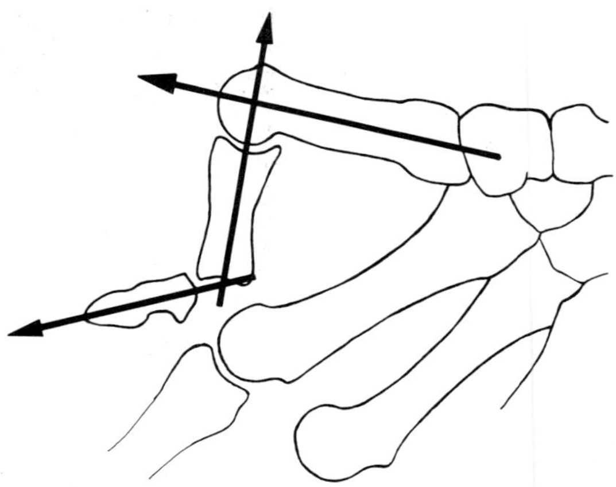

FIG. 20-11. A collapse deformity of an established boutonniere deformity is self-perpetuating.

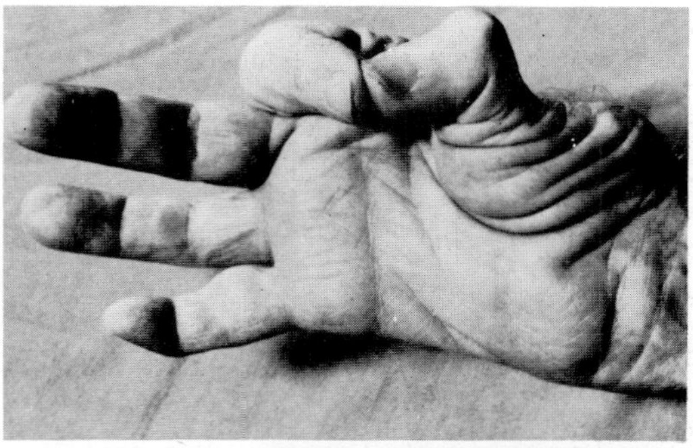

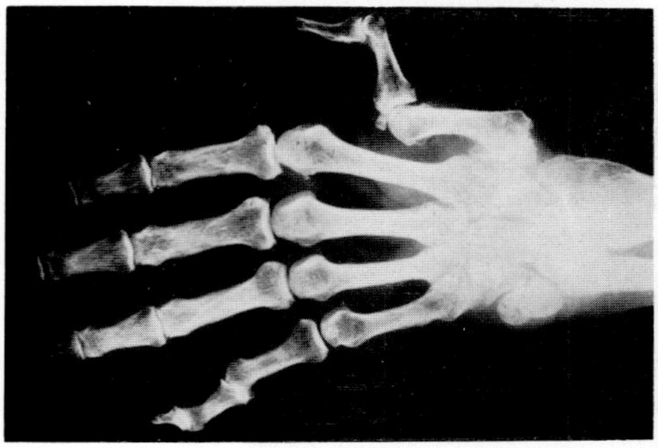

FIG. 20-12. The swan-neck deformity of the thumb is usually initiated by synovitis of the carpometacarpal joint.

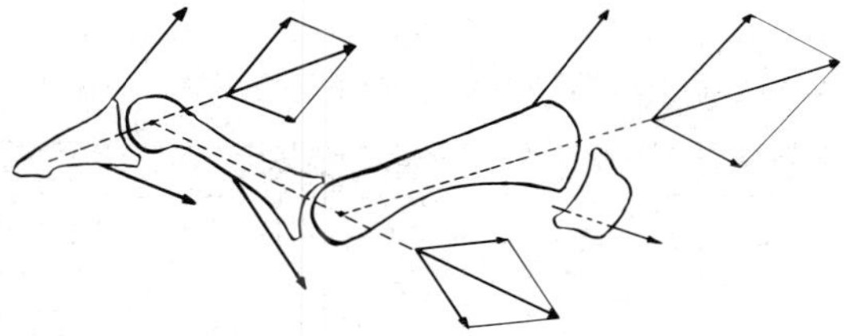

FIG. 20-13. Forces developed in a swan-neck deformity of the thumb: as deformity is increased in one segment, it aggravates associated deformities in other areas.

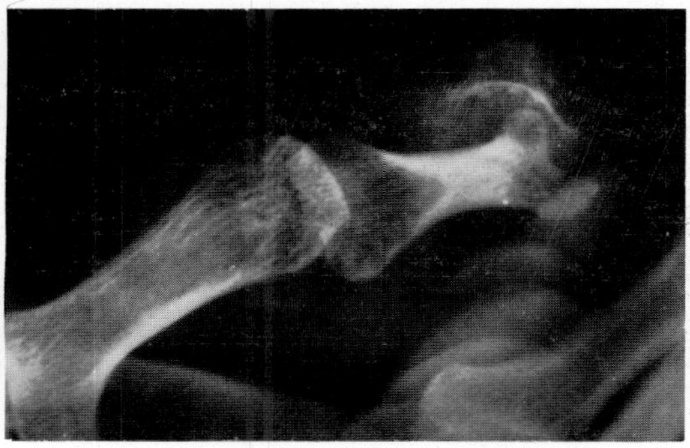

FIG. 20-14. Instability of the distal joint is the result of ligament loosening, erosive bone changes, and extrinsic forces.

of the distal joint. The pinch movements of functional adaptation accentuate the deformity so that a vicious circle is produced. A collapse deformity of the digit occurs (Fig. 20-11). The intrinsics and the long extensor apply all their power on the distal joint. There is a failure of extension of the MP joint due to loss of the extrinsic extensor power. In time, as contractures occur, the deformity becomes fixed. Further destructive joint changes compound the deformity, and joint disorganization and subluxation may occur.

The Swan-Neck Deformity. The swan-neck deformity of the thumb is usually initiated by synovitis of the carpometacarpal joint (Fig. 20-12). Stretching of the joint capsule follows, and the metacarpal may subluxate radialward. Abduction is painful, and a degree of adductor muscle spasm occurs. This imbalance of forces results in an adduction deformity of the metacarpal. A contracture of the adductor pollicis develops.

As abduction of the thumb becomes more difficult, the patient compensates by overextension of the distal joints. Hyperextension deformities of the distal joint may occur. More frequently, hyperextension occurs at the MP joint.

Once hyperextension of this joint occurs, a vicious circle of deformity ensues. Further hyperextension aggravates the adduction of the metacarpal. Adduction of the metacarpal promotes increasing lateral subluxation of the carpometacarpal joint and contracture of the adductor muscle. The distal joint flexes. This is similar to the swan-neck collapse deformity seen in the finger and the deformity is self-perpetuating. As one segment becomes more deformed, it aggravates the deformity in associated areas (Fig. 20-13). Occasionally, severe erosive changes occur in the carpometacarpal joint, and absorption of the trapezium occurs, which decompresses the joint. The digit deformity in this situation is less pronounced.

Distal Joint Instability. Instability of the distal joint may occur as an isolated deformity due to synovial invasion, erosive bone changes, and deformity accentuated by the forces applied during pinch (Fig. 20-14). This gross destruction of the distal joint may also occur in the late stages of the boutonniere deformity.

THE INCIDENCE OF DIGIT DEFORMITIES IN ADVANCED RHEUMATOID ARTHRITIS

To survey the incidence of classical rheumatoid digit deformities, a group of consecutive patients presenting for reconstructive hand surgery was reviewed. The finger deformities considered were ulnar drift, palmar subluxation of the proximal phalanx at the metacarpophalangeal joint, dislocation of the common extensor tendon, boutonniere deformity, and swan-neck deformity. The thumb deformities included boutonniere and swan-neck deformities, instability of the interphalangeal joint, and dislocation of the carpometacarpal joint. The distribution of finger deformities in the index, middle, ring and little fingers is surveyed. A correlation is made of the status of the proximal interphalangeal joint when the metacarpophalangeal joint is abnormal.

The patients were recorded on the Rheumatoid Arthritis Evaluation Record for the Upper Extremity,[35] which has been used in our clinic since 1968. To augment informa-

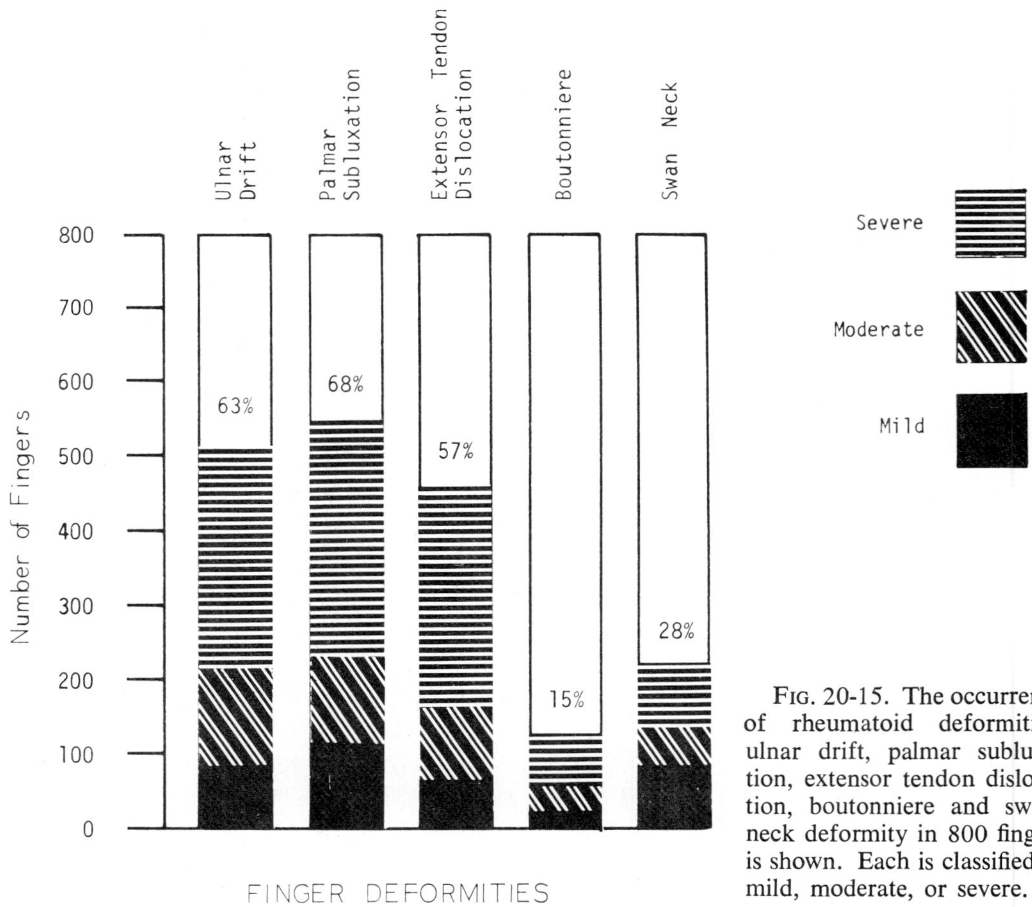

FIG. 20-15. The occurrence of rheumatoid deformities; ulnar drift, palmar subluxation, extensor tendon dislocation, boutonniere and swan-neck deformity in 800 fingers is shown. Each is classified as mild, moderate, or severe.

tion on patients, the office records, surgical dictations, and preoperative photographs and x-rays were consulted.

One hundred patients were included, giving data on 200 thumbs and 800 fingers. All had rheumatoid arthritis which had progressed to marked functional impairment of the hands. The patients were seeking help through reconstructive operative procedures. The average age at onset of arthritis was 36.7 years (range 7 to 67 years); their arthritis had been present for 17.5 years (range 4 to 49 years) at the time of the first upper extremity reconstructive procedure; and the average age at operation was 54.2 years (range 18 to 81 years).

The deformities were graded according to the severity indices specified in the Rheumatoid Arthritis Evaluation Record. Although arbitrary, this method for classifying deformity is useful in data retrieval. We feel it is valid, based on clinical experience, in the light of the purpose of this record and the desirability of a simple record system. Indicators for mild, moderate, and severe degrees of deformity were outlined. In some cases, this was evaluated according to the restricted range of motion in a joint; for example, the swan-neck deformity is associated with hyperextension of the proximal interphalangeal joint and restricted flexion. For that reason, a mild swan-neck deformity may be described as having a range of motion at the proximal interphalangeal joint of +10° to 50°; a moderate deformity, +20° to 30°; and a severe deformity, +30° to 10°. This allows the swan-neck deformity to be classified quickly. The total record, including photographs and x-rays as well as ranges of motion, describes a deformity more precisely. The severity indices are reproduced in their entirety as a reference for the evaluation of deformities in this study and as a summary of the many parameters which are evaluated (see pp. 156-157).

In the 800 fingers studied, ulnar drift was present in 507 (63 per cent), with 81 mild, 131 moderate, and 295 severe deformities

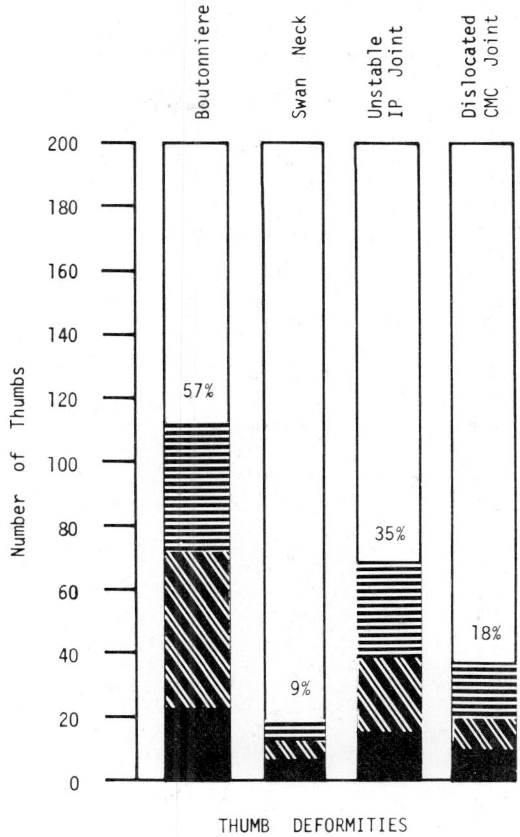

FIG. 20-16. The occurrence of rheumatoid deformities; boutonniere, swan-neck, unstable interphalangeal joint, and dislocated carpometacarpal joint in 200 thumbs is shown. Each is classified as mild, moderate or severe.

(Fig. 20-15). Palmar subluxation of the proximal phalanx at the metacarpophalangeal joint was present in 544 (68 per cent), with 112 mild, 114 moderate, and 318 severe deformities. The common extensor tendon was dislocated in 458 (57 per cent), with 63 mild, 96 moderate, and 299 severe deformities. All three deformities occurred in combination in the majority of fingers; however, variation in degree and total number of each deformity demonstrates that they do not always occur concomitantly or increase in severity at the same rate. Palmar subluxation was the most frequently occurring deformity, followed by ulnar drift and

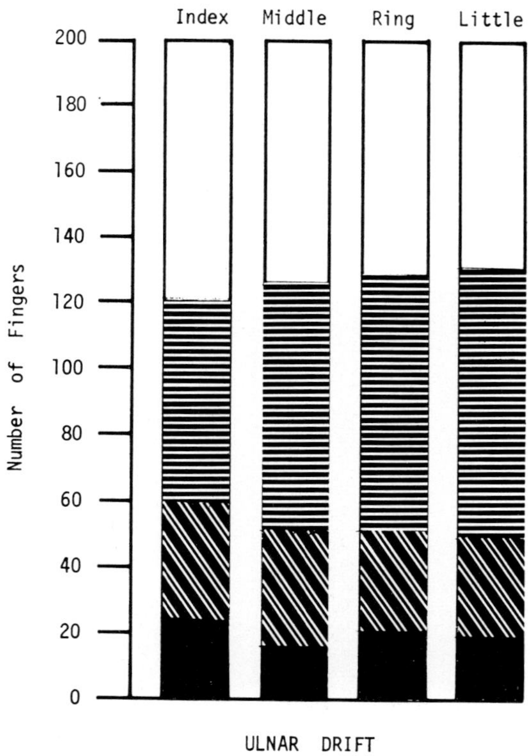

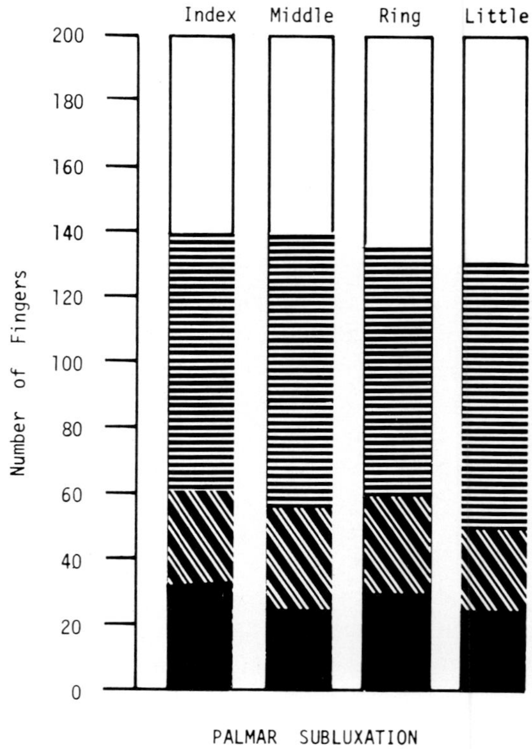

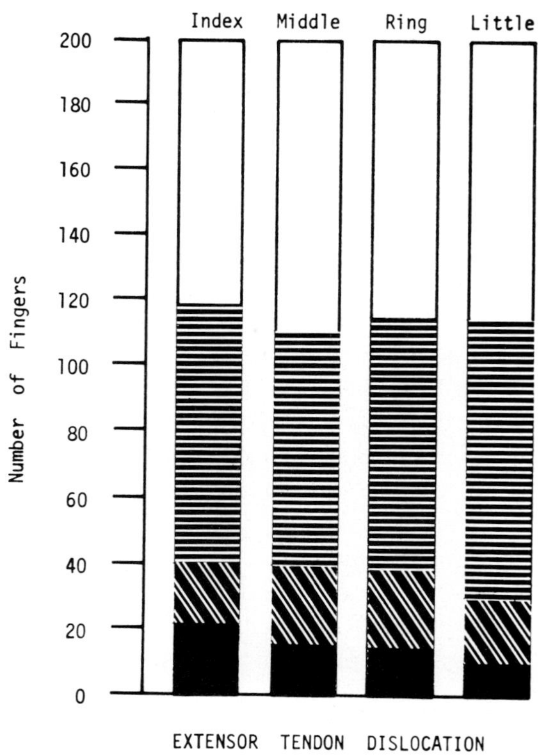

FIG. 20-17. Ulnar drift, palmar subluxation, and extensor tendon dislocation are broken down as they occurred in each of 800 fingers. Each deformity is classified as mild, moderate, or severe.

then dislocation of the common extensor tendon.

Deformity in the proximal interphalangeal joint was much less frequent than in the metacarpophalangeal joint. Boutonniere deformity was found in 123 (15 per cent), with 18 mild, 33 moderate, and 72 severe deformities. There was swan-neck deformity in 220 patients (28 per cent) with 80 mild, 48 moderate, and 92 severe cases.

In the 200 thumbs, the boutonniere deformity was the most prevalent and appeared in 113 cases (57 per cent), with 23 mild, 49 moderate, and 41 severe deformities (Fig. 20-16). Only 18 swan-neck deformities (9 per cent) were found; 7 were mild, 5, moderate, and 6, severe. Instability of the interphalangeal joint occurred 69 times (35 per cent), with 15 mild, 23 moderate, and 31 severe deformities. The carpometacarpal or trapeziometacarpal joint was dislocated in 36 cases (18 per cent); there were 9 mild, 10 moderate, and 17 severe deformities.

In the advanced rheumatoid arthritic hand, the triad of ulnar drift, palmar subluxation and extensor tendon dislocation occurred often. As can be seen in Figure 20-17, there was little variation from index to little finger, and most of the deformities fell into the severe category. There was a tendency for ulnar drift to occur more on the ulnar side of the hand (index, 122; middle, 126; ring, 128; and little, 131) and for the ulnar fingers to be the most severely involved (index, 63; middle, 74; ring, 76; little, 82 with severe degree of deformity). Palmar subluxation of the proximal phalanx was slightly more prevalent on the radial aspect of the hand (index 139, middle 139, ring 134, little 132), and no trend was noted in the degree of deformity from one finger to another. Dislocation of the common extensor tendon occurred less frequently than

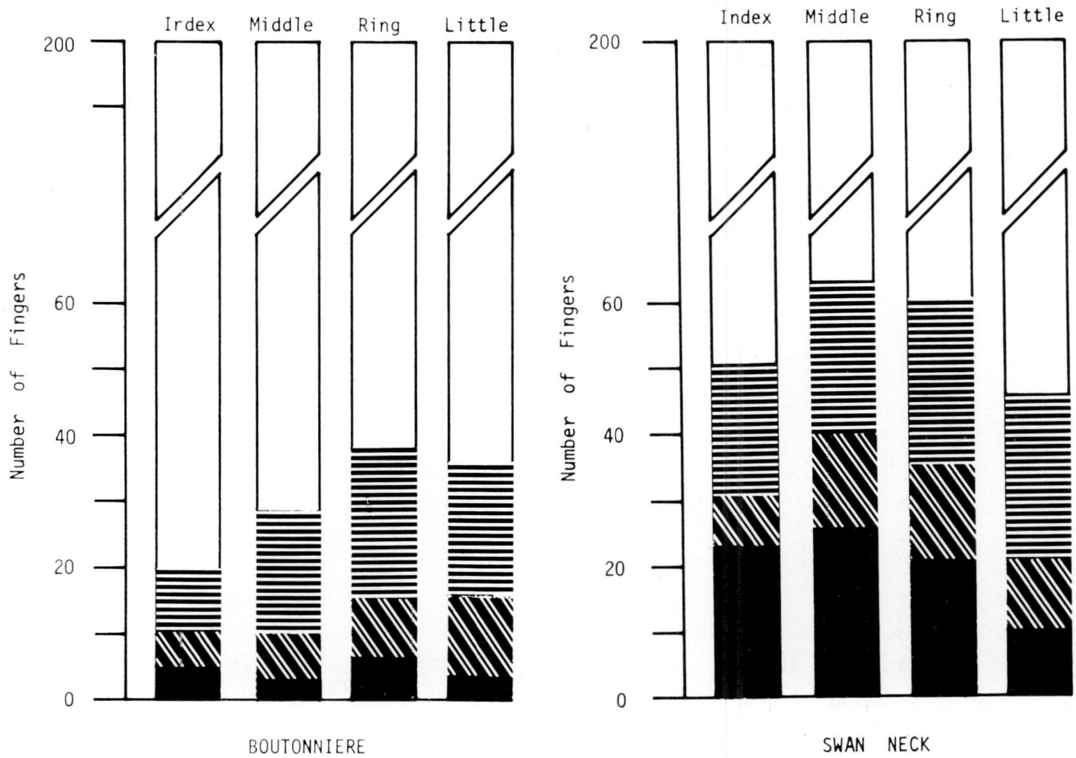

FIG. 20-18. Boutonniere and swan-neck deformities are classified as they occurred in each of 800 fingers according to degree of severity.

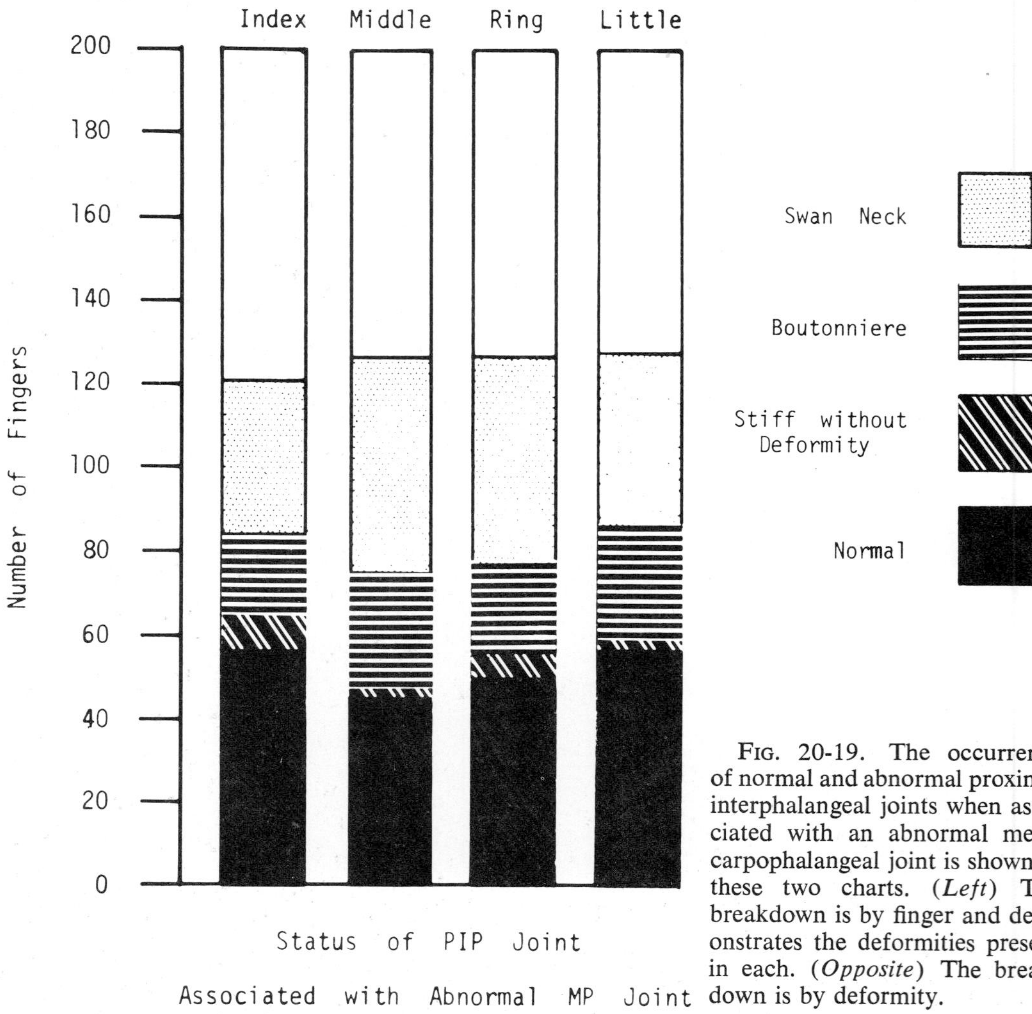

FIG. 20-19. The occurrence of normal and abnormal proximal interphalangeal joints when associated with an abnormal metacarpophalangeal joint is shown in these two charts. (*Left*) The breakdown is by finger and demonstrates the deformities present in each. (*Opposite*) The breakdown is by deformity.

other deformities; the total number was fairly constant from index to little finger. A majority of the deformities were severe; only a few were mild or moderate. Apparently, once the tendon begins to subluxate, it rapidly progresses to complete dislocation.

Compared to the abnormalities of the metacarpophalangeal joint, the proximal interphalangeal joint was less often involved (Fig. 20-18). Boutonniere deformities involved the ulnar two fingers more often than the radial fingers and were more often severe in degree of deformity than mild or moderate. The index finger was involved in 20 cases, with 5 mild, 5 moderate, and 10 severe; the middle finger in 29 cases, with 3 mild, 7 moderate and 19 severe; the ring finger in 38 cases, with 7 mild, 8 moderate, and 23 severe; and the little finger in 36 cases, with 3 mild, 13 moderate, and 20 severe. The swan-neck deformity was present much more often than the boutonniere and showed a predilection for the middle and ring fingers. Many more mild and moderate degrees of deformity existed, indicating that this deformity progresses more slowly than the boutonniere. The swan-neck deformity involved the index finger in 51 cases, with 23 mild, 9 moderate, and 19 severe; the middle finger in 63 cases, with 26 mild, 14 moderate, and

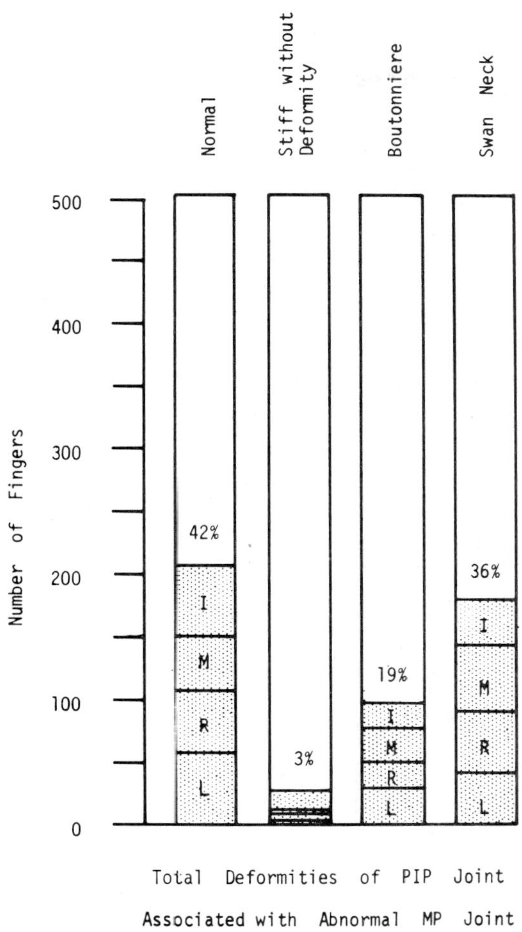

23 severe; the ring finger in 60 cases, with 21 mild, 14 moderate, and 25 severe; and the little finger in 46 cases, with 10 mild, 11 moderate, and 25 severe.

The digit is a multiarticulated structure, and preservation of a normal arch is dependent upon the integrity of the joints and a delicate interrelationship of the flexor and extensor mechanisms. Proximal alterations in joint integrity and tendon balance are often reflected in distal deformities. An analysis was done of the distal deformities in fingers which had major alterations at the metacarpophalangeal joint. The three common deformities of the metacarpophalangeal joint are ulnar drift, palmar subluxation, and extensor tendon dislocation. If two of these three were present, the joint was considered to have a major alteration, and the status of the distal finger was considered for study. No attempt was made to separate the mild, moderate, and severe deformities in this grouping.

In 800 fingers, 503 metacarpophalangeal joints (62 per cent) fulfilled the criteria for major alteration (Fig. 20-19). The index finger had slightly fewer abnormal metacarpophalangeal joints (121) compared with the middle finger (127), the ring finger (127), and the little finger (128). More normal proximal interphalangeal joints were present in the index (57) and little fingers (57) compared with the middle (45) and ring fingers (50). The swan-neck deformity predominated in the middle (53) and ring fingers (50) with the index finger (36) and little finger (41) having fewer. The tendency for boutonniere deformity in the ulnar fingers was not as strong (index finger, 21; middle finger, 27; ring finger, 22; and little finger, 28). Apparently more isolated boutonniere deformities without concomitant metacarpophalangeal abnormality occur in the ring finger. A small percentage of stiff proximal interphalangeal joints without associated boutonniere or swan-neck deformities was also present (index finger, 7; middle finger, 2; ring finger, 5; and little finger, 2).

The percentage of distal deformities in the 503 fingers is shown in Figure 20-19. Normal proximal interphalangeal joints numbered 209 (42 per cent), and only 16 (3 per cent) were stiff without deformity. Boutonniere deformity was present in 98 (19 per cent) and swan-neck deformity in 180 (36 per cent). It is interesting that despite major abnormalities at the metacarpophalangeal joint, the associated proximal interphalangeal joint was normal in 46 per cent of the cases. Conversely, when boutonniere and swan-neck deformities existed, they were frequently accompanied by proximal deformity: 98 out of 123 boutonniere deformities (80 per cent) and 180 out of 220 swan-neck deformities (82 per cent).

In summary, 200 thumbs and 800 fingers were examined in patients with advanced rheumatoid arthritis. In the fingers, ulnar drift was present in 63 per cent, palmar subluxation in 68 per cent and extensor tendon dislocation in 57 per cent. Deformities of the proximal interphalangeal joint were much less common, boutonniere deformity in 15 per cent and swan-neck deformity in 28 per cent. With major alteration of the metacarpophalangeal joint, the proximal interphalangeal joint remained normal 42 per cent of the time. However, if boutonniere or swan-neck deformity was present, the metacarpophalangeal had major abnormalities 80 per cent of the time. Boutonniere deformity was found more often in the ulnar fingers and swan-neck deformity in the middle and ring fingers. The most frequent thumb deformity was the boutonniere, present in 57 per cent of cases. Conversely, the swan-neck deformity was found in only 9 per cent of thumbs. The interphalangeal joint was unstable in 35 per cent, and there was trapeziometacarpal dislocation in 18 per cent of thumbs.

Rheumatoid Arthritis Evaluation Record Severity Indices for Clinical Abnormalities

Swan-neck, thumb—flexion limit of MCP joint ROM
Mild: +10° to 50°
Moderate: +20° to 30°
Severe: +30° to 10°

Boutonniere, thumb—extension limit MCP joint ROM
Mild: −5° to −20°
Moderate: −20° to −40°
Severe: more than −40°

Subluxation to dislocation
Mild: capable of reduction manually
Moderate: incomplete reduction manually
Severe: irreducible dislocation

Swan-neck, fingers—flexion limit of PIP joint ROM
Mild: +10° to 50°
Moderate: +20° to 30°
Severe: +30° to 10°

Boutonniere, fingers—extension limit of PIP joint ROM
Mild: −5° to −10°
Moderate: −10° to −30°
Severe: more than −30°

Intrinsic tightness—PIP flexion with MCP joint extended ROM
Mild: more than 60°
Moderate: 20° to 60°
Severe: less than 20°

Ulnar drift—joint measured in maximum active extension (measure metacarpal-phalanx angle)
Mild: 0° to 10°
Moderate: 10° to 30°
Severe: more than 30°

Radial drift—joint measured in maximum active extension (measure metacarpal-phalanx angle)
Mild: 0° to 10°
Moderate: 10° to 30°
Severe: more than 30°

Ankylosis (record angle of ankylosis under ROM)
Severe: when present

Instability (measure excess of passive medial-lateral motion compared to a normal joint)
Mild: 0° to 10°
Moderate: 10° to 20°
Severe: more than 20°

Tendon rupture
Severe: complete

Constrictive tenosynovitis
Mild: inconstant triggering during active ROM
Moderate: constant triggering during active ROM
Severe: prevents active ROM

Synovial hypertrophy—increase in joint size
Mild: visible increase
Moderate: palpable increase
Severe: more than 10% measured increase

Crepitation with motion
Mild: inconstant during active ROM
Moderate: constant during active ROM
Severe: constant during passive ROM

Extensor tendon subluxation
Mild: subluxates in MCP flexion
Moderate: tendon dislocated into intermetacarpal groove during MCP flexion but can be reduced

Severe: tendon remains in intermetacarpal groove

Rotational deformity—
Mild: 5° to 15°
Moderate: 15° to 30°
Severe: more than 30°

Erosions—x-ray exam
Mild: one
Moderate: two
Severe: three or more

Joint narrowing—x-ray exam
Mild: ⅓ narrowing
Moderate: ⅔ narrowing
Severe: obliteration of joint space

Subchondral sclerosis
Mild: when present

Painful joint with motion
Mild: pain with active motion
Moderate: pain with active motion which interferes with activity
Severe: pain at rest which prevents activity

Nerve compression—median, ulnar, or radial
Mild: sensory disturbance
Moderate: sensory disturbances and motor weakness
Severe: sensory and motor paralysis

Vasculitis
Mild: paronychial hemorrhages or subcutaneous nodules
Moderate: peripheral neuropathy
Severe: cutaneous gangrene of extremity

Nodules
Mild: one, mobile and not tender
Moderate: two, fixed and tender
Severe: more than three, fixed, tender and with skin breakdown

REFERENCES

1. American Arthritis and Rheumatism Foundation, 1969 Annual Report, New York.
2. Ansell, B. M.: Hand Assessment in Rheumatoid Arthritis. International Workshop on Artificial Finger Joints. Ann. Rheum. Dis. (Suppl.), *28*:77-80, 1969.
3. Bäckdahl, M.: The caput ulnae syndrome in rheumatoid arthritis. Acta Rheum. Scand. (Suppl.), *5*:1-75, 1963.
4. Backhouse, K. M.: Mechanical factors influencing normal and rheumatoid metacarpophalangeal joints. International Workshop on Artificial Finger Joints. Ann. Rheum. Dis. (Suppl.), *28*:15-19, 1969.
5. Boyes, J. H.: The role of the intrinsic muscles in rheumatoid arthritis. *In* Tubiana, Raoul (ed.): The Rheumatoid Hand, Group d'Etude de la Main Monograph No. 3. pp. 63-65. Paris, l'Expansion Scientifique Francaise, 1969.
6. Brand, P. W.: Paralytic claw hand. J. Bone Joint Surg. [Brit.], *40*:618-632, 1958.
7. Brewerton, D. A.: Hand deformities in rheumatoid disease. Ann. Rheum. Dis., *16*:183-197, 1957.
8. Bywater, E. G. L.: Pathogenesis of finger joint lesions in rheumatoid arthritis. International Workshop of Artificial Finger Joints. Ann. Rheum. Dis. (Suppl.), *28*:5-10, 1969.
9. Clayton, M. L.: Surgery of the thumb in rheumatoid arthritis. J. Bone Joint Surg., *44*:1376-1386, 1962.
10. Flatt, A. E.: The Care of the Rheumatoid Hand. ed. 2. St. Louis, C. V. Mosby Co., 1968.
11. Girzadas, D., Shapiro, J., Vainio, K.: Natural course of rheumatoid arthritis in the hands. In Tubiana, Raoul (ed.): The Rheumatoid Hand, G.E.M. Monograph No. 3. pp. 67-69. Paris, l'Expansion, 1969.
12. Glynn, L. E.: Aetiology of rheumatoid arthritis with regard to its chronicity. International Workshop on Artificial Finger Joints. Ann. Rheum. Dis. (Suppl.), *28*: 3-4, 1969.
13. Hakstian, R., and Tubiana, R.: Ulnar deviation of the fingers: the role of joint structure and function. J. Bone Joint Surg., *49*: 299-316, 1967.
14. Harrison, K. M.: Rheumatoid deformities of the proximal interphalangeal joints of the hand. International Workshop on Artificial Finger Joints. Ann. Rheum. Dis. (Suppl.), *28*:20-22, 1969.
15. Hollander, J. L.: Arthritis. ed. 2. Philadelphia, Lea & Febiger, 1966.
16. Kay, A.: Development of deformities in the rheumatoid hand: a preliminary report. International Workshop on Artificial Finger Joints. Ann. Rheum. Dis. (Suppl.), *28*: 95-97, 1969.
17. Kessler, I., Raunio, P., and Vainio, K.: The rheumatoid hand: a comparative study of affected sites. Acta Rheum. Scand., *11*:241-246, 1965.
18. Laine, V. A. I., Sairanen, E., and Vainio, K.: Finger deformities caused by rheumatoid arthritis. J. Bone Joint Surg., *39*:527-533, 1957.
19. Landsmeer, J. M. F.: A report on the coor-

dination of the interphalangeal joints of the human finger and its disturbances. Acta Morph. Neerl. Scand., *2*:59-84, 1960.
20. McFarlane, R. M.: Observations on the functional anatomy of the intrinsic muscles of the thumb. J. Bone Joint Surg., *44*:1073-1088, 1962.
21. Mellors, R. C., Nowoslawski, A., Korngold, L., and Sengson, B. L.: Rheumatoid factor and the pathogenesis of rheumatoid arthritis. J. Exp. Med., *113*:475-484, 1961.
22. Moberg, E., *et al.*: The early pathological changes in rheumatoid arthritis. Acta Chir. Scand. (Suppl.), *357*:142-147, 1966.
23. Nalebuff, E. A.: Restoration of balance in the rheumatoid thumb. *In* Tubiana, Raoul (ed.): The Rheumatoid Hand, G.E.M. Monograph No. 3. pp. 197-206. Paris, l'Expansion, 1969.
24. Shapiro, J. S.: A new factor in the etiology of ulnar drift. Clin. Orthop., *68*:32-43, 1970.
25. Smith, E. M., Juvinall, R. C., Bender, L. R., and Pearson, J. R.: Flexor forces and rheumatoid metacarpophalangeal deformity. J.A.M.A., *198*:130-134, 1966.
26. Smith, R. J., and Kaplan, E. B.: Rheumatoid deformities at the metacarpophalangeal joints of the fingers. J. Bone Joint Surg., *49*:31-42, 1967.
27. Sokoloff, L.: Personal communication.
28. Stack, H. G.: Muscle function in the fingers. J. Bone Joint Surg. [Brit.], *44*:899-909, 1962.
29. Steindler, A.: Arthritic deformities of the wrist and fingers. J. Bone Joint Surg., *33*: 849-862, 1951.
30. Straub, L. R.: The etiology of finger deformities in the hand affected by rheumatoid arthritis. Bull. Hosp. Joint Dis., *21*:322-329, 1960.
31. Swanson, A. B.: Surgery of the hand in cerebral palsy and the swan-neck deformity. J. Bone Joint Surg., *42*:951-964, 1960.
32. ———: The need for early treatment of the rheumatoid hand. J. Mich. State Med. Soc., *60*:348-351, 1961.
33. ———: Pathomechanics of the swan-neck deformity. J. Bone Joint Surg. (Amer.), *47*:636 (Abstract), 1965.
34. ———: Surgery of the hand in cerebral palsy and muscle origin release procedures. Surg. Clin. N. Amer., *48*:1129, 1968.
35. Swanson, A. B., Mays, J. D., and Yamauchi, Y.: A rheumatoid evaluation record for the upper extremity. Surg. Clin. N. Amer., *48*:1003-1013, 1968.
36. Tubiana, R.: The mechanisms of deformities of the fingers due to musculotendinous imbalance. *In* Tubiana, Raoul (ed.): The Rheumatoid Hand, G.E.M. Monograph No. 3. pp. 133-141. Paris, l'Expansion, 1969.
37. Tubiana, R. and Hakistan, R.: Normal and pathological ulnar deviation of the fingers. *In* Tubiana, Raoul (ed.): The Rheumatoid Hand, G.E.M. Monograph No. 3. pp. 44-50. Paris, l'Expansion, 1969.
38. Vainio, K., and Oka, M.: Ulnar deviation of the fingers. Ann. Rheum. Dis., *12*:122-124, 1953.
39. Vaughan-Jackson, O. J.: Attrition ruptures of tendons as a factor in the production of deformities in the rheumatoid hand. Proc. Roy. Soc. Med., *52*:132-134, 1959.
40. ———: Rheumatoid hand deformities as considered in the light of tendon imbalances. J. Bone Joint Surg. [Brit.], *44*:764-775, 1962.
41. Zancolli, E.: Structural and Dynamic Bases of Hand Surgery. Philadelphia, J. B. Lippincott, 1968.

CHAPTER 21

Soft Tissue Surgery of the Rheumatoid Hand

ROBERT D. MIDGLEY, M.D.C.M.

The aims of surgery in rheumatoid hand disease are: (a) to prevent further extension of the disease in the area, (b) to provide as near normal function as possible to the diseased hand, and (c) to provide a pleasing cosmetic appearance. Of these, prophylaxis against rheumatoid extension is most important. Meticulous fine instrument technique is indicated in hand surgery, particularly in rheumatoid disease, where dermal atrophy and rheumatoid vasculitis present the surgeon with thin, taut, inelastic skin that withstands trauma very poorly (Fig. 21-1). Incisions must be carefully planned and outlined with methylene blue in order to preserve as much of the lymphatic and venous drainage as possible, provide the best possible exposure, yet involve the least amount of undermining.[1] Longitudinal straight line incisions are contraindicated across any finger or hand joint. Preference is given to lazy "S" incisions (Fig. 21-2) across the metacarpophalangeal joint, lazy "S" incisions longitudinally along the dorsum of the hand, transverse incisions paralleling the crease lines on the palm of the hand, and volar digital transverse incisions with midaxial extensions on the individual fingers. Skin hooks should be used on skin edges for retraction and fine-toothed Adson forceps are used in handling the deeper tissues. Sharp dissection is less traumatic than blunt dissection and gives rise to a lower risk of hematoma formation.

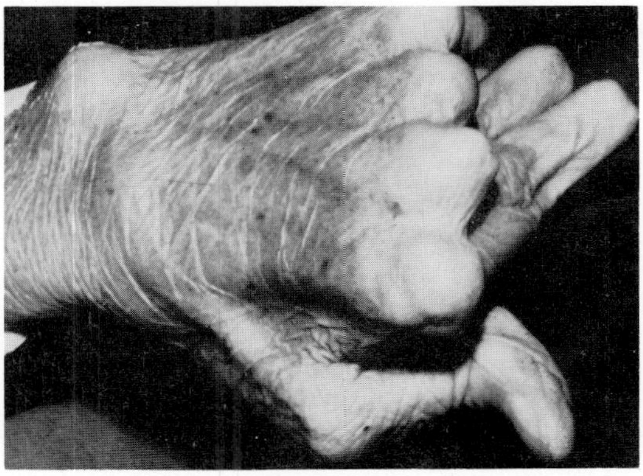

FIG. 21-1. Advanced skin changes in rheumatoid disease.

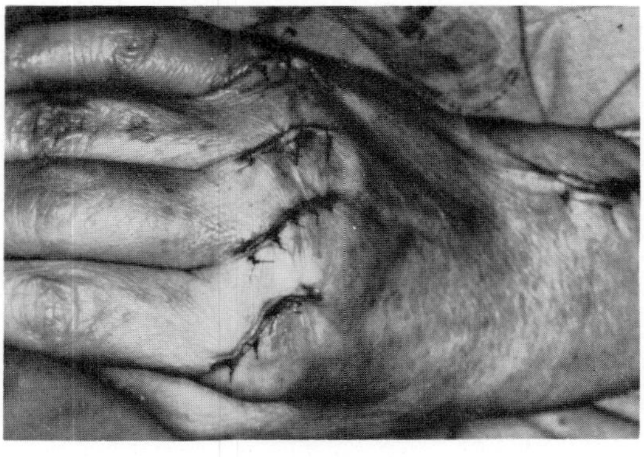

FIG. 21-2. Skin incisions over MP joints allow maximum exposure with minimum morbidity.

Operative Procedure. Rheumatoid hand surgery is performed under pneumatic tourniquet control with the limb stripped of blood by application of an Eschmarch bandage. Generally the tourniquet should be inflated for no more than 1½ hours. Upon release of the tourniquet, compression is ap-

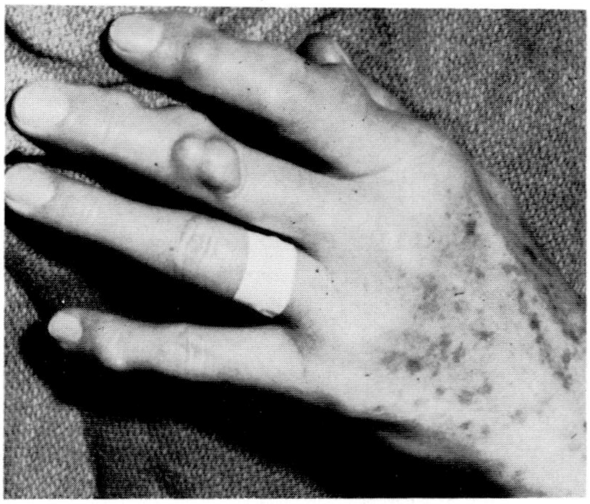

FIG. 21-3. Numerous digital rheumatoid nodules.

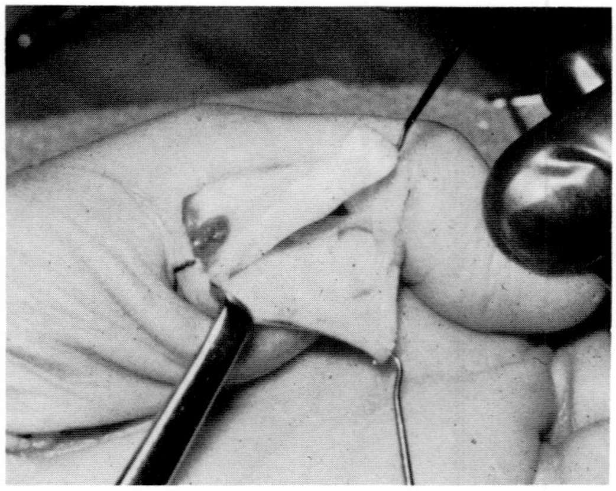

FIG. 21-4. Release of trigger thumb, showing the secondary thickening of the flexor pollicis longus tendon.

plied to the area of surgery for 5 minutes to minimize the effect of post-tourniquet vasodilatation caused by release of the endogenous histamine. Hemostasis is then secured and the wounds closed without tension. Preference is given to closure by means of interrupted horizontal mattress sutures, using fine plain catgut and non-absorbable suture material.

A well-padded hand dressing is applied with a fluff gauze bolus in the palm in order to preserve longitudinal and transverse arches. The hand is then placed in the position of function, unless the specific surgical procedure performed demands a position in which the hand may be nursed. Plaster slabs maintain the desired position and application of an elastic bandage maintains gentle compression on the operated hand. The initial dressing should remain undisturbed for at least 10 days to allow good early healing of the soft tissues.

Rheumatoid nodules. These lesions are seen in approximately 20 per cent of patients and are generally subcutaneous over bony prominences, although they may appear as nodules in sheaths of peripheral nerves (nodulous rheumarthritis perineuritis) or in tendon sheaths and on tendons. In the hand, the subcutaneous nodules tend to appear on the sides of the interphalangeal joints (Fig. 21-3). Histologically, the early nodule is comprised of nonspecific granulation tissue with the small arteries within the granulation tissue showing active inflammatory change (arteritis). As the nodule matures, it becomes relatively avascular and inert.

These nodules persist and are not responsive to cortisone therapy. They should, therefore, be excised when their location or size interferes with the function of the digit, for they are prone to trauma and undergo degenerative or inflammatory changes.

Tenosynovitis. Tenosynovitis occurs in the hand in three places where synovium-lined sheaths surround the tendons.[2] There is, therefore: (a) dorsal tenosynovitis of the long extensor tendons under the extensor retinaculum and extending distally over the dorsum of the hand, (b) volar tenosynovitis extending from the carpal tunnel area under the flexor retinaculum of the wrist and extending distally along the radial and ulnar border of the proximal palm, and (c) digital tenosynovitis. The dorsal and volar clinical presentations and therapy have been covered in Chapter 19.

Digital tenosynovitis presents early symptoms because of the unyielding nature of the surrounding fibro-osseous canals. The symptom of which patients complain is a catching or locking of the digit in movements of flexion or extension. Clinically, this is a trigger finger. The etiology may be a stenosing tenosynovitis at the level of the proximal pulley of the digital synovial sheath in the palm, which produces a secondary or sympathetic thickening and enlargement of the flexor tendon (Fig. 21-4), or trigger finger may be due to tendon nodules which increase in size and become locked in transit across the fixed pulleys of the digital fibro-osseous canal system. Variants of this type of trigger finger (primary tendon nodules) present one of two triggering phenomena, depending upon the location of the nodule with reference to the position of the finger. If the finger locks in a flexed position, the tendon nodule is in the distal palm just proximal to the proximal pulley of the fibro-osseous canal. If the finger locks in extension, the tendon nodule is on the profundus tendon distal to the sublimus decussation.

The treatment of trigger finger is surgical release of the fibro-osseous canal over the stenotic area to allow unimpeded gliding of the flexor tendon, or tendon nodulectomy and meticulous approximation of the area of nodule excision in the less common cases of primary tendon nodule trigger finger. Occasionally, when extensive tenosynovitis is present in the finger, it is advisable to make a midlateral incision on the finger and to perform a tenosynovectomy throughout the length of the finger, preserving fibrous pulleys over the middle portion of the proximal and middle phalanges.

De Quervain's disease is specific stenosing tenosynovitis involving the tendons of the abductor pollicis longus and extensor pollicis brevis at the level of the styloid process of the radius.[4] The symptom complex of painful extension and abduction of the thumb with pain and tenderness located over the distal end of the radius is classical. Treatment of rheumatoid De Quervain's disease consists of synovectomy and release of the rigid compartment beneath the extensor retinaculum through which the tendons run.

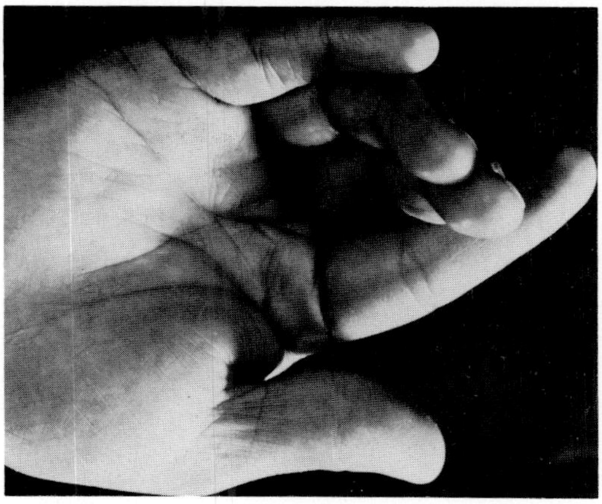

Fig. 21-5. Spontaneous rupture of sublimis with profundus to index finger and profundus to little finger.

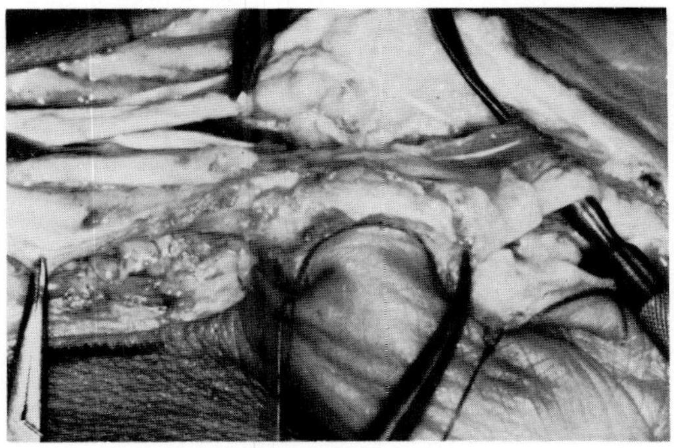

Fig. 21-6. Profound tenosynovitis with necrotic and ruptured tendons.

In digital tenosynovitis, early active digital movement is encouraged once the soft tissue has healed (about 10 days). Surgical results are excellent.

Tendon Rupture. There are two causes of tendon rupture. One is direct fibrinoid necrosis of the tendon.[5] Proliferation of tenosynovium may be so severe that the relatively avascular tendons become deprived of their blood supply, undergo necrosis, and rupture spontaneously (Figs. 21-5 and 21-6).

Tendons may rupture because of mechanical attrition over roughened spurs of bone.[6] This popular theory accounts for the rupture of the extensor pollicis longus

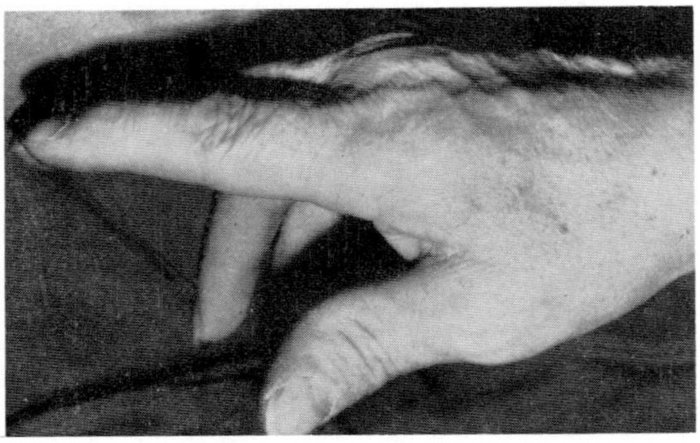

FIG. 21-7. Rupture of ulnar two extensors.

tendon as it changes direction at the level of Lister's tubercle. It also explains the progression of digital extensor tendon ruptures proceeding from ulnar to radial side, since these structures suffer attrition at the level of the bony spicule related to the subluxated ulnar head (Fig. 21-7). Further tendons said to suffer attrition rupture are the flexor pollicis longus and flexor digitorum profundus of the index finger at the level of scaphoid erosion through the wrist joint.

The management of tendon rupture is surgical with the following possible techniques[3]:

a. Transfer
b. Tendon graft
c. Anastomosis to neighboring tendon
d. Direct suture of ruptured tendon
e. Fascia lata graft
f. Arthrodesis

Rupture of the extensor pollicis longus tendon is generally readily diagnosed. Many patients give a history of a sudden snap with subsequent incomplete extension of the thumb. On examination, it is possible to have some interphalangeal joint extension because of the anatomy of the extensor apparatus. The extensor pollicis brevis is able to maintain MP extension, and the intrinsic musculature can then provide weak interphalangeal joint extension. In comparison with a normal hand, however, there is loss of normal extension of both MP and IP joints.

The treatment of extensor pollicis longus rupture favored by the author is that of the extensor indicus proprius transfer. Any tendon transfer must: (a) involve an expendable tendon with excursion equal to that of the tendon it is replacing, (b) run in a straight line, (c) possess sufficient strength and synergism, and (d) be placed subcutaneously in an unscarred bed. All of these criteria are fulfilled by extensor indicus proprius transfer to restore the thumb extension.

In this technique the extensor indicus proprius tendon is removed at its insertion through a small transverse incision over the second metacarpophalangeal joint. The tendon is run subcutaneous to the level of the anastomosis, just proximal to the thumb MP joint. The anastomosis is performed by the Bunnel technique. The thumb and wrist are splinted in a position of extension for about 4 weeks.

Rupture of the digital extensors. The surgical approach for extensor tendon rupture is usually via a lazy "S" incision over the dorsum of the hand and wrist. The ulnar end of the dorsal carpal ligament is incised longitudinally, reflected radialward, and the radial end left intact. The involved tendons are usually attenuated and frayed over a long distance, making primary approximation of healthy tendon ends impossible. Frequently, the two ends of the "ruptured tendon" are still joined by a narrow band of synovium 1 mm. to 2 mm. wide. Synovectomy should be carried out prior to tendon repair, which may be done by one of several techniques.

If a single extensor tendon has been ruptured (usually the extensor digitorum communis to the little finger), satisfactory results can be achieved by anastomosis of the distal end of this tendon to the adjacent extensor digitorum communis tendon of the ring finger. With double or multiple ruptures of the extensor tendons, the technique preferred by the author is that of tendon transfer of the extensor indicis proprius tendon to motor the ruptured tendons. Again, the prerequisite of tendon transfer must be fulfilled. The MP joints and wrist are immobilized in extension for approximately 4 weeks. In many hospitals free tendon grafts are popular. The objections to free tendon grafts are: (a) the bed in which they are placed is often in the area of previous attrition rupture, (b) the procedure takes longer to perform, and (c) donor tendons may be less than optimal in a rheumatoid patient.

In all cases of rupture of the extensor tendons of the hand, it is imperative to remove the distal 2 cm. of the ulnar head with the inevitable bony spicule, in order to prevent further attrition to the tendons which are still intact. This procedure is done at the same time as tendon transfer, tendon anastomosis, or tendon grafting.

Rupture of the flexor tendons is less common than extensor tendon rupture, possibly due to the greater bulk of the flexor structures. The sites of rupture may be in the wrist, palm, or fingers. A choice of procedure is available to the surgeon.

With rupture of the flexor pollicis longus tendon, fusion of the interphalangeal joint in 15° of flexion may be carried out, providing the patient has excellent metacarpophalangeal joint movement. If MP movement is poor, a far better technique is to motor the joints of the thumb by means of tendon graft with the proximal suture line proximal to the wrist joint. An alternative technique is transfer of flexor digitorum sublimus to motor the thumb.

Selective rupture of a digital flexor profundus in the palm is best treated by fusion of the distal interphalangeal joint of that finger. In the rare case of rupture of both sublimus and profundus tendons to the finger, the procedure of choice is to motor the distal profundus by an adjacent sublimus tendon.

In conclusion, soft tissue surgery of the hand necessitates accurate preoperative diagnosis of the often extensive pathology of rheumatoid arthritis; knowledge of the many alternative procedures to provide prophylaxis, function, and cosmesis; and meticulous technique in a bloodless field. The result of such surgery in patients suffering from rheumatoid hand deformities is rewarding.

REFERENCES

1. Calnan, J. S., and Holt, P. J. L.: Annals of the Rheumatic Diseases (International Workshop on Artificial Finger Joints), No. 5 (Suppl.), *28*:83-84, 1969.
2. Nalebuff, E. A.: Surgical treatment of rheumatoid tenosynovitis in the hand. Surg. Clin. N. Amer., *49*:799-809, 1969.
3. ———: Surgical treatment of tendon rupture in the rheumatoid hand. Surg. Clin. N. Amer., *49*:811-822, 1969.
4. Pulvertaft, R. G.: Cilnical Surgery, The Hand. pp. 203-207. London, Butterworths, 1966.
5. Straub, L. R., and Wilson, E. H., Jr.: Spontaneous rupture of extensor tendons in the hand associated with rheumatoid arthritis. J. Bone Joint Surg., *38A*:1208-1217, 1956.
6. Vaughan-Jackson, O. J.: Rupture of extensor tendons by attrition at the inferior radioulnar joint: Report of two cases. J. Bone Joint Surg., *38B*:528-530, 1948.
7. White, W. L.: Restoration of the function and balance of the wrist and hand by tendon transfers. Surg. Clin. N. Amer., *40*: 438, 1960.

CHAPTER 22

Management of Early Rheumatoid Arthritis in the Hand

MARTIN A. ENTIN, M.D.

Rheumatoid arthritis is a disease which has numerous manifestations, only some of which can be detected clinically. The disease is thought to be a result of interplay between chemical inflammatory mediators and the immune process which they evoke.[2,6] It is postulated that the early pathological changes are related to the former, while the chronicity depends upon the intensity of the latter.

The acute phase in rheumatoid arthritis begins as synovial edema and inflammatory cellular process. When the inflammatory process spills over into the joint space, joint effusion follows. Pain and tenderness are due to distention of tissues and pressure on the nerve endings. The target areas of the disease are synovia, cartilage, bone, tendons, ligaments, muscles and blood vessels.[2]

Pain causes discomfort to the patient and also muscle spasm; the patient is consequently reluctant to bend joints and to use the involved member. He usually seeks help from his doctor at this stage. Treatment must be directed toward arrest of the process and the restoration of normal function. If the process continues unchecked, anatomical alterations will take place, and only corrective surgery can be applied.

Recent consideration implicated synovial tissue as the area in which the immunological disturbance takes place. The removal of synovial tissue offers a means of reducing the area in which this process occurs, thus interrupting the inflammatory reactions.[6,11] Moreover, it is thought that it may prevent the irreversible changes of destruction of articular cartilage and underlying bone which lead to collapse of the normal architecture of the affected joints.

It is important to appreciate that the approach to various parts of the body is different. There is a difference in consideration of treatment in the upper and lower extremities. The hand is concerned with delicate fine movement, where accuracy and precision are mandatory for carrying out the tasks of one's occupation and daily requirements for personal needs.[2]

The problems associated with rheumatoid arthritis of the hands are varied in their patterns and depend primarily on what specific components of the complex structures are affected first.

RHEUMATOID ARTHRITIS IN THE FOREARM AND HAND

The forearm structures are involved in rheumatoid arthritis in several ways, and the proliferative process may involve the tendon sheath, both on the flexor and extensor aspects. The inflammatory reaction can extend from the tendon sheath into the adjacent joints; occasionally the proliferation can start in a joint and may simultaneously affect the synovium covering the tendon sheath. The clinical appearance is that of a fusiform swelling on either ulnar or dorsal aspect, proximal or distal to the extensor retinaculum; the swelling may be continuous underneath the constricting liga-

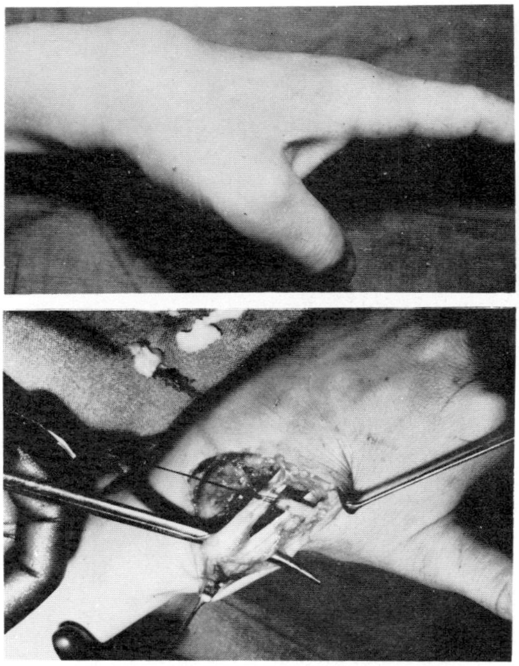

Fig. 22-1. Tenosynovitis of dorsal tendons. (*Top*) Dorsal view of the left hand showing marked swelling on either side of the extensor retinaculum. (*Bottom*) Removed synovial tissue which infiltrated around the wrist extensors is shown on the towel.

mentous structures (Fig. 22-1). It is the swelling that brings the patient to the doctor, although there is little associated pain and only slight limitation of movement. On the flexor aspect there may be involvement of the synovial sheaths. The presenting swelling may extend under the flexor retinaculum into the palm, and, occasionally, even into the volar compartments of the fingers, as a continuous mass.

Ruptured Tendons

A number of complications arise from this proliferative process, which encases the tendons and interferes with their blood supply and nutrition. There is some controversy regarding the reason for rupture of tendons: some feel that the cause is direct invasion and destruction of the tendon substance;

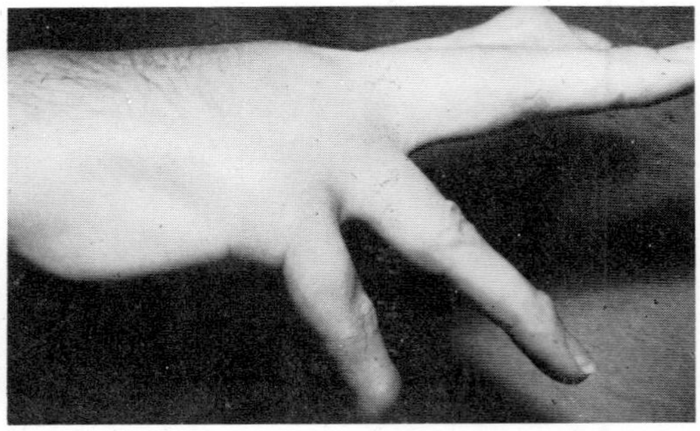

Fig. 22-2. Infiltration of extensor tendons leading to rupture.

others feel that there is attrition over the rough edges of fibro-osseous tunnels which are more prominent on the dorsum of the wrist and hand.[2,14] In these cases, synovectomy must be carried out early in order to avoid this common complication of tendon rupture (Fig. 22-2). Occasionally sharp spicules of bone are found as a result of the erosion of bone by the inflammatory process. Continuous riding of a tendon over these may cause fraying to a point where the tendon weakens and breaks. In addition, on the volar aspect of the wrist there might be compression of the median nerve within the carpal tunnel giving rise to the typical symptoms associated with median nerve compression.[2]

These sequelae of tenosynovitis compel the surgeon to carry out synovectomy at the early stages. There is a considerable amount of evidence now accumulated which suggests that some of the sequelae may be prevented after synovectomy. In a series of synovectomies carried out at Heinola, the number of ruptured tendons has been significantly decreased.[13]

Rheumatoid Arthritis in Metacarpophalangeal Joints

The MP joint is a ball-and-socket joint with two articular surfaces which permit motion in several directions. The support to the joint is provided by collateral ligaments on either side; the sagittal cam effect which is due to anterior bulging of the metacarpal head, puts the ligament on the stretch in flexion of the joint. In addition, support is provided by the dorsal extensor tendon, the sagittal band and the deep transverse metacarpal ligament, the volar flexor mechanism with the volar plate, and the buttressing of the interosseous and lumbrical tendons, which attach to the extensor mechanism (Fig. 22-3). Considerable mobility is possible at this joint, since the fingers can be adducted and circumducted.

Early involvement of the metacarpophalangeal joints of the fingers may be very moderate, but the process may go on to a distortion of normal relationships of the various parts of the finger. The changes begin with distention of the joint structures and subsequent stretching of the collateral ligaments and of the extensor expansion, more marked on the radial side. This may be associated with shortening and fibrosis of the intrinsic muscles, especially the volar interossei, which produces digital ulnar drift, and may lead to deformities of imbalance such as swan-neck, intrinsic-plus, and boutonniere. In time, stretching of the volar plate and the collateral ligaments may lead to subluxation of proximal phalanges. The sum total of these alterations is the distortion of the relationship of the various parts of the finger. Synovectomy may remove the offending inflammatory tissue, but it is not likely to restore a normal relationship and balance of the fingers. If the articular cartilaginous surfaces are well preserved, the reconstruction of the metacarpophalangeal joint entails the repair of the collateral ligaments, release of the shortened interossei, tightening of the volar plate, and repositioning of the dislocated extensor tendon in its normal site. This restoration of normal relationship of the various structures to each other is essential because it improves the function of the hand and reduces the likelihood of secondary deforming alterations.

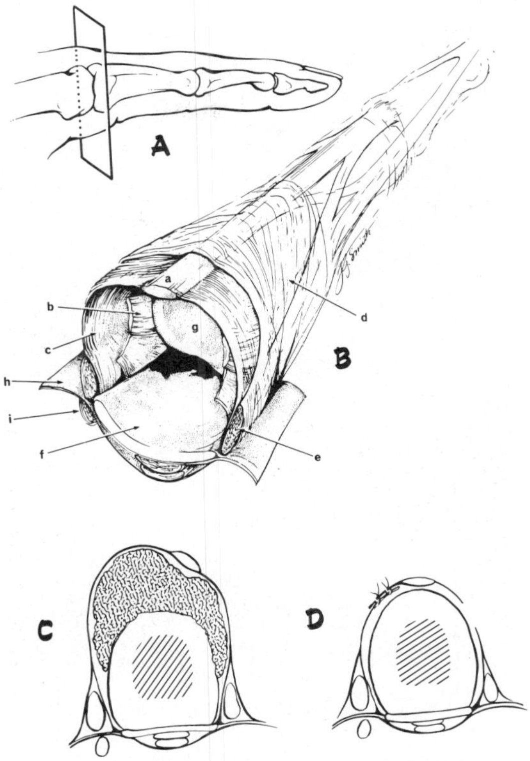

FIG. 22-3. Diagrams showing architectural features of the metacarpophalangeal joint. (*A*) Plane of section shown in detail B. (*B*) Supporting structures of joint viewed from the proximal aspect with the metacarpal head removed. The ligamentous and tendinous components keep the articular surfaces in intimate contact within the normal joint. (*a*) Extensor digitorum communis, (*b*) collateral band, (*c*) sagittal band, (*d*) extensor hood, (*e*) interosseus muscle, (*f*) volar plate with flexor tendons, (*g*) articular base of proximal phalanx, (*h*) deep transverse metacarpal ligament, (*i*) lumbrical muscle. (*C*) Cross-section of MP joint showing synovial inflammation and ligamentous stretching on radial side which permits displacement of the extensor tendon ulnarward. (*D*) Same as view C, but after removal of synovium with the inflammatory tissue. The displaced extensor tendon is repositioned in midline by overlapping and suturing the sectioned extensor hood on the radial side.

Indications for Synovectomy. Synovial membrane has been implicated as the tissue in which the active destructive process of the

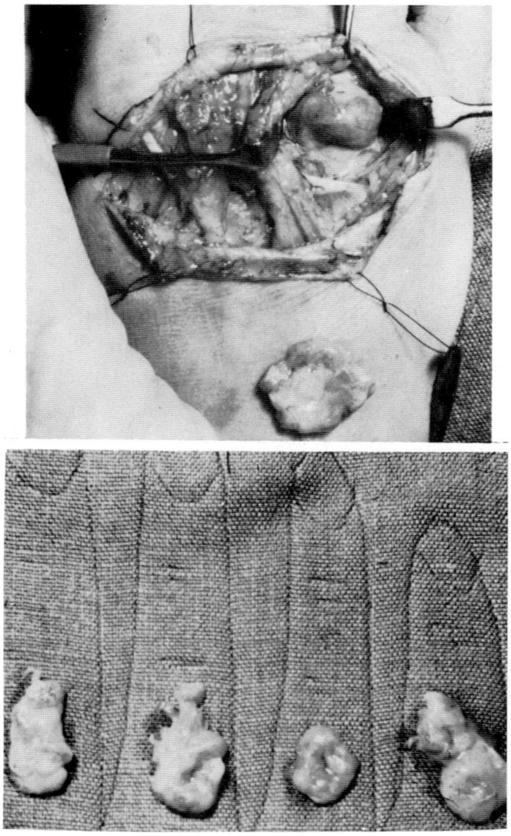

FIG. 22-4. Synovectomy in MP joints. (*Top*) Right hand of a patient with rheumatoid arthritis showing marked swelling of dorsum and of fingers. Note the synovial granulation tissue over the metacarpophalangeal joint of the ring finger. The synovial tissue on the wrist came from the long finger. (*Bottom*) The synovial tissues removed from the MP joints of the four fingers shown above.

disease occurs. The operation is indicated when an adequate medical regime does not control the disease process.

Technique of Synovectomy. Great delicacy in handling fragile structures in the hand is mandatory. Total removal of the synovial tissue is a theoretical consideration. It is not possible to remove all the involved synovia without opening the joint because a considerable amount is located in areas otherwise not accessible (Fig. 22-4). Another obvious benefit of synovectomy is the opportunity to correct the position of the deflected extensor tendons.

If the extensor digitorum communis tendon is not excessively displaced ulnarly, the approach to the joint is facilitated by longitudinal splitting of the extensor tendon (after Bunnell). This permits immediate access to the structures within the joint. Sometimes it is possible to identify the dorsal capsule (Fig. 22-4). The synovial tissue is easily accessible on the dorsal and lateral aspects. Its volar extension cannot always be easily removed. In exceptional cases, it is possible to section the radial collateral ligament on the radial side. This permits free access to the volar aspect of the joint by subluxation of the proximal phalanx. The radial collateral ligament is usually stretched by the disease process, and the repair permits tightening of this structure.

Results of Synovectomy. Because of individual variability in the pattern and course of this disease, it is difficult to evaluate the results of early synovectomies by statistical data. The task is further complicated, since very large numbers of operated patients with uniform conditions of involvement are not available in most hand centers.

Vainio and Raunio reported a well documented series of 214 operations on the PIP joints of 92 patients which were compared to non-operated controls.[13] I was able to examine some of the patients in this series. Their conclusion was that pain was reduced, range of motion was better, and swelling was less in the operated joints. The results of synovectomy were better in male patients or in patients with short duration of local disease or low activity of the systemic aspect of disease. Age of patient, length of follow-up, or the specific preoperative stage of the local condition had no effect on the final results.

While agreement has not been reached on how early one should carry out synovectomy in the hand for rheumatoid arthritis,

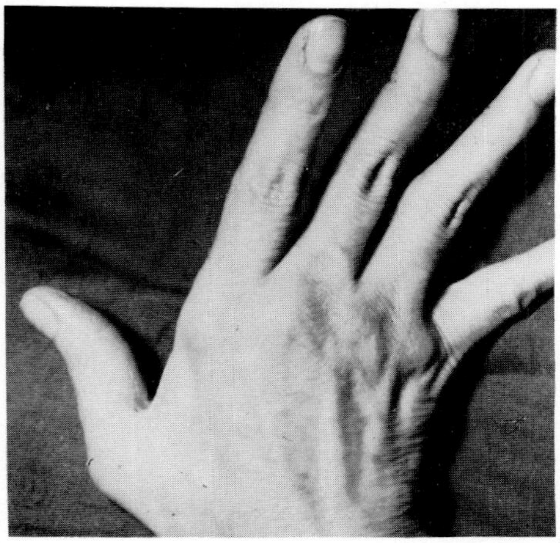

FIG. 22-5. Deforming factors in rheumatoid arthritis. Right hand of a 45-year-old woman showing the ulnar deviation of all fingers as well as swan-neck deformities. Synovial inflammation is seen about the MP joints, and there is ulnar displacement of extensor tendons.

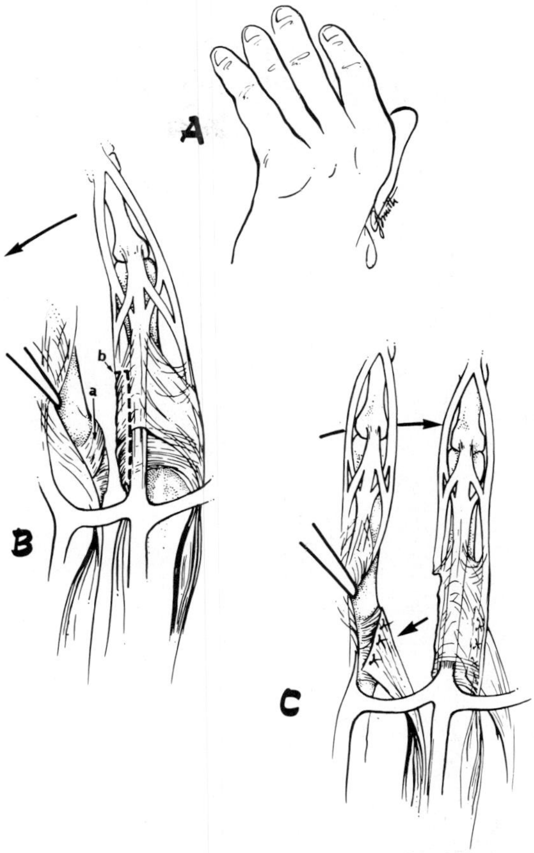

FIG. 22-6. Diagrams showing method of correcting ulnar deviation of fingers at metacarpophalangeal joints. (*A*) Dorsal view of the hand with ulnar drift of the fingers. (*B*) Dorsal aspect of the extensor mechanism showing ulnar displacement of the extensor tendon and the incision for detaching of the shortened volnar interosseus muscles on the ulnar side (b). Radial collateral ligament is shown at a. (*C*) Transfer of the detached interosseus muscle to the radial side of adjacent finger.

there is impressive evidence of its beneficial effect when done before the irreversible changes have taken place. For the best results in the hand, we find it necessary to combine synovectomy with correction of deformities and release of contractures.

Correction of Shortened Intrinsics

Usually there is a considerable amount of distortion of the relationships of the complicated anatomical structures about the metacarpophalangeal joint: there is ulnar deviation of the proximal phalanx; the extensor tendon is often displaced ulnarward; and the capsular structures, if stretched, may be displaced into the ulnar gutter between the digits (Fig. 22-5). In addition, there is shortening of the interossei tendons due to spasm[1,2,3] though Vainio questioned this concept.[12] The pathological changes that are found within the muscle and tendons undoubtedly lead to fibrosis and fixation to the periarticular structures of the metacarpophalangeal joints and may produce ulnar deviation and a swan-neck deformity.

In correcting the tight intrinsics, it is advisable to section the volar interossei on the ulnar side in order to remove the deforming force. If ulnar deviation is pronounced, the volar interosseus tendon should be shifted radially and then reattached to the base of the proximal phalanx, rather than to the lateral band. Flatt suggested attaching it to the distal portion of the collateral ligament to get the greatest advantage from its corrective action (Fig. 22-6).[4]

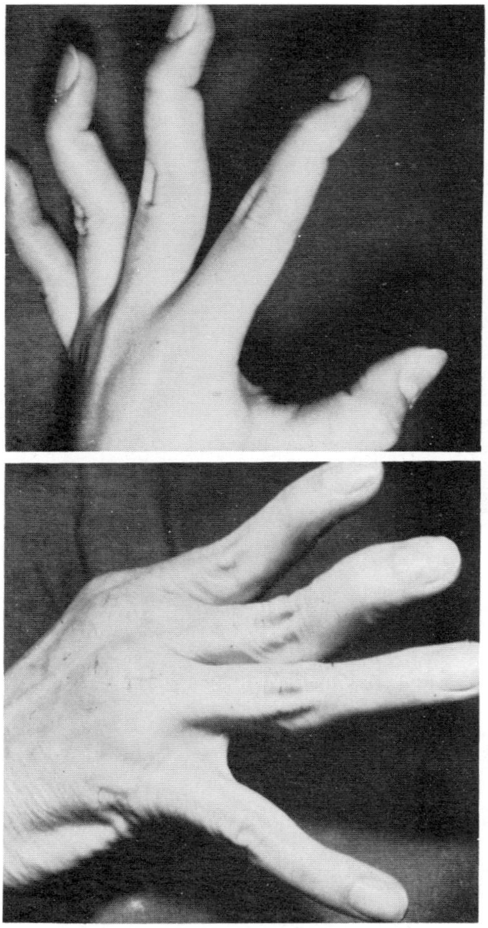

FIG. 22-7. Swan-neck deformity, showing hyperextension of the PIP joint and flexion of the DIP joint.

If the extensor tendon is displaced ulnarward, it is necessary to overcome the contraction of tissue on the ulnar side of the tendon by sectioning the oblique fibers on the extensor hood. The tendon can then be shifted to its normal anatomical position and maintained by overlapping and suturing the redundant tissue on the radial side (Fig. 22-3D).

PIP Joint in Rheumatoid Arthritis

The proximal interphalangeal joint is a uniaxial synovial joint with great congruity of the articular surfaces. The joint is supported by collateral ligaments and the volar

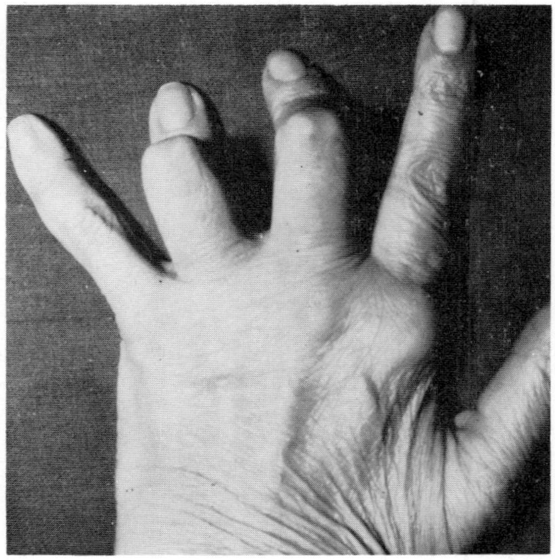

FIG. 22-8. Boutonniere deformity, demonstrating proximal joint flexion and distal joint extension.

plate. Additional stability is provided by the flexor and extensor tendon complexes. The main movement is of flexion and extension; it has very limited lateral motions. Interference with function of this joint in rheumatoid arthritis is due to synovial effusion, stretching of the ligaments and supporting structures, and secondary deformities of imbalance such as swan-neck with hyperextension of the joint (Fig. 22-7), and boutonniere deformity with acute flexion of the joint and hyperextension of the distal joint (Fig. 22-8).

Swan neck. The deformity is considered to be caused by the tightness of the volar interossei muscles and may be associated with secondary deformities of ulnar deviation of the digit and volar displacement of the proximal phalanx on the metacarpal head. The usual test for tight intrinsics does not give a true picture in hands which have marked ulnar and volar deviation of the fingers. Fowler suggested that the ulnar and volar deviation should be corrected before applying the test (Littler[7]).

The correction of swan-neck deformity (Figs. 22-9 and 22-10) is carried out by removing the force of the tight interossei by the Littler release. This involves cutting out a triangle of tissue from the proximal part of the extensor hood along with a portion of the lateral band. However, this procedure does not correct the marked recurvatum of the PIP joint associated with stretching of the collateral and volar ligaments. The most practical method of correcting the hyperextension of the PIP joint is by means of tenodesis, which will restrict the extension. Littler's method is to produce a tenodesis, either with a lateral band or by using one slip of flexor superficialis, especially, if it is inserted into the bone through a drill hole.[7] The latter is the method of choice.

Swanson's procedure of tenodesis of the whole of the superficialis tendon to a nest in the middle of the proximal phalanx (by removing the cortical bone from the volar aspect) requires maintaining the intimate contact with freshened tendon with the aide of a pull-out suture for at least 5 weeks.[9]

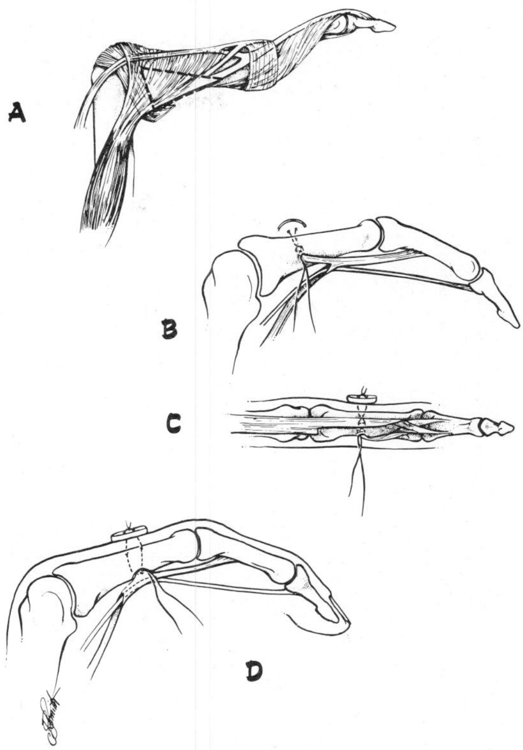

FIG. 22-9. Drawings showing methods of correcting swan-neck deformity. (*A*) Littler's release of the tight interosseus muscles (as modified by W. White). The triangle shows the extent of tissue removed. (*B, C*) Tenodesis of one limb of the superficialis tendon through a drill hole in the proximal phalanx. The pull-out wire is tied to a button (after Littler). C shows the volar aspect with profundus tendon omitted. (*D*) Swanson's tenodesis of the superficialis tendon to a nest in the proximal phalanx from which the cortical bone is removed.

Boutonniere Deformity. Stretching of the dorsal structures about the PIP joint, with the joint held in flexion, may ultimately result in tearing of the central tendon. Secondary deformities associated with stretching of the oblique fibers to the lateral bands allow slipping of the bands volar to the axis of rotation of the joint. As the lateral bands contract, they become flexors of the PIP joint and extensors of the DIP joint. This position exaggerates the action of the oblique retinacular ligament (Landsmeer's ligament) (Fig. 22-11).

This deformity is very disabling, because it interferes with the flexion of the distal phalanx and does not permit precision in handling small objects. The persistence of the deformity can cause fibrosis and ankylosis of the PIP joint that would defy reconstruction (see Fig. 22-8). Several methods are available for correcting this deformity.

Fowler suggested a simple procedure which bridges the gap between the base of the middle phalanx and the torn central tendon with the aid of a free tendon graft (Fig. 22-11B). The tendon graft is passed through a drill hole in the base of the middle phalanx and is attached to the proximal aspects of both lateral tendons, which are released from their volar displacement.[5] The graft must be sufficiently lax to allow unobstructed flexion of the PIP joint.

Another method which we find useful is to release the transverse retinacular liga-

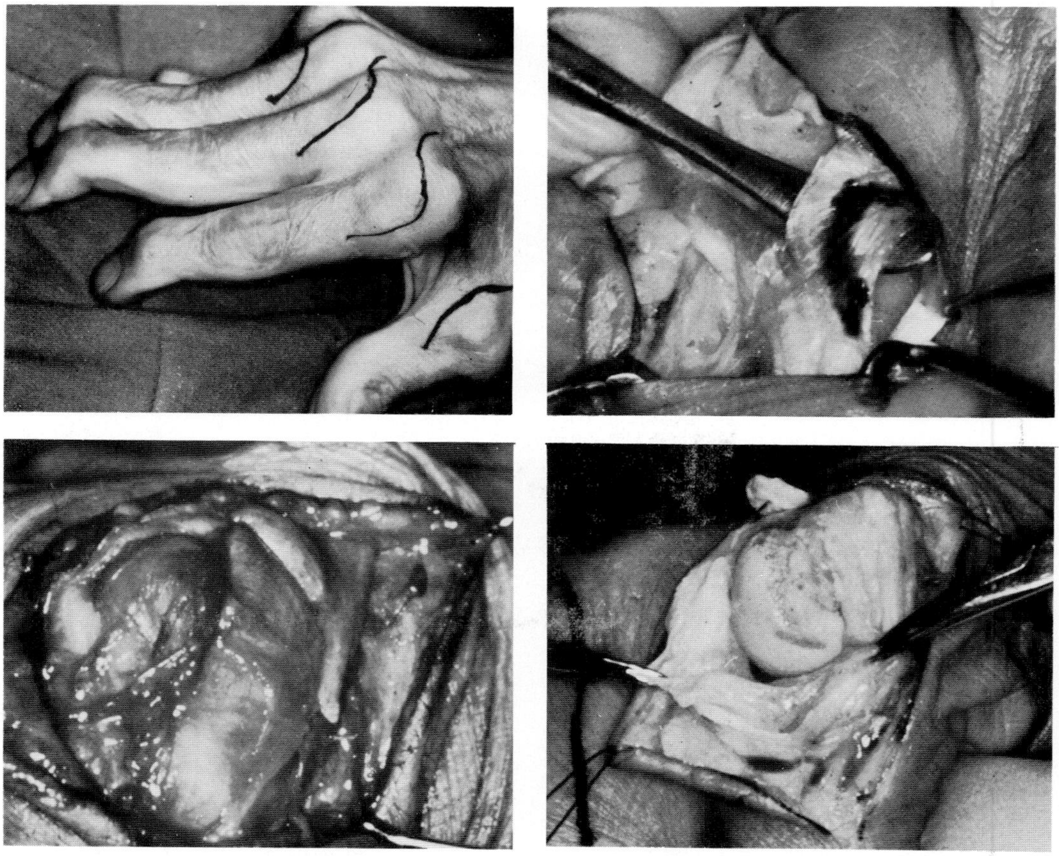

FIG. 22-10. Swan-neck deformity in rheumatoid arthritis. (*Upper left*) Right hand of 48-year-old man showing swan-neck deformities and ulnar deviation of all fingers. Ink marks delineate the incisions used. (*Upper right*) Extensor of the long finger prior to releasing tight interosseus muscle. Ink marks show the tissue to be removed. (*Lower left*) Index finger extensor tendon in corrected position. Wire pull-out sutures close the space between tendon and bone. (*Lower right*) Metacarpal head showing eroded cartilage. Reconstruction of normal joint function is impossible; joint replacement is indicated.

ment to permit displacement of the lateral bands. The procedure suggested by Littler is used[7]: the lateral band on the ulnar side is detached and passed through the central tendon. Finally, it is attached to the base of the middle phalanx through a drill hole (Fig. 22-11C).

An alternate method, which combines lengthening of the distal extensor mechanism, was suggested by Matiev[10] (Fig. 22-11D). Unless these procedures are used in the early stages of the disease, reconstruction rarely produces normal function. In long-standing boutonniere deformity complicated by joint ankylosis, it becomes more practical to arthrodese the PIP joint in a functional position.

Management of Early Thumb Deformities

The thumb architecture is somewhat different from that of the fingers because the thumb has the greatest range of motion at the carpometacarpal joint and lacks one phalanx. The early changes in rheumatoid arthritis are associated with swelling over MP joints and an adduction deformity due

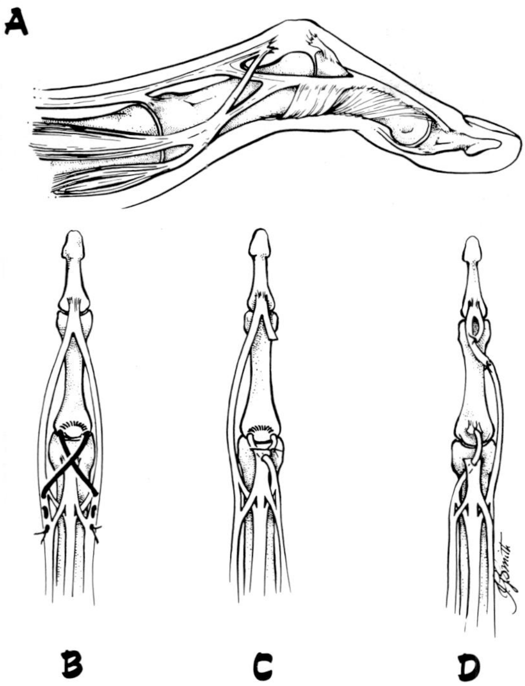

FIG. 22-11. Boutonniere deformity and methods of correction. *(A)* Lateral view. *(B)* Reconstruction of the middle slip with the aid of a free graft attached to both lateral bands proximally (Fowler). *(C)* The ulnar lateral band is severed and passed through the base of the middle phalanx activating extension of PIP (Littler). *(D)* Matiev's method utilizes the shorter ulnar lateral band to connect the middle slip to the base of the middle phalanx. The radial lateral band is severed more distally and is lengthened by crossover attachment to the longer distal stump of the ulnar lateral band.

to contraction of the adductor pollicis. Early synovectomy of the MP joint is carried out through a curved incision on the ulnar aspect of the joint. The synovial tissue is removed and the adductor muscle sectioned.

Why a specific pattern of imbalance should occur in a particular digit is not known. The hyperextension deformity of the MP joint is analogous to the effect of tight intrinsics in the fingers and is complicated by flexion deformity of the DIP. This position handicaps the patient in handling and picking up small objects. When permitted to persist, this deformity may be associated with subluxation of the carpometacarpal joint which reduces the stability. If the articular surfaces of the MP joints are intact, removing the greater multangular bone, sectioning the adductor muscle, and reefing the MP joint to prevent hyperextension will improve function.

If flexion deformity of the MP joint of the thumb is the dominant derangement, then fusion of that joint with shortening helps to control the hyperextension of the distal joint, which is quite disabling. If there is destruction of articular surfaces of the carpometacarpal joint (Fig. 22-12), replacement with Swanson silastic prosthesis can be carried out.

Postoperative Management

Meticulous attention to dressing, positioning of parts, and splinting in the correct attitude are particularly important in the postoperative period in surgery of rheumatoid hands. Especially important are the relation of various parts of the hand to each other; corrected deformities must be splinted in the desired position for the best results.

Ordinarily, splinting in a plaster cast is maintained for about 2 weeks, until the wound is healed and sutures can be removed. If combined procedures entailing synovectomy and muscle transfer have been done, graded motion may be started on some joints while the others are kept splinted.

If the skin of the hand is thin and fragile due to prolonged administration of steroids, special care must be taken during dissection and closure. Fine suture material and meticulous approximation of skin is mandatory; sutures may be left for a longer period, and intracuticular sutures may be useful.

Occasionally, in spite of postural elevation, excessive swelling of tissue and pain occur within 48 hours after operation. We have found that administration of oral steroids for 1 week, followed by gradual withdrawal, helps to control these complications.

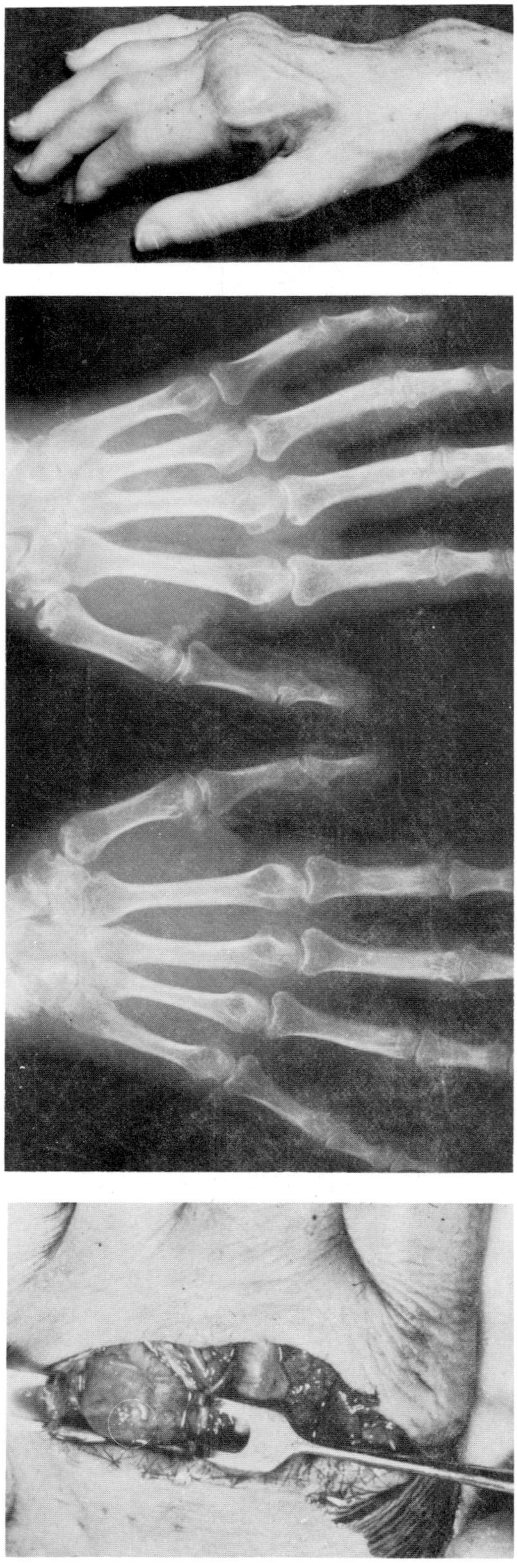

FIG. 22-12. Advanced rheumatoid arthritis with destruction of cartilage and bone in a 48-year-old woman. (*Top*) Right hand showing advanced disease despite adequate treatment and continuous steroid therapy. (*Center*) X-rays of both hands. Note erosion of bone in index-finger MP joints and bases of thumb metacarpals. (*Bottom*) Left hand at operation showing granulation tissue and underlying cartilage destruction.

Supervised daily exercises to increase the range of motion must be combined with dynamic support of the hand and fingers to maintain the desired position and to prevent recurrence of the undesirable imbalance and deformities.

CONCLUSIONS

Rheumatoid arthritis is a gradual, progressive disease which has an intermittent course characterized by remissions and relapses. Specific evolution of the disease in a given individual is unpredictable. Consequently, the early management is designed to reduce inflammation, decrease injury to the joints, and reduce atrophy of the muscles by supervised exercises, while hoping for a remission. Surgery is not an alternative method of management; it is part of the general treatment. Its purpose is to improve function, prevent further destruction, and correct deformities as they occur, before there is complete disruption of the architecture of the part.

Synovectomy should be performed early when there is distortion of the periarticular structures by inflammatory tissue or when there is interference with the function of the hand and pain. To be beneficial, synovectomy should be done as soon as it is apparent that medical treatment does not control the disease process. The efficacy of late synovectomy is difficult to assess: usually it is carried out when the process of disease is associated with changes of architecture, erosion of cartilage, or even bone.

The success of early intervention is predicated on the deployment of a careful postoperative regime with proper positioning of the hand and fingers and careful supervision during the rehabilitation period.

Other surgical intervention in the hand is indicated for alleviation of persistent pain, repair of ruptured tendons, relief of compression of nerves, and correction of imbalance of joint deformities. When complete destrucion of the joint surfaces leads to skeletal collapse, only salvaging procedures are possible.

REFERENCES

1. Bunnell, S.: Surgery of the rheumatoid hand. J. Bone Joint Surg., *37A*:759-766, 1955.
2. Entin, M. A.: Surgical treatment of rheumatoid arthritis. Surg. Clin. N. Amer., *44*:1081, 1964.
3. Flatt, A. E.: The Care of Rheumatoid Hand. St. Louis, C. V. Mosby, 1963.
4. ———: American Society for Surgery of the Hand. Membership Letter, March 16, 1970.
5. Fowler, S. B.: Extensor apparatus of the digits. J. Bone Joint Surg., *31B*:477, 1949.
6. Jakubowski, S.: Synovectomy in rheumatoid arthritis. *In* Chapchal, G. (ed.): Second International Symposium on Rheumatoid Arthritis. p. 4. Thieme, Stuttgart, 1967.
7. Littler, J. W.: Principles of reconstructive surgery of the hand. *In* Converse, J. M. (ed.): Reconstructive Plastic Surgery. vol. 4. pp. 1612-1672. W. B. Saunders, Philadelphia, 1964.
8. Savill, D. L.: Synovectomy on the metacarpo-phalangeal joint in rheumatoid arthritis. 2nd International Symposium, Basle, Switzerland, Editor G. Chapchal, 1967, p. 107.
9. Swanson, A. B.: The need for early treatment of the rheumatoid hand. J. Mich. State Med. Soc., *60*:348-351, 1961.
10. Tubiana, R., and Hakstian, R.: La Main Rheumatismale. Paris, Expansion Scientifique Francaise, 1966.
11. Vainio, K.: The role of surgery in the rehabilitation of rheumatoid arthritis patients. Proc. 4th European Rheum. Congress, 1959, p. 223.
12. ———: Indication and contraindication for surgery in rheumatoid arthritis. Rheumatism, *22*:10-15, 1966.
13. Vainio, K., and Raunio, P.: Synovectomy of PIP joints. Report presented at combined meeting of American and Scandinavian Hand Societies, Heinola, Finland, April 30, 1970.
14. Vaughan-Jackson, O. J.: Rupture of extensor tendon by attrition at the inferior radioulnar joint. J. Bone Joint Surg., *30B*:528, 1948.
15. ———: Rheumatoid hand deformities considered in the light of tendon imbalance. J. Bone Joint Surg., *44B*:764-775, 1962.

CHAPTER 23

Surgery of Established Rheumatoid Deformities in the Hand

ALFRED B. SWANSON, M.D.

Restoring function to unstable, stiff or dislocated finger joints continues to be one of the most difficult and intriguing problems in reconstructive surgery of the hand.[2,3,5,14,29,35,33,51] During recent years, a vast amount of knowledge on this subject has been obtained through the large experience gained in surgical treatment of arthritis.[1,8,12,13,15,20,23,49,52,53] Efforts have concentrated mainly on the metacarpophalangeal (MP) joint as the key joint for finger function. The deformities of this joint are especially noticeable and unsightly and are most amenable to arthroplasty. However, all of the joints of the digit are important in functional adaptations because of the interdependence of one joint on the other. Continuing deformity at the proximal interphalangeal (PIP) joint or even the distal interphalangeal (DIP) joint negatively affects the long-term results of surgery on the MP joints in rheumatoid patients. Balance at one finger joint is always dependent upon good balance of the associated joints.[19,21] In order to obtain the best possible adaptations of grip and pinch, treatment of all of the joints of the digits should be considered.[38] Appropriate treatment includes synovectomy, tendon and joint releases, tendon reconstruction, arthroplasty, and arthrodesis.[16,18,26,32]

ARCHITECTURAL CONSIDERATIONS

The normal architecture of the hand must be appreciated in order to understand the bio-mechanical disturbances which occur following the collapse of the bone and joint system in late rheumatoid arthritis.

The form of the hand has a certain unique elegance. The skeleton provides the lever arms, the mobile joints, and the stabilizing points around which functional adaptations of the hand take place. A great number of units are compacted into a small area through which great power and precision can be applied. The arches of this complex enable the digits to bring into and control objects in the hand. The bony architecture of the hand is arranged in three arches: one longitudinal and two transverse. The proximal transverse arch passes through the carpal area with its center at the capitate bone. The distal transverse arch is developed across the metacarpal heads, its center being the head of the third metacarpal. The fourth and fifth digital rays offer mobility of the ulnar aspect of the hand around this fixed point. The thumb ray provides mobility around the radial aspect. The digits make up the longitudinal arches with their apex at the metacarpophalangeal joints. A loss of integrity of this arch system through deformity or contracture will consequently diminish normal function. A break in the longitudinal arch system of the digit may result in a collapse deformity of the multi-articulated structure. Stiffness or deformity of the joints will disturb the normal flexion sequence of the digit with its resultant disturbance of functional adaptations.

The ligament system of the finger joints is arranged so that stability is provided as flexion occurs. When the joints are in extension, the collateral ligaments are relatively lax. If the digit is held in extension, these ligaments may tighten, and flexion will be limited. Therefore, an important dictum in treating the injured or diseased part must be to place the hand in the functional position with its joints in a semiflexed position.

The fingers rotate slightly around the third "metacarpal keystone" to converge toward the scaphoid. Only the middle finger lies in a longitudinal axis of its own. Care must therefore be given to align the reconstructed digits according to this convergence; otherwise the fingers may overlap each other on grasping.

JOINT REPLACEMENT PROBLEMS

The development of synthetic materials which can be used in the human body has given the researcher tools for human engineering.[4,33,54] They have opened up extraordinary possibilities for joint reconstruction. The concept of total joint replacement, in which the function of the joint is completely substituted by a mechanical model, is a new and popular approach.[7,28,30] This has certain attractive possibilities from the engineering standpoint. A problem remains, however, with the total dependency upon insubstantial synthetic materials and the interface or boundary between the artificial material and human tissue. There must always be this boundary separation, and as a result, any implant device is only as successful as its biomechanical and biologic tolerance by the human host tissue.

The use of flexible materials provides a new approach to joint reconstruction, especially in the upper extremity. It allows us to take an easier alternative, to help nature build her own new joint system through the resection arthroplasty concept.[41-46,48] Silicone rubber (Silastic*) has been used in our research department since 1962 in efforts to find a suitable joint-space orientation device for resection arthroplasties.† We have designed, developed, and tested 21 devices to be used in reconstructive surgery of the limbs since that time (Fig. 23-1).

* Dow Corning Corporation, Midland, Michigan.

† Research was done in the Orthopaedic Research Department of Blodgett Memorial Hospital, Grand Rapids, Michigan under a grant from the John A. Hartford Foundation.

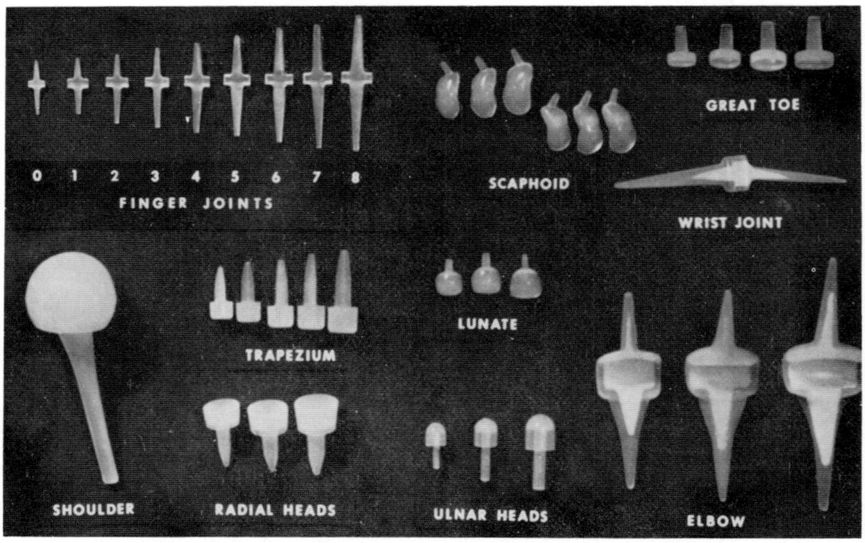

FIG. 23-1. The ten most frequently used silicone rubber implants in resection arthroplasties of the extremities.

The most popular implant has been the finger joint (Fig. 23-2). It has been used in more than 4,000 patients in most countries of the world.

Obtaining the perfect implant depends on proper design and the development of the ideal implant material. The ideal arthroplasty should be mobile, stable, and pain-free. It can be obtained by proper use of a good implant and proper handling of associated tissues operatively and post-operatively.

The aims of the finger joint implant arthroplasty should be to: (1) obtain more predictable results immediately and later, (2) improve range of motion, especially extension, (3) provide better pain relief, (4) provide better stability, and (5) facilitate rehabilitation. Efficient use of implants in finger arthroplasty must consider all of the goals mentioned above. An intelligent compromise between mobility and stability is necessary in these reconstructions.

Principles of Implant Resection Arthroplasty

Any implant design requires a compromised balance of:

1. Engineering principles
2. Anatomical factors
3. Physical characteristics of material
4. Patient's needs

Design characteristics of finger joint implants should follow these considerations:

1. Maintain postoperative bony alignment, AP and LAT
2. Maintain joint space
3. Orient encapsulation
4. Support joint capsule
5. Provide non-reactive implant surface
6. Follow gliding principle of the implant
7. Respect homogeneity of material
8. Provide longest flex-life of implant models
9. Provide stiffness-flexibility balance
10. Note center axis of joint rotation
11. Note compression-tension force distribution
12. Design for proper distribution of material in midsection
13. Provide anatomical sizing: length, height, width

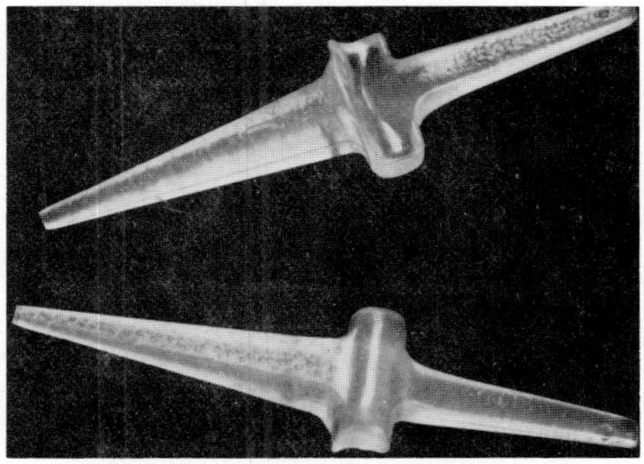

FIG. 23-2. Intramedullary stemmed heat-molded silicone rubber finger joint implants, available in nine anatomical sizes. This implant has been used successfully in finger joint arthroplasties in more than 4,000 cases.

An increased range of motion in any arthroplasty may be obtained by:

1. Widened joint space
2. Non-contracted ligaments
3. Non-contracted palmar plate
4. Loose capsule
5. Minimal articular scarring
6. Mobile cutaneous coverage
7. Decreased pain and swelling
8. Accurate bony alignment, AP and LAT
9. Active flexors and extensors
10. Early postoperative movement
11. Flexible implant
12. Non-fixating implant stems
13. Balanced associated joints
14. Adequate range of motion of associated joints

Lateral stability in a joint arthroplasty may be obtained by:

1. Narrower width of the joint space
2. Tight ligamentous system
3. Tight capsule
4. Active contraction of balanced intrinsics and extrinsics
5. Limited range of motion
6. Proper shape of the implant
7. Increased implant rigidity
8. Good tendon balance and alignment
9. Solid, immediate implant fixation
10. Neighboring lateral digit support
11. Normal associated joint angles
12. Altering external forces in habits of hand function

Arthroplasty in reconstructive surgery of the upper limb requires consideration of the following general indications used for any implant arthroplasty:

1. Good condition of the patient
2. Good neurovascular status
3. Adequate skin cover
4. Adequate bone stock
5. Possibility of a functional muscle-tendon system
6. Availability of good postoperative therapy
7. A cooperative patient

Silicone Rubber Implant Characteristics

Eight years experience in the development of flexible implants for reconstructive procedures in the extremities, utilizing laboratory animals, laboratory testing of the materials for fatigue, and clinical evaluation, has shown silicone rubber to meet many of the requirements for the ideal implant material.

Silicone rubber is a unique material belonging to the family of silicones, which are a combination of organic and inorganic materials. By utilizing a chain of silicone and oxygen atoms to which organic groups are attached, the chemist is able to blend the inertness of quartz with the ability of plastics to be fabricated. The silicone rubbers are heat-stable, do not appear to deteriorate with time, and have no adhesive characteristics. They have excellent flexion characteristics and force-dampening properties, but will tear easily if a laceration occurs in the surface.[40] Correct design of the prosthesis can greatly improve the flexural durability of the silicone rubber implant. Machine testing has shown that a one-piece heat-vulcanized implant has much better wear advantages than a hand-carved or hand-molded implant. The implant will flex longer if it is of a single material. Attempts to reinforce it with Dacron or other materials, in fact, result in earlier breakdown at the interface between the two substances. The medical-grade silicones with which we are dealing do not produce tissue reaction when properly sterilized and should not be confused with industrial silicones that have potentially toxic additives. They are as biologically inert as any material known and, being softer than bone, they are not so likely to stimulate resorption as metal implants.

The implants are made of a heat-vulcanized medical-grade silicone elastomer stock. They are formed in a mold at approximately 250° F and under pressure of 325 pounds per square inch. They are then cured for several hours at a high temperature in an air-circulated oven. The type of silicone elastomer stock from which the implants are manufactured is extremely important. The material of choice must provide adequate implant flexibility and have enough strength to maintain joint stability. Various silicone elastomer stocks were evaluated in the development of a joint replacement implant to determine the stock that would best satisfy the requirements of implant strength and flexibility.

The development of a flexible, heat-molded joint implant of silicone rubber for phalangeal arthroplasties in the rheumatoid arthritic hand has proceeded through many changes in design (Fig. 23-3). The intramedullary-stemmed one-piece design has satisfactorily fulfilled the specified requirements for joint replacement. It provides a satisfactory degree of stability and, because of its intrinsic flex qualities, can be used as a flexible hinge. Six years of testing were involved in the development of this final design. The present model has been machine-tested for more than 400 million flexions without evidence of breakdown (Fig. 23-4). The implant is relatively inexpensive and is easy to handle; it is made in a variety of sizes and can be sterilized by autoclaving.

Silicone rubber causes very little reaction, and therefore minimal foreign body activity takes place around the implant itself. Scar tissue does fill in around the implant and between the bone ends and the ligamentous and capsular system. The movement of the implant after insertion

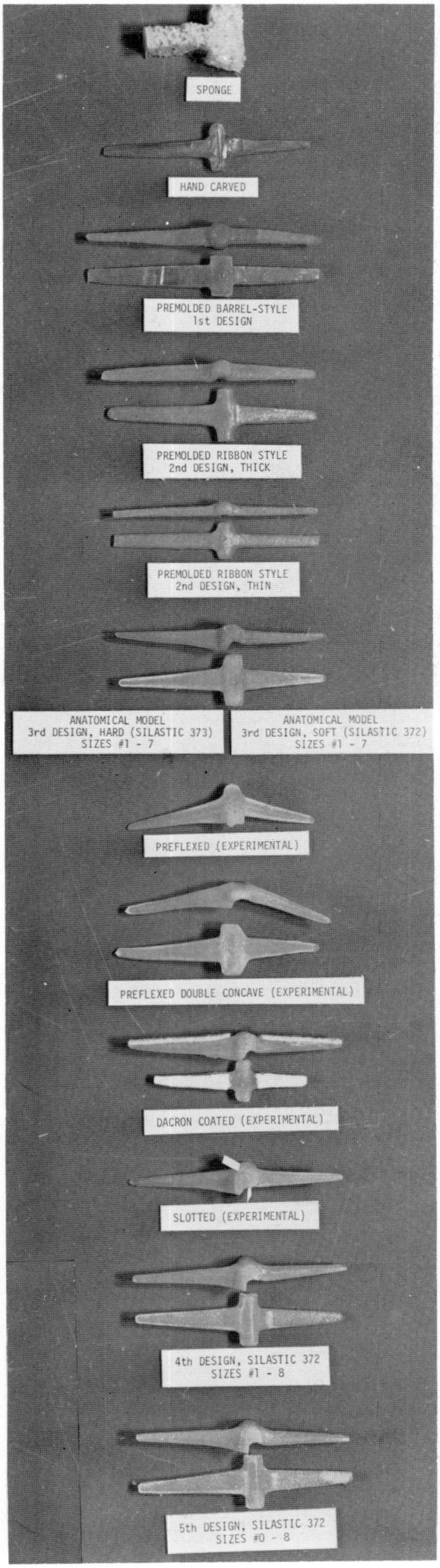

FIG. 23-3. Design stages in the development of finger joint implant. The latest model is the result of 8 years effort to find a suitable space orientor device for resection arthroplasties.

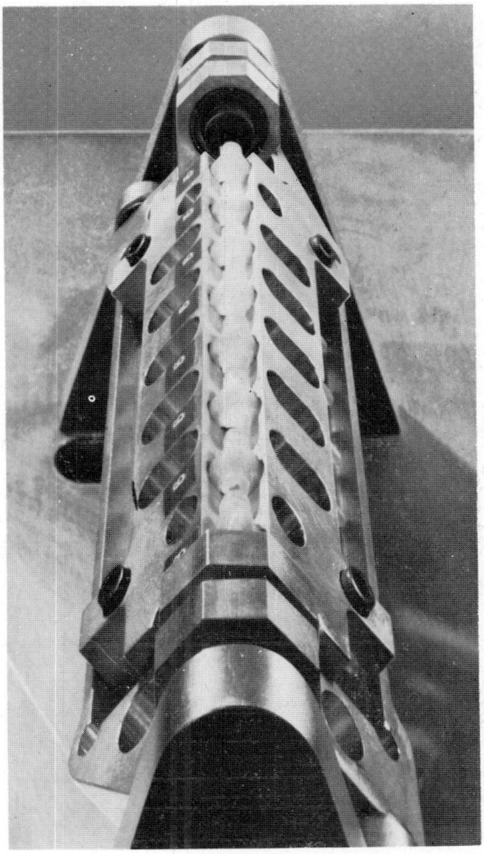

FIG. 23-4. Test machine which flexes the finger joint implant at 90° 50 million times a month. The present model has been machine tested for more than 400 million flexes without evidence of breakdown.

should be protected until this surrounding fibrous capsule has formed. Silicone rubber should not be placed immediately beneath the skin but under fat, a protective ligament, tendon, or fascia.

Preparation of the Implant

Medical-grade silicone elastomers are extremely inert, but if contaminated by lint, fingerprints, and other foreign materials, they can cause a foreign-body reaction. It is therefore important that the implant be thoroughly cleaned before sterilization. The material is heat-resistant and can be autoclaved, but every effort should be made to eliminate the chances of contamination with other foreign bodies throughout the entire procedure. The implants should be handled

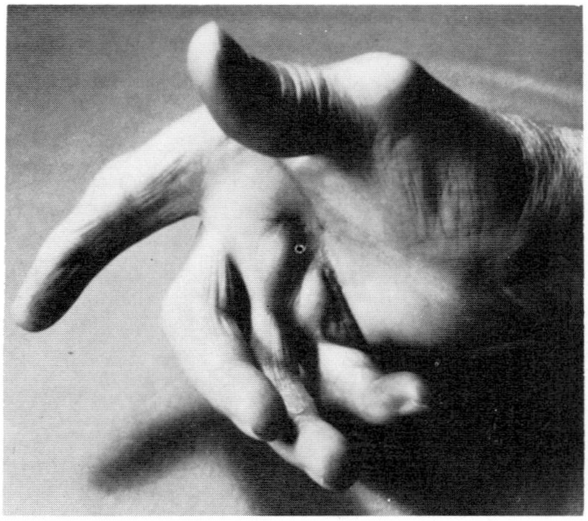

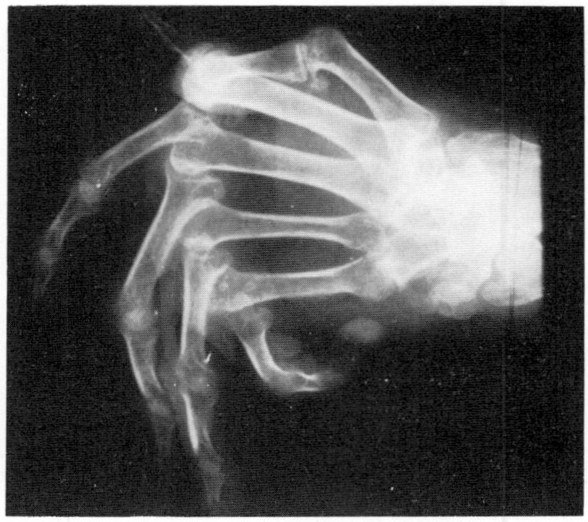

FIG. 23-5. (*Left*) Preoperative condition of a rheumatoid hand with severe ulnar drift and dislocation of the MP joints and boutonniere deformity of the thumb. (*Right*) The preoperative roentgenogram shows the severe deformities at the MP joints.

FIG. 23-6. (*Left*) One year postoperative roentgenogram of hand shown in Figure 23-5: the deformities are corrected, and there is excellent tolerance of the bone to the implants. The thumb MP joint has been fused. (*Top, right*) The correction of the deformities with good extension of the digits 1 year postoperatively. (*Bottom, right*) Range of finger joints flexion. The patient has stable, mobile, pain-free MP joints with excellent functional restoration.

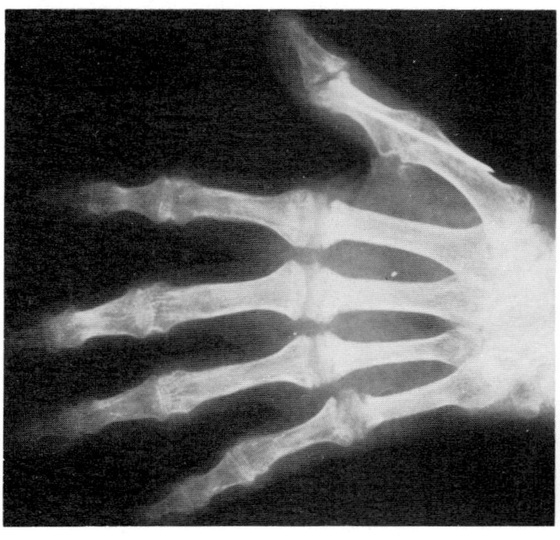

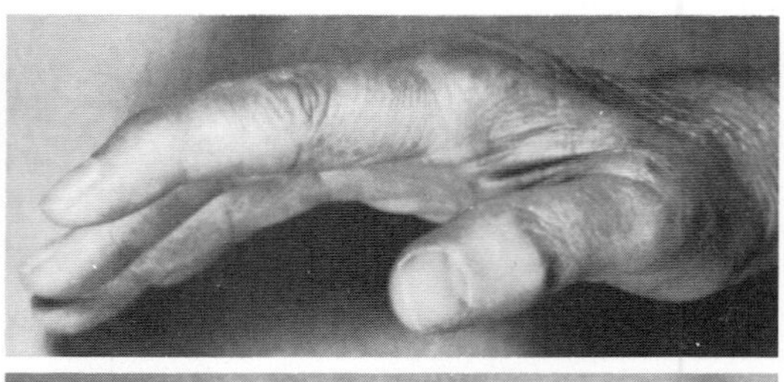

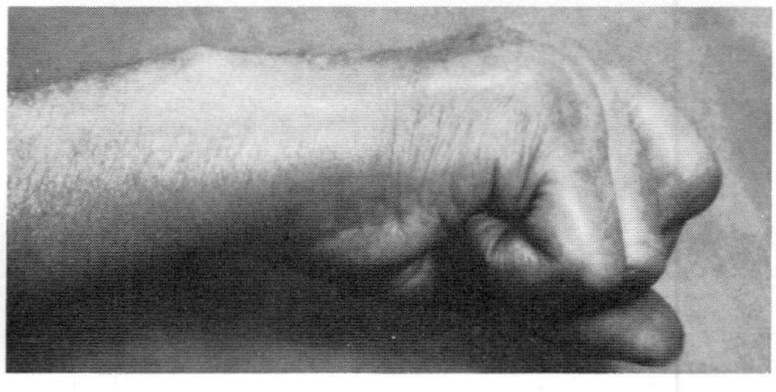

with instruments rather than gloves. The following cleaning and sterilization procedure is recommended if the implants become contaminated or are not sterilized before packaging:

> Boil the implants with distilled water and a non-oily mild soap for 20 minutes. Rinse thoroughly in distilled water. Wrap in a lint-free cloth or place on a clean open tray and autoclave by one of the following methods: (1) high-speed instrument sterilizer—3 minutes at 270° F, (2) standard gravity sterilizer—30 minutes at 250° F, or (3) pre-vacuum high-temperature sterilizer—normal cycle at 250° F.

Concept of Fixation by Encapsulation

Regular joint resection arthroplasty works well in the hand, if the joint space and alignment can be maintained. This frequently requires excessive postoperative fixation with pins and external support. The fixation, if overused, will compromise the expected range of motion. In a considerable number of these cases, the joint space gradually narrows, and stiffness and subluxation may result. Exceptional results do occur, however, and are related to the development of a supportive fibrous joint capsule organized during the time when a guarded range of motion is allowed. In the finger joint arthroplasty, the proper amount of flexion-extension, appropriate lateral movement, and reduction of dorsopalmar subluxation are difficult to obtain but necessary for a good result. Therefore, one of the most important functions of a successful implant is to maintain proper joint alignment internally while allowing early motion as this new, functionally adapted fibrous capsule matures. By continuing to support the important fibrous capsule and acting to keep the joint surfaces apart, the implant serves a further purpose in the postoperative course.

The intramedullary stems of the implant help to maintain alignment and prevent joint displacement. Orientation of the proper capsule is extremely important in the early stages of healing. The immediate postoperative positioning and control of joint movement during the 6 to 8-week rehabilitation period are as important as the surgery itself. These are achieved by dynamic bracing and physiotherapy.

Stability of the arthroplasty for both correction of ulnar drift and palmar subluxation has not been a problem in the many cases reviewed (Figs. 23-5 to 23-8). As long as the postoperative positioning maintains the anatomical position, there have been no significant recurrences of deformity. Rotation of the index and middle fingers, which frequently occurs in the rheumatoid hand, can also be improved in the early postoperative phase with a dynamic brace. It should be emphasized that other surgical procedures necessary to balance the hand are as important in implant arthroplasties as in any arthroplasty.

The implant is so well stabilized by the encapsulation process that no other fixation is required. In fact, any other fixation of a flexible implant is contraindicated. Attempts at fixing an implant with cross pins, gluing, or with a Dacron cover on the intramedullary stems[22] have led to early breakage of the implant at the junction of the stem and central portion. This has also occurred during the machine tests in the laboratory. It would appear that a slight amount of piston movement actually improves the life of the implant. Forces which are developed around the implant on flexion and extension are, therefore, not concentrated in one particular area but are spread over a broader section. Gliding of the implant also allows a greater range of motion to occur. Gliding permits the flexible implant to find the center of axis of rotation of the joint. A rigid implant or one fixed tightly would not have this advantage. The gliding, flexible implant has less stress on it and causes less stress to surrounding bone.

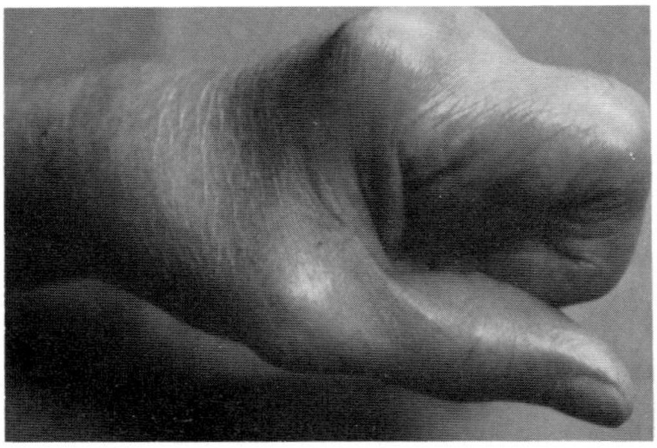

FIG. 23-7. Preoperative photo of hand showing palmar dislocation of MP joints.

THE METACARPOPHALANGEAL JOINT

Conditions which indicate MP joint implant arthroplasty are: (1) fixed or stiff MP joints; (2) x-ray evidence of joint destruction or subluxation; (3) ulnar drift, not correctable by surgery of soft tissues alone; (4) contracted intrinsic and extrinsic musculature or (5) associated stiff interphalangeal joints.

MP joint arthroplasty is contraindicated when too much shortening will be necessary to release severe soft tissue contracture. In such circumstances a classical arthroplasty is indicated.

Surgical Procedure

This technique is for a typical rheumatoid hand (Figs. 23-9 to 23-12). A long transverse skin incision is made on the dorsum of the hand over the necks of the metacarpals. The dissection is carried down through subcutaneous tissue to expose the extensor tendons. The dorsal veins that lie between the metatarsal heads are carefully released by blunt longitudinal dissection and are retraced carefully away from the underlying tendon and joint. The extensor hood is exposed to the base of the proximal phalanx. The radial portion of the hood is

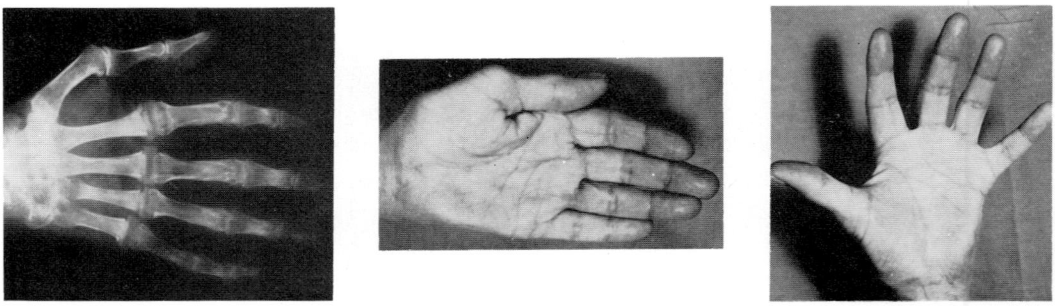

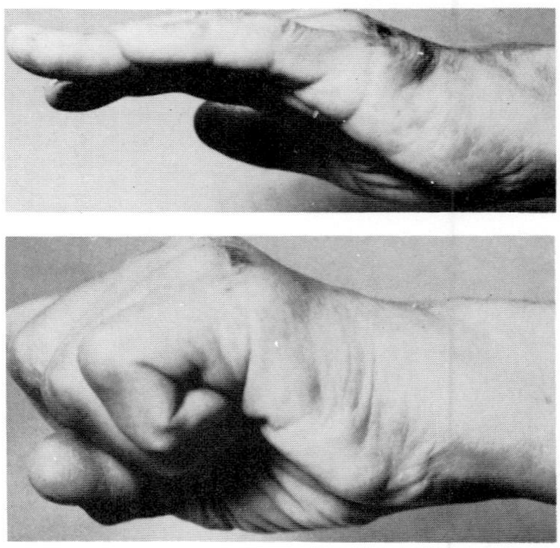

FIG. 23-8. (*Clockwise from top left*) Roentgenogram of hand shown in Figure 23-7 4 years postoperatively: implants tolerated well by bone; adduction; abduction essentially normal; extension; flexion. The flexible implant arthroplasty allows abduction-adduction movements as well as flexion-extension. This patient has a hand with near normal function. She is an executive secretary and can type 60 words per minute.

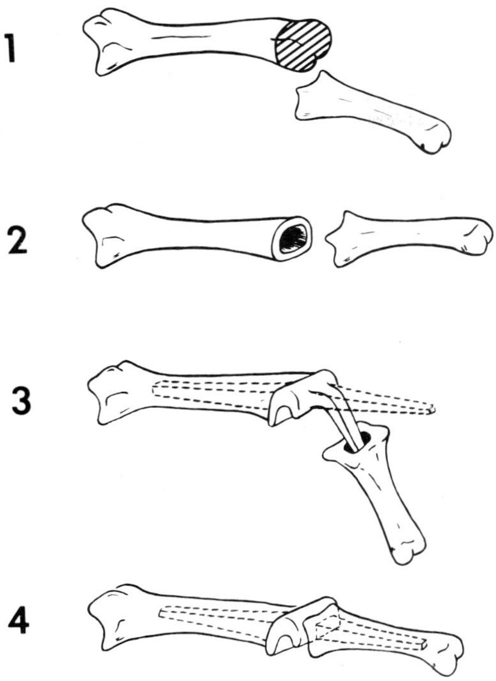

FIG. 23-9. Resection of head of the metacarpal and intramedullary insertion of stems of implant. The largest implant that can be well-seated should be used. A comprehensive soft tissue release procedure must be done so that the base of the proximal phalanx can be displaced dorsally above the metacarpal.

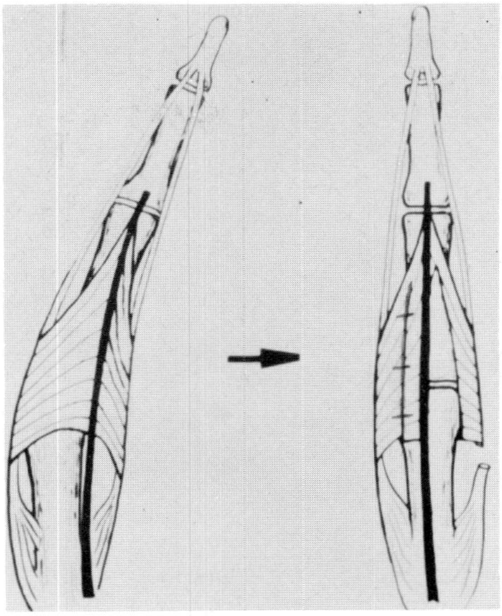

FIG. 23-10. The dislocated extensor tendon is released by incision on its ulnar border. The ulnar intrinsics are usually released. The sagittal fibers of the dorsal hood are reefed on the radial side to maintain the correction.

usually stretched out and the extensor tendon dislocated ulnarward. A longitudinal incision is made in the extensor hood fibers parallel to the extensor tendon on its ulnar aspect. The hood fibers and capsule are carefully dissected from the underlying synovium and retracted to the radial side. The joint is exposed and the head of the metacarpal identified. The neck of the metacarpal is dissected subperiosteally and transected with an air drill, motor saw, or bone cutting forceps. Care should be taken to avoid splintering the bone. The head of the metacarpal is grasped, and the collateral ligament and capsule attachments are incised. The head of the metacarpal, along with the hypertrophied synovial material is thereby removed *en masse*. Any remaining involved synovium of the joint cavity and surrounding tissues is removed. A pituitary rongeur is useful for this purpose.

A comprehensive soft tissue release procedure must be done at this stage so that the base of the proximal phalanx can be displaced dorsally above the metacarpal. This may require incision of the palmar plate and collateral ligament attachments from the proximal phalanx. This should be done symmetrically so that the release will be complete. The ulnar intrinsic tendon, seeking its insertion into the extensor mechanism, is identified. If it is tight, it is pulled up into the wound with a blunt hook and sectioned at the myotendonous junction.

In some patients who have evidence of a flexor synovitis, the flexor sheath will be incised longitudinally in its dorsal aspect and the long flexor tendons can be identified and pulled up gently into the wound with a blunt hook. The degree of involvement of the flexor tendons can be evaluated. In some of our cases, we have done a partial synovectomy and tendon sheath release or

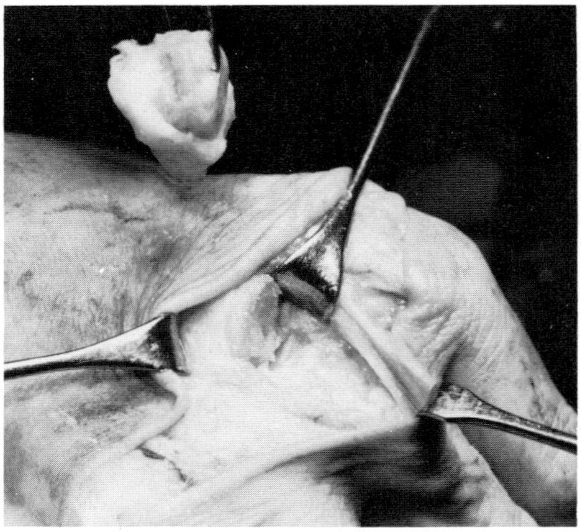

FIG. 23-11. The transverse skin incision is used. The longitudinal veins are protected in the intermetacarpal space. The head of the metacarpal, along with hypertrophied synovia, is removed.

injection of hydrocortisone through this incision.

The tendons of the abductor digiti minimi and flexor digiti minimi are exposed on the ulnar aspect of the fifth MP joint. The tendons are pulled up into the wound with a blunt hook and sectioned. Care should be taken to avoid the ulnar digital nerve in this dissection. It is our opinion that these tendons eventually reattach but in a lengthened position.

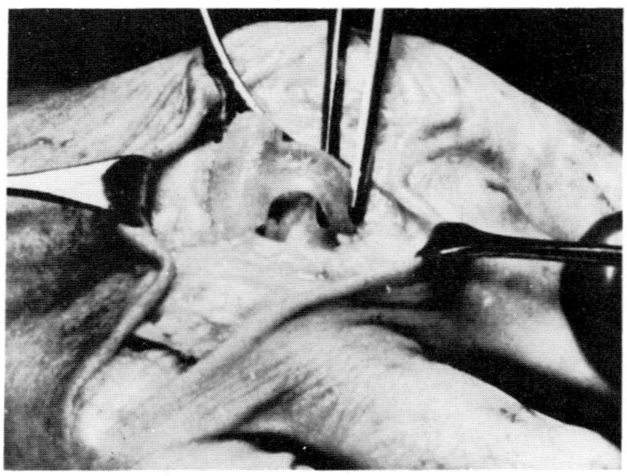

FIG. 23-12. The intramedullary stemmed implant is inserted into the canal of the proximal phalanx and the metacarpal. The canals are carefully prepared with curettes, broach, or air drill.

Usually, no bony resection of the base of the proximal phalanx is performed, except for marginal osteophytes which might interfere with the implant. Occasionally in patients with osteoporosis and long-standing dislocation, deformities of the base of the proximal phalanx will be severe. In these cases, a shaping of the base of the phalanx may be necessary.

The intramedullary canal of the metacarpal may be prepared with a curette, broach, or, as we prefer, an air drill with a special burr that prevents cutting through the shaft of the metacarpal. These burrs have a smooth leader point which helps keep them in the canal. Occasionally the canal is constricted in its proximal third; this can easily be enlarged with the burr. Care should be taken to avoid too much reaming of the canal, especially in patients with thin bones. Test implants are used to select the proper size. The stem of the implant should fit well down into the canal so that the transverse midsection of the implant abuts against the bone end. The largest implant possible should be used. (Implants of sizes 4 through 8 are used.)

A rectangular hole is then made in the joint surface of the proximal phalanx with an osteotome, knife, broach, or air drill. The intramedullary canal is reamed, in the same fashion as for the metacarpal, for the appropriate size of the distal stem of the implant that has been chosen for the metacarpal.

This procedure is repeated for all of the digits. The intramedullary canal of the ring metacarpal is frequently quite small and requires careful preparation. The ends of the metacarpals should be free of any sharp points and should be appropriately smoothed. The joints are thoroughly irrigated with saline to remove debris. The silicone finger joint implants are inserted with a no-touch technique, using blunt instruments. The implant is first firmly

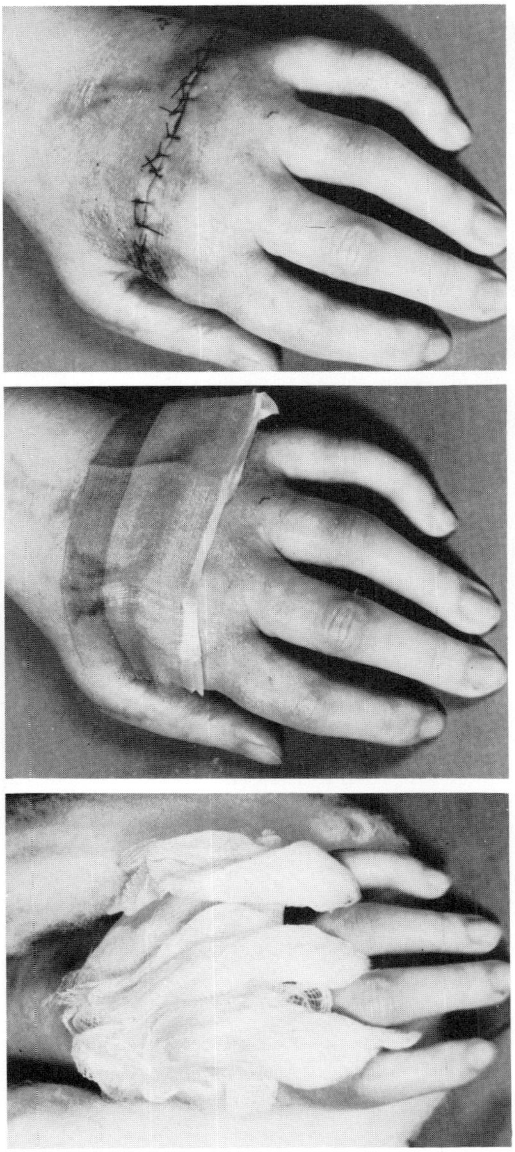

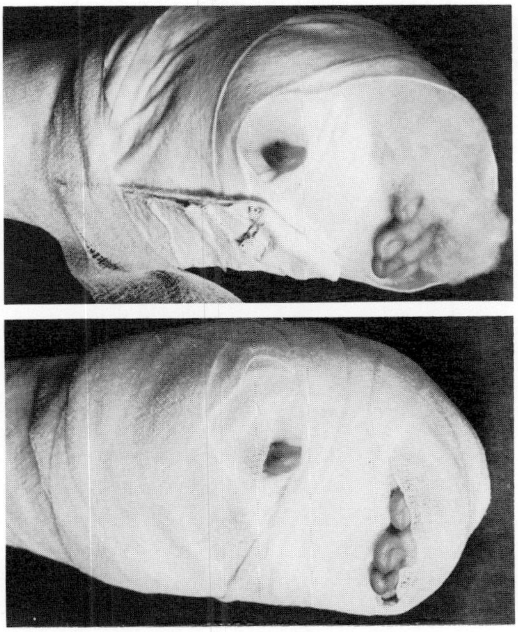

FIG. 23-13. Application of postoperative dressing. Bare hand shows level of the transverse incision (*top left*). The incision is dressed with rayon gauze covered by Furacin gauze or a similar lubricated product (*center left*). Gauze fluffs are placed between the fingers. Care should be taken not to push the gauze too deeply into the clefts lest this embarrass circulation. Dacron batting (available as pillow filling in most department stores) is used to develop a bulky conforming pressure dressing (*bottom left*). The batting is placed across the palm and on the dorsal and palmar aspects of the hand, wrist, and forearm. The dressing is wrapped with Webril. A short palmar splint is applied. A non-elastic bandage such as Kling is used to secure the dressing (*top right*). The completed dressing should support the wrist and fingers in a functional position (*bottom, right*). The limb is elevated postoperatively, and the dressing is worn for 3 to 5 days.

inserted into the intramedullary canal of the metacarpal and then, by slight traction on the finger, the joint is distracted and the implant flexed so that the distal stem can easily be inserted into the proximal phalanx. With the joint in extension, there should be no impingement of the implant. If there is, an inadequate soft tissue release or bone resection has been done.

The radial portion of the sagittal fibers of each extensor hood mechanism is reefed in an overlapping fashion so that the extensor tendon is brought slightly to the radial side of the center of the joint. Three to five 4-0 Dacron sutures with a buried-knot technique are used.

Occasionally in patients who have an inadequate first dorsal interosseus muscle or a tendency for pronation deformity of the index finger, a reconstruction of the radial collateral ligament has been done. A distally based flap is made of the radial portion of the palmar plate and collateral ligament, which is separated from the underlying intrinsic muscles and tendon. This 1½-cm. to 2-cm. flap is attached around the radial aspect of the neck of the metacarpal to a hole in the dorsal radial portion of the neck of the bone. It does not appear to interfere with the use of the implant. This procedure has seemed to be important in correction of pronation deformities and provides some improved lateral stability for pinch. This has been done on the last 20 patients, and though it seems to decrease flexion of the index MP joint, it seems to improve rotational deformity and may be important in certain cases.

The skin incision is closed with interrupted 5-0 nylon sutures; two small drains of strips of silicone rubber sheeting are inserted into the wound under the skin. A non-adherent dressing, such as rayon, is applied over the wound along with a Furacin or other type gauze overlay. A voluminous hand conforming pressure dressing is applied after gauze has been placed between the fingers (not into the clefts, since this might cause vascular constriction). A roll of Dacron batting is placed across the palm, and Dacron batting is layered across the dorsal and palmar aspects of the forearm, wrist, hand and fingers. Sheet wadding or Webril is then applied over this. A narrow plaster splint is applied to the palmar aspect, and the entire dressing is wrapped in a conforming bandage, such as Kling (Fig. 23-13). The extremity is then placed in a special sling, which may be attached to an IV stand. This maintains the hand and forearm in the elevated position during the postoperative course.

It is not wise to operate on a rheumatoid extremity for longer than 1½ to 2 hours, and finger joint implant arthroplasties can usually be done in 1 hour. Frequently, other reconstructive procedures can be carried out for thumb, finger PIP and DIP deformities, wrist joint synovectomy or distal radio-ulnar reconstructions, or, occasionally, radial head implant arthroplasty and synovectomy of the elbow, depending on the time involved. Other small joints may also be injected with hydrocortisone and Thio-tepa during the anesthetic period. Frequently other affected joints, such as knee or foot, will be simultaneously operated on by another surgical team.

The wound is checked on the second day and the drains removed. Swelling is usually minimal, so the dynamic brace can be used on the third to fifth postoperative day. A light dressing is applied to the hand and forearm, and the dynamic brace is fitted and adjusted so that the patient can start finger movements in a protected arc (Fig. 23-14). The brace must be carefully readjusted as necessary, so that a range of movement from 0° of extension to 90° of flexion is possible. Goniometer readings of joint flexion should be recorded. The joints have a tendency to tighten up in the second postoperative week. The patient is encouraged to flex his joints within the limits of pain and fatigue. If there is difficulty obtaining or maintaining 70° of movement, the rubber band slings are removed part time or the flexion cuff is used part time to assist joint flexion passively. The extension part of the brace is usually worn night and day for 3 weeks, except by patients who may require intermittent flexion assistance. It is then worn at night for approximately 3 weeks. Patients who have a tendency for extensor tendon lag or recurrent deformity may need it longer. A carefully controlled follow-up and rehabilitation program should be provided for these patients for at least 3 months postoperatively.

Objectives of Implant Arthroplasty

1. Complete release of contractures of ligaments and capsule, palmar plate, and ulnar intrinsics.

2. Adequate bone preparation: sufficient bone resection and shaping of the intramedullary canal.
3. Proper selection of implant size.
4. Reefing of extensor mechanism.
5. Rebalance of longitudinal arch of hand: wrist joint, collapse deformities of digits, temporary Kirschner wire fixation.
6. Proper postoperative dressing must be: voluminous but avoid transverse constriction and must include an anterior plaster splint. It should prevent hematoma and swelling, maintain functional position of the parts, and elevate the limb.
7. Rehabilitative measures: dynamic bracing, early mobilization, alternating movements. Extension-flexion progress should be measured. Rehabilitation seeks to correct angulation and rotation and maintain what correction has been achieved.

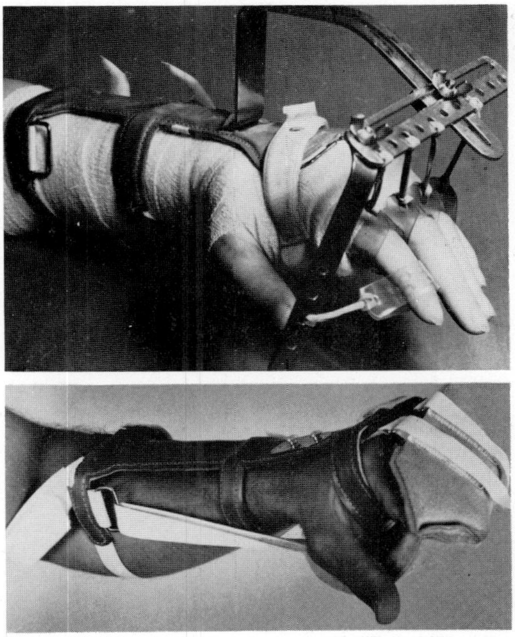

FIG. 23-14. The adjustable dynamic brace is placed over a slightly padded dressing between the third and fifth days. The patient is encouraged to flex his joints within the limits of his pain and fatigue. Proper use of bracing is essential to ensure an adequate range of motion. The flexion cuff (*bottom*) may be used intermittently to assist flexion movements.

Associated Flexor Tendon Involvement

Synovitis of the flexor sheaths in rheumatoid arthritis occurs frequently and is painful and disabling.[25,31,34] Because the patient is unable to pull the tendons through the sheaths, either because of pain or mechanical block, the finger joints will not flex properly. Extension deformities of the interphalangeal joints are the most common result. Trigger-finger phenomena may occur. The flexor tendon synovial hypertrophy may be palpated between the examiner's fingers at the sheath over the proximal phalanx. The tendons can be felt to crepitate on movement in the fingers, palm, and wrist. Hyperextension at the PIP joint and swan-neck deformities may occur. These patients frequently have associated MP joint and PIP joint deformities which require implant surgery. The flexor tendons should be released before this surgery is contemplated. Associated median or ulnar nerve compression also may be present in these cases.

Procedures for tendon release. The tendon release procedure should begin with an incision starting in the palm and wrist, similar to the approach for a carpal tunnel release. The transverse carpal ligament is incised, and the flexor tendons are identified. Traction on them will demonstrate their degree of restriction. The synovium is carefully removed without damage to the tendon surface. If the fingers cannot be easily pulled down into the palm and the joints are passively movable, distal restriction must be exposed. A transverse incision is made distal to the distal palmar crease, and the sheath and the flexor tendons for the four digits are identified. If necessary, the proximal pulley is cut longitudinally on the radial aspect. The tendons are then pulled down. If severe synovitis is occurring in the finger and pulling on the tendons still does not affect interphalangeal joint flexion, a lateral finger approach is used to isolate the flexor sheath. Usually, if the finger is involved, the sublimis tendon, which most often has the severest attritional change, should be removed. Invasion of the tendon and formation of nodules within the tendon substance may be seen. Occasionally these nodules can be carefully excised and 6-0 sutures used to close the tendon. If the sublimis has to be removed and hyperextension deformity of the PIP joint of more than 10° is present, one slip of the sublimis can be used as a tenodesis to hold the PIP joint in approximately 20° of flexion.[37] The tendon is sutured to the capsular structures and periosteum of the neck of the proximal phalanx with 4-0 Dacron sutures. A small Kirschner wire may then be placed across the PIP joint to hold it in flexion for 2 weeks. Sometimes the ulnar nerve will have to be decompressed in the Guyon's canal and a synovectomy done in this area.

The wounds are closed in the usual manner, and a voluminous pressure hand dressing is applied. The patient is usually placed in a dynamic brace during the postoperative course. He is encouraged to use his flexor tendons on a programmed basis, within the limits of his fatigue and pain tolerance. Tendon release for adhesions and synovectomy in rheumatoid arthritic patients is much more successful than it is for the residuals of trauma. Surgical reconstruction of joints is usually done 6 or 8 weeks after the patient has recovered from his flexor tendon surgery.

THE INTERPHALANGEAL JOINTS

The interphalangeal joints are commonly disabled in rheumatoid, degenerative, and traumatic arthritis. The deformities are usually of three basic types: (1) collapse into swan-neck deformity, (2) collapse into boutonniere deformity, and (3) flexion or extension stiffness.

The restoration of function of the PIP joint has been more or less neglected, because an arthrodesis of this joint does not appear to impair hand function significantly.[17] The distal interphalangeal joint also has been ignored, because its function has not been adequately appreciated. Difficulty in treatment of these deformities is

(Text continues on page 192)

Classification of Treatment of Collapse Deformities of Fingers

I. THE SWAN-NECK PIP JOINT

Without MP Joint Involvement

The Initial PIP Deformity

Local injections—corticosteroids, Thio-tepa.
Flexor tendon synovectomy with or without sublimis tenodesis.
Intrinsic release with or without flexor tendon synovectomy.

The Flexible PIP Deformity

Dermodesis of the PIP joint.
Lateral tendon relocation with or without central tendon elongation.
Sublimis tenodesis and flexor tendon synovectomy.

The Rigid, Subluxated or Dislocated PIP Joint

Joint resection and lateral tendon relocation and implant.
Joint resection and fusion.

DIP Joint Treatment, if Required:

Temporary pinning in neutral position if passively corrected.
Fusion if severely flexed or damaged.

WITH MP JOINT INVOLVEMENT

MP Joint Treatment	*PIP Joint Treatment*
The Flexible PIP Deformity	
Synovectomy and proximal intrinsic release.	Manipulation and K-wire temporary fixation in flexion, if required.
Relocation subluxated joint and proximal intrinsic release.	Manipulation and K-wire temporary fixation in flexion, if required. Dermodesis.
Resection and proximal intrinsic release and implant.	Manipulation to 50° flexion with temporary fixation. Relocation of lateral tendons with or without central tendon elongation.
The Rigid, Subluxated or Dislocated PIP Joint	
Resection and implant.	Relocation of lateral tendons and central tendon elongation. Resection and fusion. Resection and implant.

DIP Joint Treatment, if Required:

Temporary pinning in neutral position if passively corrected.
Fusion if severely flexed or damaged.

II. THE BOUTONNIERE PIP JOINT

The Initial PIP Deformity

Local injections, corticosteroids, Thio-tepa, splinting.
Synovectomy.

*The Flexible PIP Deformity**

Reconstruction of the central tendon.
Elongation of the lateral tendons.
Both of above procedures.

* with or without synovectomy

The Rigid PIP Joint without Bone Erosions

Joint release and reconstruction of the central tendon and elongation of the lateral tendons.
Joint resection and reconstruction of the central tendon, with or without implant.
Distal lateral tendons release.

The Rigid PIP Joint with Bone Erosions

Joint resection and reconstruction of the central tendon, with or without implant.
Joint resection and fusion.

The Subluxated or Dislocated PIP Joint

Joint resection and reconstruction of the central tendon + implant.
Joint resection and fusion.

DIP Joint Treatment, if Required:

Distal lateral tendons release.
Fusion.

III. THE STIFF OSTEOARTHRITIC PIP JOINT

The Non-Dislocated PIP Joint

Joint resection and implant.

The Subluxated or Dislocated PIP Joint

Joint resection and implant.
Joint resection and fusion.

DIP Joint Treatment, if Required:

Fusion.

compounded not only by the joint destruction but also by the accompanying muscle imbalance from contiguous joint malpositioning.[6,9] Treatment of the PIP joint disability should be considered if reasonable hand-function potential is to be achieved. The longitudinal arch of the digit must be reestablished. Though emphasis must be placed on MP joint restoration, PIP joint reconstruction obtains some stable pain-free movement and should always be considered. The distal joint should also be placed in the position for best function.

The treatment of the PIP and distal interphalangeal (DIP) joints varies according to the degree of disability and other associated joint disturbances. Long experience in surgery of these joints has led us to attempt to classify their treatment.[47]

THE PROXIMAL INTERPHALANGEAL JOINT

Resection implant arthroplasty for the proximal interphalangeal joint has been done for destroyed or subluxed joints and for stiffened joints in which soft tissue release alone would be inadequate. Resection arthroplasty for severe disabilities of the PIP joint, using an intramedullary stemmed heat-molded medical-grade Silastic implant, is successful if enough bone stock is present and if an adequate tendon mechanism can be reconstructed. Points of importance in the successful implant arthroplasty include proper release of contractures; sufficient bone resection; careful preparation of the intramedullary canals, preferably with an air drill; selection of the proper sized implant; meticulous tendon reconstruction; and a well-planned postoperative program including early movement.

Operative Procedure for the Stiff PIP Joint

A longitudinal gentle S-shaped incision is made over the dorsum of the joint, protecting the dorsal veins whenever possible (Fig. 23-15). The extensor mechanism is exposed by blunt dissection, with care to avoid injury to its surface. The central tendon is identified and incised longitudinally in a proximal fashion from its insertion at the base of the middle phalanx through the distal two-thirds of the proximal phalanx. In flexible deformities of the PIP joint, the extensor mechanism can be gently dislocated palmarward as the joint is flexed. The collateral ligaments are incised from their attachment to the proximal phalanx. The insertion of the central tendon into the middle phalanx should not be disturbed. If the joint is contracted the extensor mechanism cannot be readily dislocated, and the head of the proximal phalanx may be removed first. It is cut transversely at the neck with an air drill and then removed piecemeal. The collateral ligaments and accessory collateral ligaments are completely released from the proximal phalanx. They will relocate and reattach during healing. Adequate release of the joint is essential for good arthroplasty. If the joint is contracted, the palmar plate must be released. This is done by incising it at its membranous insertion proximally, so that the joint is completely loosened. If there is a severe contracture of the joint, the collateral ligaments, accessory collateral ligaments, and palmar plate are carefully and completely excised.

After resection of the head of the proximal phalanx, the intramedullary canal is carefully reamed with an air drill. A special

FIG. 23-15. Technique of implant arthroplasty in a stiff non-deformed arthritic joint. (A) Longitudinal S-shaped incision is made over dorsum of PIP joint. (B) Extensor mechanism is incised longitudinally from base of middle phalanx proximally. Care is taken to maintain insertion of tendon on base of middle phalanx. (C) Split extensor tendon is retracted laterally. Collateral ligaments are incised, and head of proximal phalanx is exposed. (D) Head of proximal phalanx is sectioned through neck with an air drill and

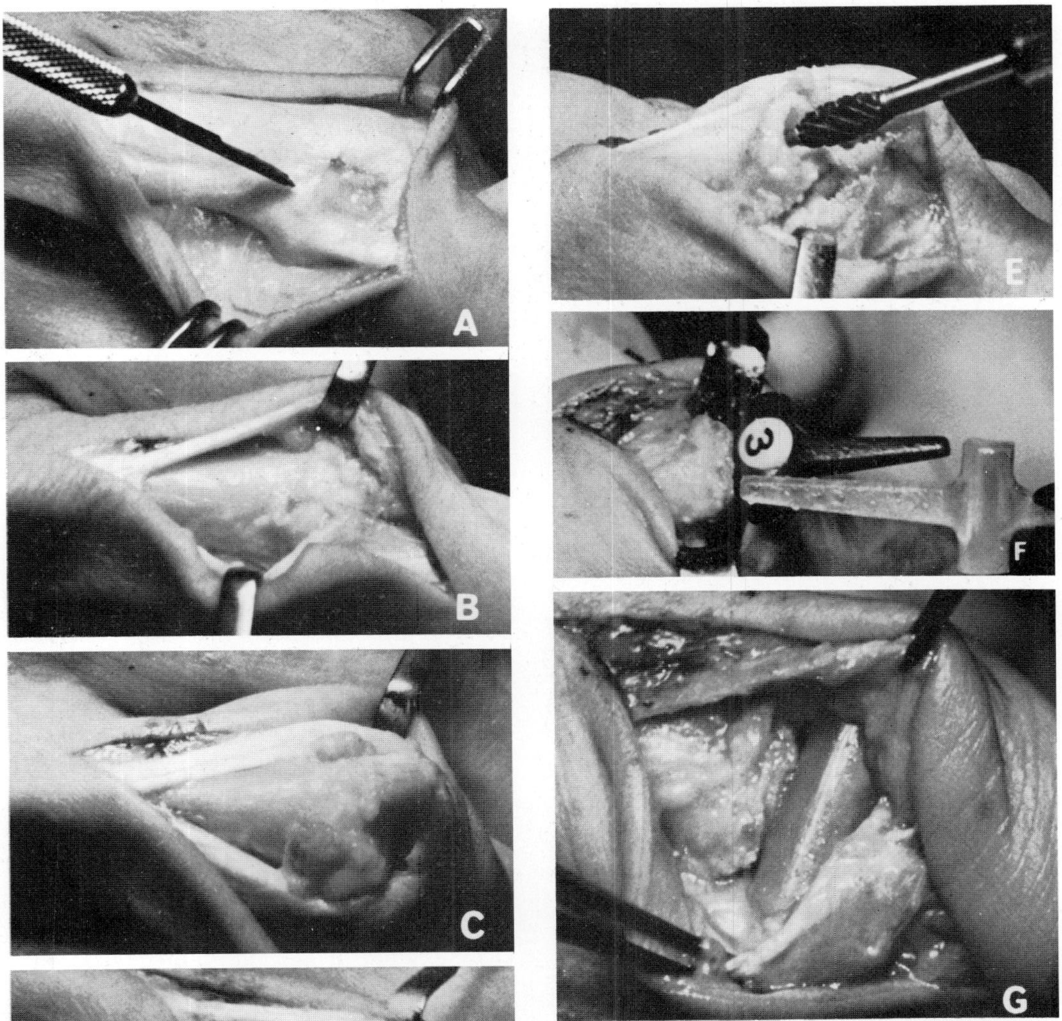

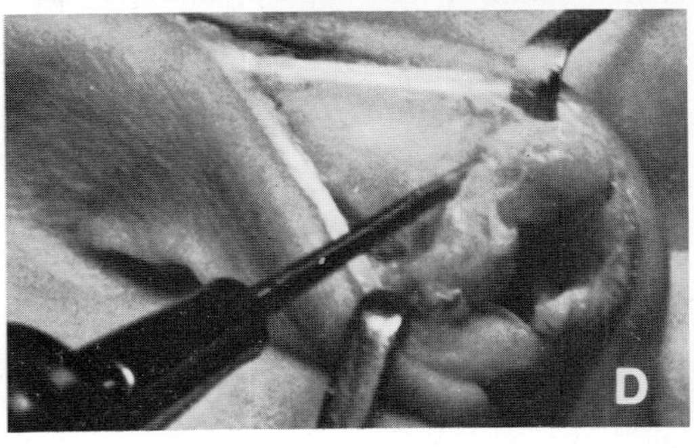

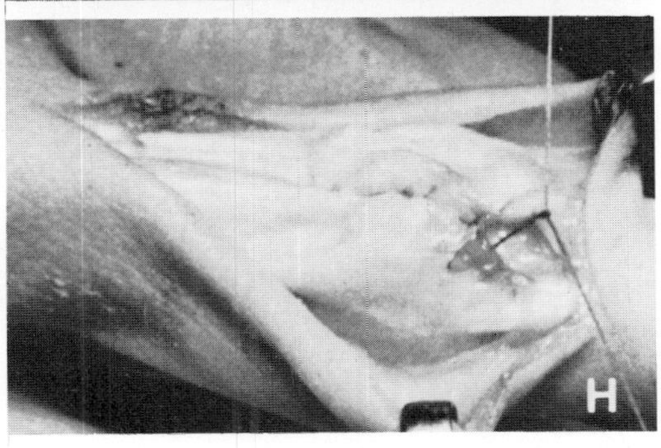

removed. When joint is extremely tight, the bone may have to be removed piecemeal before tendon can be safely retracted. (E) A special burr, with a smooth tip extension to avoid perforation of cortex of phalanx, is used to prepare the intramedullary canal. (F) A test implant is used to determine correct implant size. Implant sizes 0, 1, 2, and 3 are usually used for PIP arthroplasty. (G) Implant is in place with finger in extension. Proper bone removal and soft tissue release must be done so that on extension there is enough space for midsection of implant. (H) Extensor mechanism is reapproximated with 3 to 5 Dacron sutures with an inverted knot technique. Arthroplasty for boutonniere and swan-neck deformities usually requires an individualized tendon reconstruction.

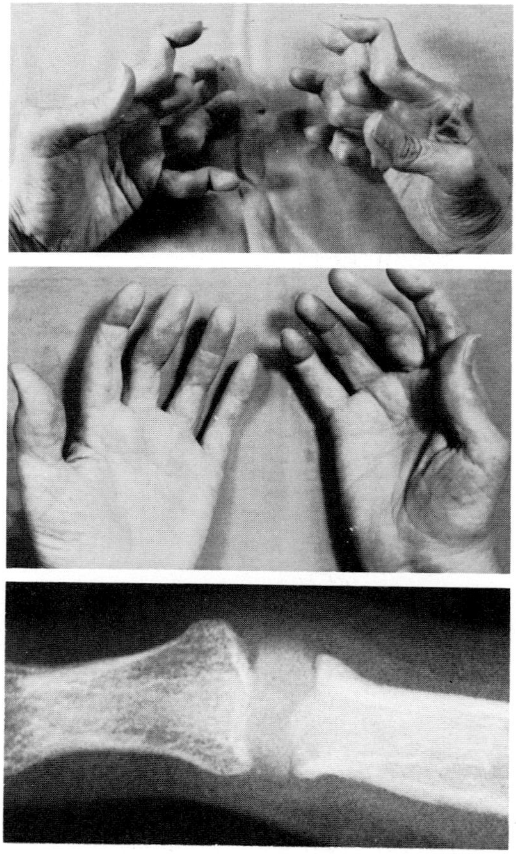

FIG. 23-16. (*Top*) Severe swan-neck deformities in a rheumatoid patient with dorsal dislocation of the middle of the proximal phalanx. (*Middle*) Postoperative result following reconstructive surgical procedures including PIP implant arthroplasties. (*Bottom*) Roentgenogram three years after implant arthroplasty for swan-neck deformity. Note the acceptance of the implant by the bone.

burr with a smooth tip extension is used to avoid perforating the cortex of the phalanx. The canal should be shaped to accept the rectangular stem of the implant. The intramedullary canal of the middle phalanx is prepared in a similar fashion. The base of the middle phalanx is not resected; any osteophytes are trimmed. The proximal stem of the implant is inserted first. With the joint in flexion, the distal stem is inserted in the prepared intramedullary canal of the middle phalanx. Implant sizes 0, 1, 2, and 3 are most frequently used for PIP-joint arthroplasty. The largest acceptable size is selected. The midsection of the implant should seat well against the bone surfaces of the phalanges. The bone ends should be trimmed smoothly to avoid sharp edges cutting into the implant. The joint is extended. If the implant midsection is impinged by the bone ends, more soft tissue release or more bone removal from the proximal phalanx or the middle phalanx should be done. The incised extensor mechanism is brought together and sutured with 4-0 or 5-0 Dacron or other nonabsorbable sutures using an inverted knot technique. A small drain is placed in the wound, and a voluminous pressure dressing is applied. Active movements are allowed on the third postoperative day. An exercise program is prescribed. The proximal phalanx is supported by a brace, cast, or exercise device. The patient is encouraged to flex and extend the digit fully, short of causing pain and swelling in the finger. Small aluminum splints are taped on the fingers in the extension position at night for 3 to 6 weeks. Occasionally, a flexion cuff device or a dorsal strap is used to gently force flexion, if necessary, after 3 weeks.

Swan-Neck Deformity

Implant arthroplasty for stiff swan-neck deformities has been used successfully in our clinic (Fig. 23-16). The technique differs slightly from that for the non-deformed stiff PIP joint. On exposure of the joint, the central tendon is separated from the dorsally displaced lateral tendons, which are allowed to displace volarward. The central tendon is cut transversely and dissected up over the proximal phalanx, thereby lengthening it. Occasionally, a severely flexed distal joint is held in extension with an intramedullary small Kirschner wire. This will improve flexion forces at the PIP joint in the postoperative period. The proximal phalangeal joint is held in approximately 20° of flexion in a small taped-on aluminum splint for approximately 10 days. Active movements are encouraged, usually on the tenth day. Flexion movements are encouraged supporting the proximal phalanx. Care is taken to avoid hyperextension of these joints in the first 3 to 6 weeks. A slight flexion contracture will then develop, and correction of the deformity will be maintained.[39]

Boutonniere Deformity

In the boutonniere deformity of rheumatoid arthritis, the central tendon has usually been lengthened due to severe stretching of the capsule and attrition of the capsulary and bony attachments of the central tendon to the middle phalanx. The lateral tendons are usually palmarly displaced, and the connecting fibers are stretched out. Implant joint reconstruction in these severe cases also requires reconstruction of the extensor mechanism.[10,11,24,27,50,55] Two methods have been used. One is a repair of the central tendon attachment to the base of the middle phalanx. The stretched-out central tendon is sutured through a very small drill hole in the base of the middle phalanx. The lateral tendon also can be used to reconstruct the central tendon by attaching the ulnar tendon to the insertion of the central tendon. Release of the radial lateral tendon for correction of hyperextension deformities of the distal joint may be required if passive flexion cannot be accomplished after reconstruction. This is usually done proximally to the insertion of the fibers of Landsmeer's ligament. The finger is immobilized for approximately 10 days in extension in a taped-on aluminum finger splint. Guarded flexion movements are then allowed. The PIP joint is held in extension for from 3 to 6 weeks, part time, depending upon the degree of extensor lag that is demonstrated.

The results of implant arthroplasty for the PIP joint have been very rewarding. We have performed this procedure in 146 arthritic fingers with severe stiffness or deformity in the past 6 years. The range of flexion movement was 20° to 100°, with an average of 65°. There was a range of extension from 0° to —20°, depending on the type of case. Some severe boutonniere cases had a full range of movement from 0° to 90°. No patients complained of lack of stability. Though the index digit demonstrated some weakness in lateral pinch, the patients either supported the index with the middle digit or used pulp pinch. There were no implant failures or infections. In several cases of recurrent stiffness, the joint was further released and a smaller implant inserted. This usually resulted in 20° to 30° more motion.

RESULTS

A recent statistical evaluation of results of MP joint implant arthroplasty, done in our clinic and in a participating field clinic, showed that in nearly all of the patients, function and cosmetic appearance were subsequently improved and there was good acceptance of the implant by the host tissue. The results impress us as far superior to our previous experience with other techniques of joint arthroplasty in the arthritic patient.

A comparative study was done in April, 1970, between this clinic and 112 participating field clinics using similar implants and surgical technique. It is felt the variation in the results of range of motion in different clinics derives from the different types of cases selected for surgery and, most important, from the differences in postoperative care. Those who mobilized their patients' hands with a dynamic brace postoperatively had better results. The implant resection arthroplasty for severe MP and PIP joint impairment appears to hold promise for these difficult reconstructive problems of the rheumatoid arthritic patient.

SILASTIC IMPLANT ARTHROPLASTY IN MP JOINTS*

Grand Rapids Clinic, April 1970
Complications in 358 Implants—
6 Months to 5 Years Follow-Up

Complication	*No.*	*%*
Fracture	7	1.95
Dislocation	3	0.83
Infection	2	0.56
Implant removed	2	0.56

MP Implant Arthroplasty
Average Extension/Flexion

Digit	*Extension*	*Flexion†*
2	−2.9°	61.6°
3	−2.2°	63.9°
4	−2.6°	66.8°
5	−2.4°	62.3°
Average	−2.5°	63.6°

† Range of flexion was from 30° to 100°, most cases were between 50° and 70°.

Correction of Alignment in 358 Fingers

Deformity	*%*
Ulnar drift	96.8
MP dislocation	98.9

Field Clinic Study, April 1970
Complications in 3,409 Implants

Complication	*No.*	*%*
Fracture	30	0.88
Dislocation	29	0.85
Infection	25	0.73
Implant removed	3	0.08

Correction of Alignment in 3,004 Fingers

Deformity	*No.*	*%*
Ulnar drift	2948	98.1
MP dislocation	2974	99.5

* Different numbers of fingers in various tables reflect the degree of completeness with which postoperative questionnaires were filled out.

Implant Arthroplasty in 2,544 Fingers

Average extension	−4°
Average flexion	57°

Average Range of MP Joint Flexion in 2736 Fingers‡

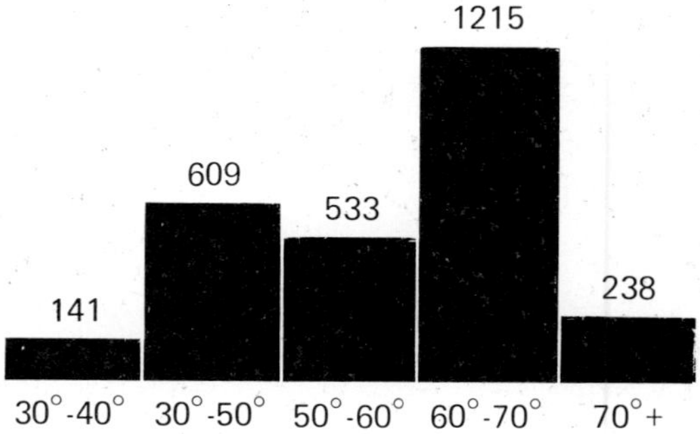

‡ Data collected from various clinics; average flexion = 57.9°.

REFERENCES

1. American Arthritis and Rheumatism Foundation. 1969 Annual Report. Arthritis Manual. New York, 1969.
2. Barron, J. N.: Assessment of suitability for surgery in general: Timing of operation. International Workshop on Artificial Finger Joints. Ann. Rheum. Dis. Suppl. [Brit.], *28*:74-76, 1969.
3. Boyes, J. H.: Bunnell's Surgery of the Hand. ed. 5. Philadelphia, J. B. Lippincott, 1970.
4. Braley, S.: The silicones as tools in biological engineering. Med. Electron. Biol. Engin., *3*:127-136, 1965.
5. Bunnell, S.: Surgery of the rheumatoid hand. J. Bone Joint Surg., *37A*:759-766, 1955.
6. Carroll, R. E., and Taber, T. H.: Digital arthroplasty of the proximal interphalangeal joint. J. Bone Joint Surg., *36A*:912-920, 1954.
7. Charnley, J.: A biomechanical analysis of the use of cement to anchor the femoral head prosthesis. J. Bone Joint Surg. [Brit.], *47B*:354-363, 1965.
8. Clayton, M. L.: Surgery of the thumb in rheumatoid arthritis. J. Bone Joint Surg., *44A*:1376-1386, 1962.
9. Curtis, R. M.: Capsulectomy of the interphalangeal joints of the fingers. J. Bone Joint Surg., *36A*:1219-1232, 1954.

10. Dolphin, J. A.: Extensor tenotomy for chronic boutonniere deformity of the finger. J. Bone Joint Surg., *47*:161-164, 1965.
11. Elliot, R.: Injuries to extensor mechanism of the hand. Orth. Clin. N. Amer., *1*:335-354, 1970.
12. Entin, M. A.: Surgical treatment of rheumatoid arthritis. Surg. Clin. N. Amer., *44*: 1081-1090, 1964.
13. Flatt, A. E.: The Care of the Rheumatoid Hand. ed. 2. St. Louis, C. V. Mosby Co., 1968.
14. Fowler, S. B.: Instructional Course Lectures. American Academy of Orthopaedic Surgeons, 1958.
15. Fowler, S. B., and Riordan, D. C.: Surgical treatment of rheumatoid deformities of the hand. J. Bone Joint Surg., *40*:1431-1432, 1958.
16. Gschwend, N.: Die Operative Behandlung der Progressive Chronischen Polyarthritis. Stuttgart, George Thieme Verlag, 1968.
17. Granowitz, S., and Vainio, K.: Proximal interphalangeal joint arthrodesis in rheumatoid arthritis. Acta Orthop. Scand., *37*:301-310, 1966.
18. Hollander, J. L.: Arthritis. ed. 7. Philadelphia, Lea & Febiger, 1966.
19. Kaplan, E. B.: Functional and Surgical Anatomy of the Hand. ed. 2. Philadelphia, J. B. Lippincott, 1965.
20. Laine, V. A. I., Sairanen, E., and Vainio, K.: Finger deformities caused by rheumatoid arthritis. J. Bone Joint Surg., *39*:527-533, 1957.
21. Landsmeer, J. M. F.: A report on the coordination of the interphalangeal joints of the human finger and its disturbances. Acta Morph. Neerl. Scand., *2*:59-84, 1960.
22. Liotta, D.: Personal communication.
23. Lipscomb, P. R., and Henderson, E. D.: Surgical treatment of the rheumatoid hand. J.A.M.A., *175*:431-436, 1961.
24. Littler, J. W., and Eaton, R. G.: Redistribution of forces in the correction of the boutonniere deformity. J. Bone Joint Surg., *49*:1267-1274, 1969.
25. Mannerfelt, L.: On formation of bony spurs in the rheumatoid hand. *In* Tubiana, Raoul (ed.): Group d'Etude de la Main Monograph No. 3. The Rheumatoid Hand. pp. 117-121. Paris, l'Expansion Scientifique Francaise, 1969.
26. Marmor, L.: Surgery of Rheumatoid Arthritis. Philadelphia, Lea & Febiger, 1967.
27. Matev, I. B.: Transposition of the lateral slips of the aponeurosis in treatment of long-standing boutonniere deformity. Brit. J. Plast. Surg., *17*:281-286, 1964.
28. McKee, G. K., Watson-Farrar, J.: Replacement of arthritic hips by the McKee-Farrar prosthesis. J. Bone Joint Surg. [Brit.], *48*: 245-259, 1966.
29. Moberg, E., *et al.*: The early pathological changes in rheumatoid arthritis. Acta Chir. Scand. (Suppl.), *357*:142-147, 1966.
30. Müller, M. E.: Hüftkopf und Total Prosthesen in der Hüftchirurgie. Laugenbeck Arch. Klin. Chir., *305*:48-52, 1968.
31. Nalebuff, E. A.: Nature and management of flexor tendon nodules in the rheumatoid hand. *In* Tubiana, Raoul (ed.): G.E.M. Monograph No. 3. The Rheumatoid Hand. pp. 123-128. Paris, l'Expansion, 1969.
32. Preston, R. L.: The Surgical Management of Rheumatoid Arthritis. Philadelphia, W. B. Saunders, 1968.
33. Roberts, A. C.: Silicones and their applications as implant materials. Biomed. Engin., *3*:156-160, 1967.
34. Savill, D. L.: Some Aspects of Rheumatoid Hand Surgery. *In* Tubiana, Raoul (ed.): G.E.M. Monograph No. 3. The Rheumatoid Hand. pp. 107-110. Paris, l'Expansion, 1969.
35. Steindler, A.: Arthritic deformities of the wrist and fingers. J. Bone Joint Surg., *33*: 849-862, 1951.
36. Straub, L. R.: The rheumatoid hand. Clin. Orthop., *15*:127-138, 1959.
37. Swanson, A. B.: Surgery of the hand in cerebral palsy and the swan-neck deformity. J. Bone Joint Surg., *42A*:951-964, 1960.
38. ———: The need for early treatment of the rheumatoid hand. J. Mich. State Med. Soc., *60*:348-351, 1961.
39. ———: Pathomechanics of the swan-neck deformity. J. Bone Joint Surg., *47*:636 (Abstract), 1965.
40. ———: Improving end-bearing characteristics of lower extremity amputation stumps. New York University Inter-Clin. Inform. Bull., *5*:1-7, 1966.
41. ———: A flexible implant for replacement of arthritic or destroyed joints in the hand. New York University Inter-Clin. Inform. Bull., *6*:16-19, 1966.
42. ———: Silicone rubber implants for replacement of arthritic or destroyed joints in the hand. Surg. Clin. N. Amer., *48*:1113-1127, 1968.

43. ———: Finger joint replacement by silicone rubber implants and the concept of implant fixation by encapsulation. International Workshop on Artificial Finger Joints, Ann. Rheum. Dis. Suppl. [Brit.], *28*:47-55, 1969.
44. ———: Silicone rubber arthroplasty for arthritic problems at the base of the thumb. American Society for Surgery of the Hand, Jan. 1969.
45. ———: Silicone rubber implants for replacement of arthritic or destroyed joints in the hand. *In* Tubiana, Raoul (ed.): G.E.M. Monograph No. 3. The Rheumatoid Hand. pp. 176-189. Paris, l'Expansion, 1969.
46. ———: Arthroplasty in traumatic arthritic joints in the hand. Orthop. Clin. N. Amer., *1*:285-298, 1970.
47. Swanson, A. B., and Matev, I. B.: The proximal interphalangeal joint in arthritic disabilities and experiences in the use of silicone rubber implant arthroplasty in the upper extremity. Scientific Exhibit, American Academy of Orthopaedic Surgeons, Chicago, Jan. 1970.
48. Swanson, A. B., and Yamauchi, Y.: Silicone rubber implants for replacement of arthritic or destroyed joints. Scientific Exhibit, American Academy of Orthopaedic Surgeons, Chicago, Jan. 1968.
49. Tsuge, K., Sanada, M. D., and Nagayama, Y.: Surgical treatment of rheumatoid hand. Hiroshima J. Med. Sci., *15*:103-120, 1966.
50. Tubiana, R.: Surgical repair of the extensor apparatus of the fingers. Surg. Clin. N. Amer., *48*:1015-1031, 1968.
51. Vainio, K.: Surgery of Arthritis. Baltimore, Williams & Wilkins, 1964.
52. Vainio, K., Reiman, I., and Pulkki, T.: Results of arthroplasty of the metacarpophalangeal joints in rheumatoid arthritis. Reconstr. Surg. Traumat., *9*:1-7, 1967.
53. Vaughan-Jackson, O. J.: Rheumatoid hand deformities as considered in the light of tendon imbalances. J. Bone Joint Surg. [Brit.], *44*:764, 1962.
54. Wesolowski, S. A., Martinez, A., and McMahon, J. D.: Use of artificial materials in surgery. *In* Current Problems in Surgery. Chicago, Year Book Medical Publishers, Inc., Dec. 1966.
55. Zancolli, E.: Structural and Dynamic Bases of Hand Surgery. Philadelphia, Lippincott, 1968.

CHAPTER 24

A Dynamic Brace for Finger Joint Reconstruction in Arthritis

ALFRED B. SWANSON, M.D.

The advent of flexible implants for internal stabilization of finger joint arthroplasties has opened up new possibilities for successful reconstructive surgery of the hand.[7,8,9] A dynamic brace has been developed to facilitate early postoperative motion in these cases.[9,12] Its use has greatly improved the anatomical and functional results.

The requirements for a successful arthroplasty are stability, mobility, and freedom from pain. In well-done resection arthroplasties, soft tissues must be released sufficiently to correct the frequently associated contracture, subluxation, or angulation deformities.[1] After adequate release, the joint is unstable in the early postoperative period. Internal fixation with wires has usually been needed to maintain the restored anatomy.[4] Early motion has therefore not been possible. Since the preoperative dislocation or angulation tends to recur, mobility must be sacrificed to stability.

The use of flexible heat-molded silicone rubber implants as an adjunct to resection arthroplasty has allowed the desired early motion to be realized. The implant acts as an internal splint that separates incongruous bone ends, decreases the tendency for recurrent subluxation, and provides a mold for the development of a new joint capsule. Once the released ligaments and scar have healed, they will stabilize the joint in a fashion similar to normal ligaments.[10]

Controlled Early Motion

As with simple resection arthroplasty, if motion is restricted during this healing phase, there will be poor mobility. Controlled motion during this period will train the new capsule to have sufficient looseness for flexion and extension with sufficient tightness in the medial-lateral plane for rotational and angular stability. An adjustable dynamic brace is therefore necessary to encourage the joint to move in desired

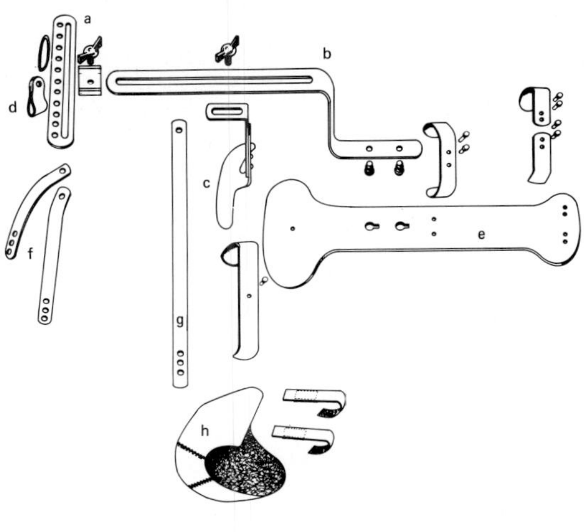

FIG. 24-1. Basic brace of lightweight aluminum, exploded view. (a) Transverse adjustable bar for rubberband dynamic finger loops (d), (b) longitudinal bar, (c) lumbrical bar, (e) basic wrist splint, (f) finger rotation bars, (g) thumb outrigger bar, (h) sheepskin flexion cuff.

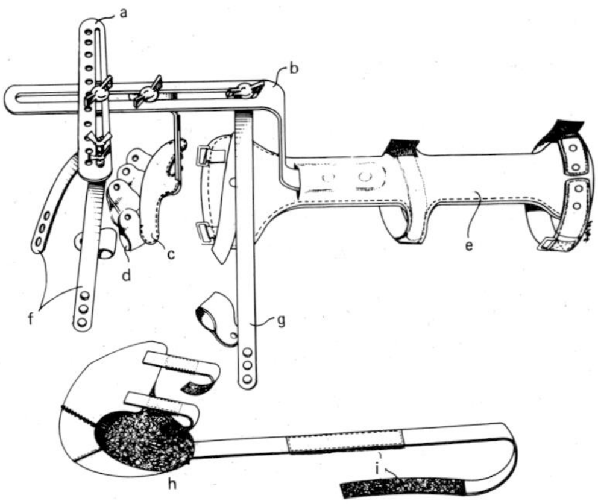

FIG. 24-2. Finished splint, covered with leather, has Velcro straps (i), plastic finger loops. Brace is available in three sizes. (See Fig. 24-1 for key to labels.)

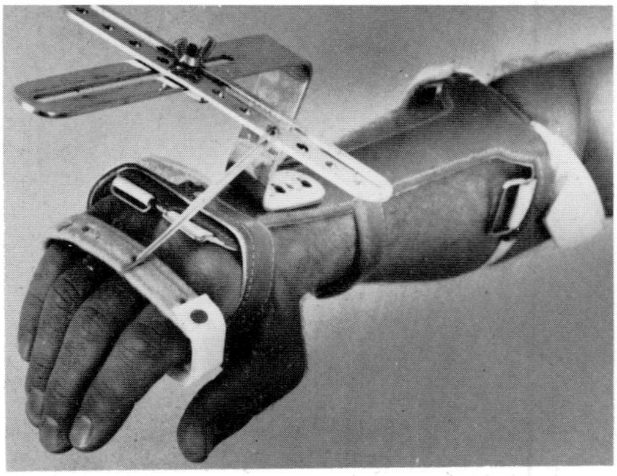

FIG. 24-4. The C bar is an alternative method for holding the fingers to rubber band suspension. Most cases require individual finger sling control.

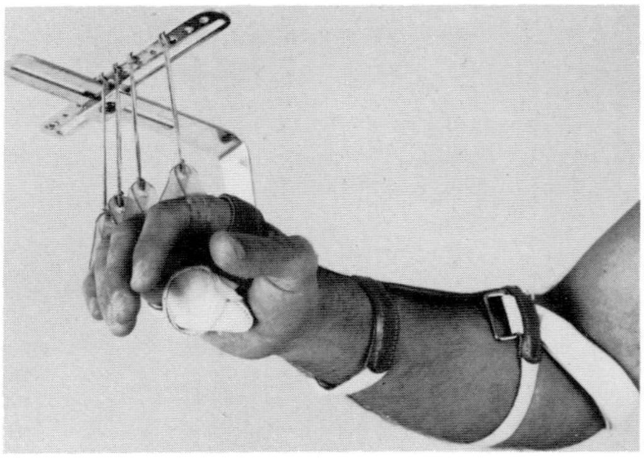

FIG. 24-3. Fitted brace shows palmar pad, which maintains arch of hand and helps prevent rotation of the device. Stability is provided for the wrist. The finger slings assist MP joint extension by lifting the proximal phalanx and prevent ulnar drift by pulling from the radial side. The rubber bands should be loose enough to permit 90° of flexion, especially in the little finger. If flexion strength is weak, the slings must be periodically removed to allow a full range of joint flexion.

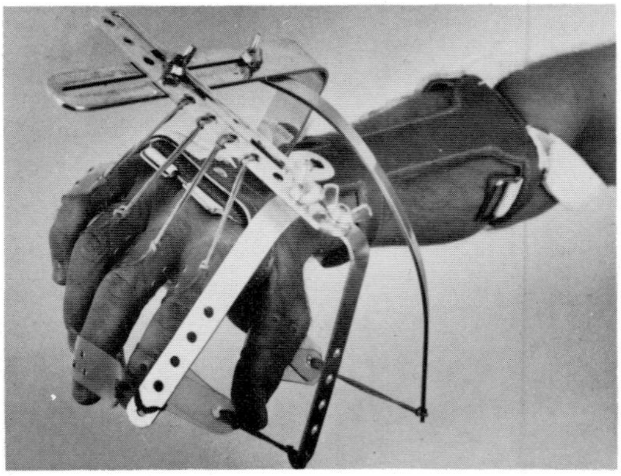

FIG. 24-5. Outrigger bars to index and middle fingers can help control the frequent tendency for pronation deformity of these digits. By pulling laterally on the slightly flexed digit, a supinatory corrective force is produced. The long outrigger bar can be used if assistive abduction of the thumb is desired.

planes and to prevent recurrences of deformity during the early postoperative course. The brace will prevent undue stretching of associated reconstructed tendons and ligaments. It will also assist the extensors and flexors of the digits, which are frequently weak due to long-standing deformity, accompanying tenosynovitis, and fibrosis. The dynamic brace has three major functions: (1) to provide complete and adjustable correction of residual deformity, (2) to control motion in the desired range, and (3) to assist flexor and extensor power in insuring an adequate alternation of complete extensor and flexor ranges of joint movement.

Brace Construction

The basic brace is a dorsal splint which provides a stable base for outriggers and support for the weak or deficient wrist joint.[2,3,5,6,11] A transverse bar to which finger slings are attached is fitted onto the dorsal arm. The slings are of soft plastic with multiple perforations and are connected to the bar with rubber bands (Figs. 24-1 to 24-4). Small radially placed outriggers may be added for correction of the pronation deformity often present in the index and middle fingers (Fig. 24-5). A longer bar can be used to increase thumb abduction. All of these outriggers are attached with thumb screws. The position of the transverse bar can be adjusted in all three planes.

When weakness of the flexors is present, a flexion cuff is used to insure that the joint is carried through an adequate range of motion (Fig. 24-6). This sheepskin cuff is attached to the dorsal molds and around the digits and is drawn into flexion by a Velcro strap which is run through a loop on the proximal portion of the brace. With this cuff, the finger joints can be passively brought into flexion for prescribed periods of time during the day. An elbow strap is used to prevent distal migration of the brace when the cuff is used. The brace is held in position with two adjustable Velcro straps on the forearm and a narrow Velcro strap across the palm. A palmar pad is used to help maintain the arches of the hand and prevent rotation of the brace.

The brace is available in three basic sizes.* The brace should be obtained before surgery so that it can be applied on the third to fifth postoperative days. The voluminous operative pressure dressing is removed, and light padding is applied to the hand, wrist, and forearm. Small dressings may be applied to individual digit wounds. The metal portions of the straps are relatively flexible and can be easily adjusted to the patient's size. The brace is adjusted so

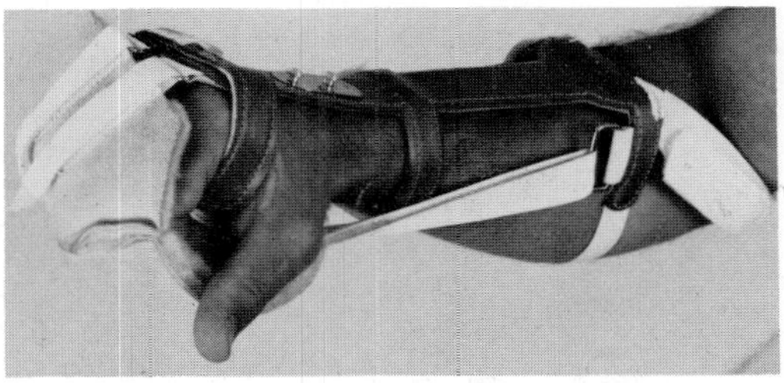

FIG. 24-6. A sheepskin finger cuff is used to obtain passive finger joint flexion in cases of flexor weakness. The elbow strap helps prevent distal migration of the brace. The elbow strap may also be placed as a figure-eight around the arm.

that the rubber band loops hold the fingers in distal extension and slight radial deviation. If there is a tendency for pronation of the index and middle fingers, extra loops are applied laterally to the distal phalanx. A suppinatory rotation can be achieved in this manner. The tension of the rubber bands should not be so great that the patient cannot accomplish flexion to 90°. This is especially true of the fifth digit. The patient is encouraged to flex and extend his digits frequently, within his fatigue and pain tolerance. He is also asked to elevate the extremity and move the elbow and shoulder. The brace may require adjustment once or twice a day in the early postoperative course.

Postoperative Applications

The extension portion of the brace is worn continuously for the first week. In the second postoperative week, the patient is allowed to remove the rubber bands to achieve greater flexion of the MP joints. This is usually allowed 1 to 2 hours twice a day. A range of motion from 0° to 70° of flexion is the goal. If the patient appears not to be obtaining 70° of flexion, the flexion cuff is worn 1 to 2 hours twice a day. The extension portion of the brace is used at least for 3 weeks continuously, night and day. The extension portion of the brace is then usually worn just at night for another

* Pope Brace Foundation, Kankakee, Illinois.

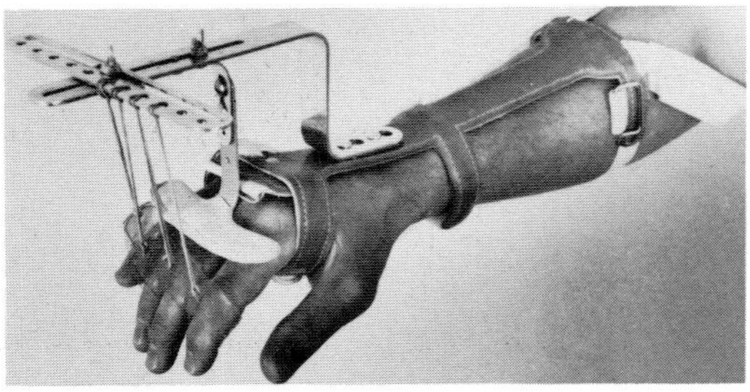

FIG. 24-7. This brace is used to stretch PIP joints or long flexor tendons. The lumbrical bar prevents hyperextension of the MP joints. This adaptation should not be used after MP joint arthroplasty because it may produce a palmarward subluxation of the proximal phalanx.

3 weeks. In a certain few cases, where there is a persistent extensor lag or a tendency for deviation of the digits, continued support by the brace must be prescribed for several more weeks. A flexion cuff may also be applied during this period if it appears that the desired range of flexion is not being achieved. The range of motion should be measured with a goniometer and recorded for evaluation of progress. The patient should have a prescribed exercise and stretching program for at least the first 3 months. After this time, the final range of motion will usually be reached. Collagen maturity and scar contraction differ from patient to patient.* The associated tendon deficiencies also vary. Therefore, the use of the brace in the postoperative period requires the careful attention of the operating surgeon.

The brace is designed so that, after simple adjustment, it can be used for either the right or left hand. It has also been modified so that it can be valuable in a variety of other conditions. A lumbrical bar is supplied for patients who need pre- or postoperative PIP joint extension (Fig. 24-7). Care must be taken when using this device for patients who have had recent MP joint arthroplasty, because in these cases the proximal phalanx has a tendency to subluxate palmarwards on the metacarpal, if too much force is applied. The brace has also been used for patients who have undergone proximal interphalangeal joint arthroplasties. When the proximal phalanx is supported with the slings, selective PIP joint active motion is encouraged. The flexion cuff can be applied to assist in improving the flexion of the proximal interphalangeal joints. The brace has also been used after simple synovectomy of the finger joints in arthritis and following release of contracted finger joints in traumatic injuries.

The dynamic brace, which was developed in the Orthopaedic Research Department at the Blodgett Memorial Hospital and used for the past six years, has been used in more than 200 patients.† Its application has never been refused by any patient. It forms an extremely important adjunct in arthroplasty surgery of the digits. In our opinion, it is absolutely necessary in the postoperative period if the full potential for functional restoration is to be achieved. It fulfills its role, inasmuch as it is versatile, adjustable, and allows the patient the freedom of motion he desires and needs.

* Peacock, E. E., and Madden, J. W. Personal communication.

REFERENCES

1. Boyes, J. H.: Bunnell's Surgery of the Hand. ed. 5. Philadelphia, J. B. Lippincott, 1970.
2. Bunnell, S.: Splinting the hand. American Academy of Orthopaedic Surgeons Instructional Course Lectures, vol. IX, p. 233. Ann Arbor, J. W. Edwards, 1952.
3. Evans, E. B.: Orthopaedic measures in the treatment of severe burns. J. Bone Joint Surg., *48*:643, 1966.
4. Flatt, A. E.: The Care of the Rheumatoid Hand. ed. 2. St. Louis, C. V. Mosby, 1968.

† Recognition is given to the kind assistance in the development of this brace by orthotists, Mr. A. Oostindie and Mr. B. Stegman of Grand Rapids, Michigan.

5. Moberg, E.: Dressings, splints and postoperative care in hand surgery. Surg. Clin. N. Amer., *44*:941-949, 1964.
6. Nickel, V. L., Perry, J., and Garrett, A.: Development of useful function in the severely paralyzed hand. J. Bone Joint Surg., *45*:933-952, 1963.
7. Swanson, A. B.: The need for early treatment of the rheumatoid hand. J. Mich. State Med. Soc., *60*:348-351, 1961.
8. ———: A flexible implant for the replacement of arthritic or destroyed joints in the hand. New York Univ. Inter-Clin. Inform. Bull., *6*:16-19, 1966.
9. ———: Silicone rubber implants for the replacement of arthritic or destroyed joints of the hand. Surg. Clin. N. Amer., *48*:1113-1127, 1968.
10. ———: Finger joint replacement by silicone rubber implants and the concept of implant fixation by encapsulation. International Workshop on Artificial Finger Joints. Ann. Rheum. Dis. (Suppl.), *28*:47-55, 1969.
11. Swanson, A. B., and Coleman, J. D.: Corrective bracing needs of the rheumatoid arthritic wrist. Amer. J. Occup. Ther., *20*: 38-40, 1966.
12. Swanson, A. B., and Yamauchi, Y.: Silicone rubber implants for replacement of arthritic or destroyed joints. Scientific Exhibit. Amer. Academy of Orthopaedic Surgeons, Chicago, Jan. 1968.

Index

Numbers in *italics* indicate illustrations.